RELIEF AT LAST!

Neutralization for Food Allergy and Other Illnesses

Diplomate American Board of Allergy and Immunology, a conjoint board of the American Board of Internal Medicine and the American Board of Pediatrics
Diplomate American Board of Pediatrics
Fellow American Academy of Allergy and Immunology
Fellow American College of Allergists
Fellow American Association of Certified Allergists
Fellow American Association for Clinical Immunology and Allergy
Fellow American Academy of Environmental Medicine
Fellow American Academy of Pediatrics
Member American College of Physicians
President, The Miller Foundation, Inc.
Director, Seminars on Food and Chemical Sensitivity in Human Disease
Consultant, Department of Pediatrics, University of South Alabama Medical School
Research Associate, Spring Hill College, Mobile, Alabama
Author of book, Food Allergy: Provocative Testing and Injection Therapy
Contributor of eight chapters to books edited by other allergists, and of thirty medical journal articles

RELIEF AT LAST!

Neutralization for Food Allergy and Other Illnesses

FOOD ALLERGY.
MIGRAINE. ASTHMA.
UNEXPLAINED FLUID RETENTION.
OBESITY CAUSED BY ALLERGIC FOOD CRAVINGS.
MOUTH ULCERS. NERVOUS STOMACH. IRRITABLE BOWEL.
COLON ALLERGY. ULCERATIVE COLITIS. CROHN'S DISEASE.
ALLERGY OF NOSE, SINUS, EAR, BREATHING PASSAGES, SKIN.
REPEATED INFECTIONS OF SINUS, EAR, BREATHING PASSAGES.
BRAIN ALLERGY. HYPERACTIVITY. LEARNING/BEHAVIOR DISORDERS.
YEAST INFECTION. ARTHRITIS. MUSCLE/JOINT PAIN. POISON IVY/OAK.
PREMENSTRUAL SYNDROME. MENSTRUAL CRAMPS. ENDOMETRIOSIS. BREAST PAIN.
HERPES I & II. SHINGLES. INFLUENZA. MONONUCLEOSIS. E-B VIRUS INFECTIONS.

By

JOSEPH B. MILLER, M.D.

CHARLES C THOMAS • PUBLISHER
Springfield • Illinois • U.S.A.

Published and Distributed Throughout the World by

CHARLES C THOMAS • PUBLISHER
2600 South First Street
Springfield, Illinois 62717

ISBN 0-398-05283-2

Library of Congress Catalog Card Number: 86-19170

With THOMAS BOOKS *careful attention is given to all details of manufacturing and design. It is the Publisher's desire to present books that are satisfactory as to their physical qualities and artistic possibilities and appropriate for their particular use.* THOMAS BOOKS *will be true to those laws of quality that assure a good name and good will.*

Printed in the United States of America
SC-R-3

Library of Congress Cataloging-in-Publication Data

Miller, Joseph B., 1921–
Relief at last!

Bibliography: p.
Includes index.
1. Allergy—Popular works. 2. Food allergy—Popular works. 3. Nutritionally induced diseases—Popular works. I. Title. [DNLM: 1. Allergy and Immunology—popular works. WD 300 M6485r]
RC584.M55 1987 616.97 86-19170
ISBN 0-398-05283-2

This book is dedicated to
GREATER RELIEF OF HUMAN SUFFERING
and
PROGRESS IN THE PRACTICE
OF MEDICINE

*"Days pass and the years vanish, and we walk sightless among miracles. Lord, fill our eyes with seeing and our minds with knowing; let there be moments when your Presence, like lightning, illumines the darkness in which we walk."**

*Excerpted from *Gates of Prayer,* Copyright 1975 by the Central Conference of American Rabbis and the Union of Liberal and Progressive Synagogues; reprinted by permission.

PREFACE

I wrote this book to bring good news to you and to millions of needlessly suffering patients. Welcome relief for many of your "hopeless" medical problems is now available. A newly developed medical procedure, NEUTRALIZATION THERAPY, can quickly reduce or entirely eliminate many severe ailments for which little or no relief could be offered previously.

I did not acquire this information from test tubes, guinea pigs, or isolated laboratory research. Neither is this book an academic treatise on technical aspects of rare diseases. Rather, the breakthroughs described here have been made in the offices of practicing physicians treating fellow human beings who confront them daily with certain "hopeless, idiopathic, psychosomatic, or intractable" medical problems.

I have tried to write a simple, factual account for the nonprofessional reader of how thousands of physicians—including myself—are successfully helping millions of patients with a wide variety of common, serious, persistent illnesses. These illnesses are usually caused by *inappropriate reactions of the patients' own bodies* to substances in their internal or external environment. Many of these patients had been suffering for years and had felt doomed to continue in misery the rest of their lives.

For those who wish additional information, I have included references to other publications where the need seemed indicated. Hopefully, we can all join together to bring greater relief to additional millions of suffering people and promote further progress in the science and art of medicine.

ACKNOWLEDGMENTS

I wish to gratefully acknowledge the commitment to my profession initiated in me by the late Father Patrick Henry Yancey, S.J., Chairman of Pre-Medical Education at Spring Hill College in Mobile, Alabama; the specific interest in allergy, immunology, food sensitivity, and clinical research awakened in me by the late Dr. Bret Ratner during my training and research years at Seaview and Bellevue Hospitals in New York; the ingenuity of Dr. Carleton H. Lee of St. Joseph, Missouri, who discovered and developed neutralization therapy; and the depth and breadth of knowledge of Dr. Theron Randolph of Chicago concerning the impingement on the human organism of hidden food sensitivities and noxious chemicals in our air, food, and water long before they came to be recognized by society or the profession. It is from the strength and spirit of these giants of medicine that I have drawn over the years.

My special thanks go to my associate in practice, Dr. Leonard Caputo, a skillful and dedicated physician with a fine artistic gift which he freely shared in the development of the illustrations for this book. I would also like to express deep appreciation to many friends and colleagues for their advice, encouragement, and constructive criticisms.

Every effort has been made to obtain permission to reprint copyrighted passages, and I believe that I have done so. If any errors or omissions are pointed out, I will be pleased to correct them in subsequent editions.

I would also like to express gratitude to my diligent secretaries, Margaret Murray and Linda Fell, and the other members of my staff who helped in innumerable ways in the development of this book:

Pearl Bringhurst, Patricia Davis, Ann Doss, Phoenie Everett, Sybil Franklin, Beatrice Grimes, Cindy Lane, Cynthia Locke, Karyn Lyle, Angela Natale, Suzanne Odom, Robin Pool, Barbara Ryan, Leona Shivers, Susan Sylvia, Gaylene Sollie, Sharon Tourné, Malinda Williford, Kelly Ziebach.

I particularly wish to acknowledge the critical role played by my many patients who, over decades of practice, have put their trust in me and honored me by choosing me as their physician. I have learned more from them than from all my teachers and texts. My greatest pleasure has been from their smiles of relief—and sometimes exclamations of delight—when I have been able to help them quickly through a particularly obscure or persistent health problem.

My appreciation extends to the many hours of pleasant distraction from the chores of writing and working provided by my children, Joan, Paige, Bruce, and Carol, and my grandchildren, Michael and Beth. My final and foremost wish is to express my personal dedication to my wife, Annice, for sharing her love, time, effort, support, and constancy through nearly a half-century of being there whenever I needed her.

CONTENTS

RELIEF AT LAST!

Neutralization for Food Allergy and Other Illnesses

IMPORTANT NOTICE

I have presented this book to serve only as a general informational guide and reference source for the understanding of nonprofessional and professional readers. Obviously, I cannot assume medical or legal responsibility for having the contents of this book considered as a prescription for anyone or an instruction manual for professionals.

Treatment of illness must be supervised by an appropriate physician. Responsibility for uses made of any knowledge acquired from this book must be taken by the patient and the physician who employ it.

Chapter 1

DISCOVERY OF THE RAPID RELIEF RESPONSE: HOW NEUTRALIZATION THERAPY BEGAN

Allergists have always known that an occasional patient would respond almost immediately to an injection of a given dose of *inhalant* allergy extract. Such an extract is made from inhaled allergenic particles such as dusts, molds, and pollens.[1]

After each treatment injection, these patients would note relief in about thirty minutes. Usually, the relief would continue for nearly a week.

Such a patient might come in about a week later and ask the allergist: "Please give me another injection like the last one you gave me. That one provided great relief of my symptoms and now it's wearing off."

Allergists have long been puzzled by this rapid-relief phenomenon. It did not occur in the majority of their patients and did not fit accepted concepts of allergy injection therapy.

According to orthodox theory, benefit was supposed to come very slowly over many months or years as a cumulative effect of a large total summation of gradually increasing allergen dosage.[2] Some allergists undoubtedly chalked up the rapid-relief phenomenon to psychological or placebo factors, a laying-on-of-hands response.

Until recently, we had no technique for deliberately reproducing this rapid-relief effect. We even tended to doubt its existence despite the clear testimonials of some patients.

THE FIRST BREAKTHROUGH

Then in 1957, Dr. Carleton H. Lee of St. Joseph, Missouri made the breakthrough.[3] It all began when Dr. Lee determined to find a way to protect his wife from her severe asthma attacks brought on by eating many common foods.

She could only remain free of her food-caused asthma by limiting her diet exclusively to chicken and rice. Although beefsteak was her favorite food, eating a minute amount of beef was sufficient to bring on a severe adrenalin-requiring attack.

For nearly a century, allergists have believed that food extract skin tests were of little value and that food extract injection therapy was useless. Yet, Dr. Lee persisted.

He reasoned: "Food allergen molecules are not qualitatively different from inhalant allergen molecules. If extract injection therapy against inhaled substances like ragweed can be effective, why should extract injection therapy not be effective for foods also?"

After many attempts, Dr. Lee discovered that he could produce mild asthma within ten minutes by injecting into the most superficial layer of the skin (*intradermally*) one carefully chosen concentration of a food extract. He could then relieve (*"neutralize"*) the asthma in ten minutes with an intradermal injection of a different carefully chosen concentration of the same food extract. He also found that he could keep his wife virtually free of food-caused asthma with twice-weekly treatment injections under the skin (*subcutaneously*) of a solution containing the neutralizing doses of all her symptom-causing foods.

In like manner, he was able to provide relief for his other food-sensitive patients, including those with many symptoms that had not even been recognized previously as being caused by foods or even by allergic sensitivity. He first termed this procedure "the provocative method."

In the ensuing years he and others have refined the procedure so that definitive (neutralizing) doses usually can now be determined with much less or no provocation of symptoms. Therefore, the terms "relief-dose therapy," "neutralizing dose therapy," "definitive dose therapy," or "individualized treatment dose therapy" have been used at various times.

The term most commonly used today is probably "neutralizing therapy." This describes the most prominent part of the procedure, namely neutralization of the patients' symptoms.

It was thus through concern for his wife that this ingenious man developed the neutralizing method of testing and treatment for food allergy. He next applied the new procedure to extracts of other materials including inhalants such as dusts, molds, and pollens. He found that by changing the procedure slightly, he could reproduce the quick relief regularly and reliably for illnesses caused by these inhalants and a wide variety of other substances.

With inhalants, the relief after each neutralizing treatment injection usually turned out to begin in about thirty minutes and last nearly a week. This fitted well the rapid-relief phenomenon reported by the occasional patient on orthodox inhalant allergy therapy. My experiences with both procedures have convinced me that the dose which resulted in the rapid-relief phenomenon in orthodox therapy often happened to be the neutralizing dose for at least one of the major allergens in the treatment solution.

MY ENTRY INTO NEUTRALIZATION THERAPY

My first contact with this new method of treatment occurred in 1965. I heard a paper delivered by Dr. Lee at a meeting of the American College of Allergists in Chicago.

He listed a large number of illnesses which he had found to respond well to his system of food extract treatment. Migraine was high on his list.

His mention of migraine secured my intense and undivided attention. For three years I had been suffering painful daily migraine attacks and had sought relief from all the usual specialists to no avail. So despite my natural skepticism for what sounded like a panacea, I was personally motivated to learn more.

After Dr. Lee's lecture I asked him many questions, and learned the basics of the procedure. I immediately went to the seminar exhibit hall, where various allergy extract companies had exhibit booths, and ordered extracts of my most frequently eaten foods. Although I did not know that any foods bothered me, it was these foods which Dr. Lee assured me would be the most likely culprits of my chronic daily migraine.

About two weeks later the extracts arrived in my office. I immediately directed my nurse to start testing me. Much to my surprise, I found that I could often turn my migraine on in miniature form with one intradermally injected concentration of a given food extract and turn it off in minutes with a different intradermally injected concentration, just as Dr. Lee had described.

Then I started giving myself subcutaneous treatment injections of a food extract solution containing the foods which had produced my symptoms during testing. My migraine virtually disappeared within two weeks, just as had occurred in many of Dr. Lee's patients. I found myself to be sensitive to many of my most frequently eaten foods; but milk, corn, wheat, and chocolate were the worst.

Until then I had considered myself quite a capable allergist, keeping up to date on all the most modern treatments available. My migraine response convinced me that I still had much to learn.

As patients continued to come to me for treatment day by day I began to realize that I, like other allergists, had been satisfied to help only a very limited number of health problems such as nasal allergy and asthma. I had not considered the relief of migraine and many other "nonallergic" illnesses as within the scope of allergy practice.

Although I continued using my older methods for another three years, I simultaneously began using food extract injections. I treated many patients with migraine and a host of other syndromes described by Dr. Lee as being caused by foods. Under my unbelieving eyes, I observed one major "intractable" illness after another respond in similar fashion.

My original skepticism steadily changed to conviction. Over a three-year comparative study, neutralization therapy won hands down.

I continued to pile one dramatic success on top of another. When I used the same food treatment procedure in patients with resistant rhinitis and asthma, which had not responded sufficiently to inhalant injections and other treatment measures, many improved markedly and rapidly.

The previously incomplete response of some was due to the fact that they had had food as well as inhalant sensitivities. I had not treated the foods or even been aware that foods had been contributing to the illness.

Then I switched some of my slowly or poorly responding *inhalant* patients from orthodox inhalant dosage to neutralizing inhalant dosage. Many with persistent hay fever, chronic nose and sinus allergy, and resistant asthma improved greatly.

In some patients with both food and inhalant syndromes, inhalant neutralization treatment gave great relief for their inhalant allergies, while food neutralization treatment in some cases increased their relief from these "inhalant" symptoms (such as nasal congestion) and also, as a bonus, relieved many unsuspected food-caused illnesses.

SYMPTOMS AND SYNDROMES RESPONDING TO NEUTRALIZATION THERAPY

A symptom is a *single* sensation subjectively recognized by the patient. A syndrome is a *combination* of symptoms commonly occurring together so as to constitute a distinct clinical picture, condition, or illness. At times these terms are used interchangeably.

The food-caused conditions which responded to food extract injection therapy included headache, dizziness (vertigo), swelling of the vocal cords (laryngeal edema), irritable bowel syndrome, spastic colon, chronic ulcerative colitis, Crohn's disease (ileo-colitis), muscle and joint pain, eczema (atopic dermatitis), chronic hives (urticaria), hyperactivity, learning difficulties, behavior problems, "brain-fogginess," and many others. I rapidly found myself successfully treating and relieving not just the few illnesses which had constituted almost my entire previous allergy practice, but dozens of additional formerly resistant conditions.

It was at this point that the great cost-effectiveness, as well as the human relief, provided by neutralization therapy began to dawn on me. Many patients who had been coming to me for allergic rhinitis or asthma had also been going to several other specialists for multiple additional problems.

When I neutralized these patients for inhalants, not only their allergic ear, nose, throat, and bronchial symptoms responded but also many others. These included symptoms such as vertigo, ear-ringing, fluctuating hearing loss, fainting tendencies, and other symptoms which had not responded to treatment by other specialists.

When I then neutralized them for foods, I was able to provide relief for many additional symptoms. These included headaches, stomachaches, diarrhea, bloating, hyperactivity, depression, fatigue, compulsive drowsiness, floating sensations, impaired ability to think clearly, poor memory, joint pains, itchings, swellings, rashes, and many others. Their many symptoms had previously required regular care by several other specialists, including pediatricians, internists, gastroenterologists, neurologists, dermatologists, cardiologists, psychologists, and psychiatrists.

Many had been undergoing repeated extensive diagnostic testing by one specialist after another. Some had had repeated hospitalizations and even surgical procedures, and many were burdened with multiple heavy pharmacy expenses. So my treatments were saving most of them a great deal of money as well as misery.

On the other hand, I must remind you that some symptoms which at first glance might seem to be caused by allergy may not necessarily be so. There are instances where the ruling out of other kinds of diseases by other specialists is appropriate.

MY FURTHER STUDIES

You must not assume that I swallowed these new concepts and procedures without a great deal of skepticism, soul searching, and critical trials. I deliberately sought to challenge and possibly disprove all of Dr. Lee's concepts and procedures which sounded so unbelievably effective.

Rather than disproving them, I confirmed them solidly, over and over again. I also made additional discoveries which have broadened the field of allergy and neutralization still further.

One of the tasks I assigned myself was to attempt to simplify, organize, and objectify the procedures for my own understanding. At first they had seemed to me to be somewhat subjective and mysterious.

Working closely with Dr. Lee, I learned a great deal about objective observation of physical changes in test patients and the whealing response of the skin. Once I had a firm grasp on the innumerable fine points of techniques which make this system highly effective and objective, I was moved to teach it to others.

To further this goal, I have published a series of papers on the procedure and its uses in medical journals.[4–13] I have also presented it at many internationally attended medical seminars.

In 1972 I published a book for physicians and allergy technicians entitled *Food Allergy: Provocative Testing and Injection Therapy*.[14] It provides physicians who have a background in allergy and environmental medicine the basic knowledge required to get started into this procedure.

Several books[15–21] edited by other physicians contain chapters contributed by me. I have also lectured at many seminars of the American College of Allergists and other international, national, regional, and local seminars of allergy societies and other medical organizations. As well, I have provided physicians with cassette courses.

I published the first double-blind controlled study comparing placebo with food extract injections using doses determined by intradermal neutralizing testing.[8] Hundreds of individual allergists have attended one-week courses in my office to supplement these other educational materials and to see the innumerable details and fine points that can only be learned at first hand.

My point is simply that I have tried very hard to make the benefits of this procedure widely available. I have personally instructed nearly 3,000 physicians from the United States and many other countries, and have lectured to many thousands more.

Therefore the concepts in this book, while possibly new to many nonallergists and suffering patients, are not bolts from the blue. For nearly two decades, I have provided numerous instructive opportunities and materials for allergists, medical environmentalists, and others who might wish to learn them.

Chapter 2

WHAT IS NEUTRALIZATION?

I have described how neutralization therapy began. Now let us take a closer look at the procedure itself.

THE DIAGNOSTIC FEATURE

Neutralization has both diagnostic and therapeutic features. The diagnostic part of neutralization is based on a skin test system very similar to the well-established *intradermal* (within the skin) test procedure used by allergists the world over for nearly a century. However, diagnosis by neutralization is also useful in instances other than allergic diseases.

THE TREATMENT FEATURE

What is new about intradermal neutralizing testing is that it enables the physician to determine with a high degree of precision for each individual patient the best *treatment* dose of an allergenic extract, a hormone, a virus vaccine, or other treatment material *right at the moment of testing.* When this best treatment dose is then injected *subcutaneously* (under the skin) at regular intervals it can quickly relieve and protect many patients from a large number of both allergic and nonallergic illnesses.

The subcutaneous injections constitute the treatment part of the method. They provide relief to a degree and with a rapidity, reliability, and safety rarely experienced before in medical therapy.

Buildup of dosage over months or years of treatment is not required since the full optimal treatment dose of each individual substance for each individual patient is determined during the test procedure. Treatment *begins* with the full "just right" treatment dose of all the substances simultaneously.

GENERAL APPLICATIONS

Neutralization is effective in a great many allergic illnesses, inflammatory diseases, hormonal imbalances, and infectious processes. For many of these, no accurate diagnostic procedure and no effective treatment were previously available. Some of these illnesses constitute major causes of suffering and disability for literally millions of people.

FOODS

To be specific, one major breakthrough has come in the field of food allergy, or more broadly food "sensitivity." "Allergy" is used by some to define a particular type of immunologic response. Sensitivity is a more general term utilized by some to designate all four types of harmful immunologic responses. Since the term "allergy" is more familiar to most readers and we want to instruct rather than confuse, it may at times be used in this book even in instances where the broader term, "sensitivity," might be scientifically more accurate. It will also be used at times when it is not certain whether a given response is immunologic or nonimmunologic. However, it will not be used to include responses due to enzyme deficiencies, toxins, food aversions, or other responses obviously not due to sensitivity.

WHICH FOOD-CAUSED ILLNESSES CAN BE NEUTRALIZED?

Extracts of *inhaled* substances have been in use for nearly a century, but the equally reasonable use of *food* extract injections has been almost totally overlooked. Since food sensitivity is far more common than inhalant sensitivity, the remarkable effectiveness of neutralizing injections of food extracts has come as a much needed and greatly welcomed surprise.

Outstanding examples of highly neutralizable illnesses usually due to unrecognized food sensitivity are

(1) Severe *headache,* particularly vascular headache such as migraine.

(2) A number of common misery-causing dysfunctions of the *gastrointestinal* tract. These may be manifested by such symptoms as nausea, vomiting, gassiness, bloating, abdominal pain, diarrhea, or constipation. There may be ulcers of the mucous membrane of the mouth, small intestine, or colon.

GENERAL APPLICATIONS OF NEUTRALIZATION

1. FOOD ALLERGY
   a) Migraine Headache
   b) Digestive symptoms
   c) Skin diseases
   d) Pain in muscles and joints
   e) Brain allergy
      i. Increased brain activity
      ii. Decreased brain activity
      iii. Inappropriate activity
2. INHALANT ALLERGY
   a) Hay fever
   b) Asthma
   c) Allergy and recurrent infection of the eyes, nose, sinuses, throat, ears, bronchial tubes, and lungs
3. CHEMICAL SENSITIVITY
4. CANDIDA YEASTS AND OTHER FUNGI
5. HORMONES
   a) Premenstrual syndrome
   b) Menstrual cramps
   c) Endometriosis
   d) Nausea and vomiting of pregnancy
   e) Intolerance to birth control pills
   f) Fibrocystic breast disease
   g) Menopausal symptoms
6. VIRUSES
   a) Influenza
   b) Herpes
      i. Herpes Simplex I
      ii. Herpes Simplex II
      iii. Shingles
      iv. Postherpetic pain
      v. Chickenpox
      vi. Infectious mononucleosis
      vii. Epstein-Barr Virus Syndrome

Patients with these "digestive" symptoms are often diagnosed as having one or more of a variety of conditions. These include nervous stomach, irritable bowel, spastic colon, colitis, canker sores of the mouth (recurrent aphthous ulcers or aphthous stomatitis), chronic ulcerative colitis, or Crohn's Disease (ulceration of the colon and part of the small intestine).

(3) Certain *skin* diseases such as adult acne, eczema (atopic dermatitis),

chronic hives (urticaria), localized allergic swellings (angioedema), and generalized periodic swelling of the entire body (cyclic edema).

(4) The pain, stiffness, and inflammatory swellings of certain *muscle and joint syndromes.*

(5) Certain *mental symptoms* such as periodically increased, decreased, or bizarre mental activity. These seem to be caused by allergic swellings in various parts of the brain.

Increased brain activity due to food sensitivity may be manifested as nervousness, insomnia, restlessness, hyperactivity, inability to concentrate, short attention span, learning disability, and behavior disorders. *Decreased* brain activity may range from difficulty in reading or writing, mild lethargy, unusual fatigue, periodically impaired ability to think clearly ("brain-fogginess"), or compulsive drowsiness, to "psychiatric" depression. There may also be periodic episodes or continuous manifestations of *bizarre* or inappropriate thinking and behavior.

In children, these mental symptoms occur in various combinations and under various labels, such as dyslexia and minimal brain dysfunction. They are now usually lumped together under the diagnosis of "Attention Deficit Disorder."

As occurs so often in medicine, the diseases and symptoms remain; only the name of the illness changes. And the symptoms are common in adults as well. However, adults have often learned ways of "covering up" so that the problem is not always perceived as such by others. Even the victim does not often make the "food connection," and struggles on.

INHALANTS

A second major breakthrough has come in the field of allergy to inhaled particles such as dusts, mold spores, pollen grains, feathers, and skin scales (danders) of fur-bearing animals. These are the inhalant allergens that cause much hay fever; allergic eye, nose, sinus, and ear disease; and asthma.

These conditions have long been treated successfully with injections ("allergy shots") of allergenic extracts made from the causative inhalable substances. When *neutralizing* doses of inhalant extracts are used, such allergies typically respond to an unusually great degree and with striking frequency, rapidity, and safety. Relief usually comes within one to three weeks, rather than after months or years of ordinary buildup allergy injection therapy.

CHEMICALS

A third category of responding illnesses consists of those caused by manmade chemicals, whether ingested or inhaled. These chemicals include artificial food colors, flavors, preservatives, and thousands of other food additives. They also include fumes, smokes, perfumes, solvents, plastics, textiles, foam rubber, insulating materials, chlorine, formaldehyde, and insecticides. These manufactured molecules are often of petrochemical origin. They are found in the air, food, water, medicines, clothing, structural materials of buildings, and other things which make up our new synthetic environment.

Chemical susceptibility is a complex and fairly recently recognized problem, and much research remains to be done. It can be extraordinarily severe in some patients. Not all such patients can be protected by neutralization alone at the present time.

However, in some patients neutralization with food and inhalant extracts and with the few chemical extracts currently available can often provide much relief. This reduces the total burden on the immune system and often allows it to handle chemicals more successfully.

Additional relief can be provided when needed by careful instruction in avoidance of hidden or excessive chemical exposures. Clearly, much interaction between chemists and allergists will be needed to clarify this picture further so we can provide more relief.

CANDIDA YEASTS AND OTHER FUNGI

Also responsive are allergic *and infectious* illnesses caused by certain living yeasts, molds, and other fungi which take up residence in and on our bodies. These microorganisms may become infectious invaders of our tissues or they may induce allergic and toxic reactions to their cellular products.

An outstanding example of this group of organisms is the candida or monilia yeast that causes infections such as yeast vaginitis, yeast dermatitis, and oral thrush. Thrush has long been a problem for infants. In recent years it has also become a common and serious problem in many adults as well.

Favorable conditions for the overgrowth of yeasts have been provided by modern technology and life styles. These include the increasing use of antibiotics, birth control pills, chemotherapeutic agents, immunosuppressives, cortisone products, and sugary diets.

Certain allergic skin reactions to the cellular products of these yeast organisms are called "id" reactions. Id reactions often show up first as tiny water blisters on the palms of the hands, or scaly, itchy lesions in other areas.

Yeast dermatitis can readily become secondarily infected. This can result in severe dermatitis of the hands, ear canals, and other skin and mucous membrane surfaces. For example, "detergent dermatitis" in women is often an irritative or inflammatory reaction secondary to allergic yeast reactions of the hands.

Aside from such localized reactions, less obvious systemic reactions can occur. The extra burden on defense mechanisms of the absorbed products of the yeasts that live in our colon and in other body cavities and surfaces is now becoming recognized as a cause of serious dysfunction of many internal organs including the brain.

HORMONES AND OTHER SELF-PRODUCED SUBSTANCES

Surprisingly, neutralization treatment using specific extracts is not only effective for reactions to foreign substances entering from the external environment, but also for symptoms caused by some of our own *self-produced* natural substances, such as hormones. Our bodies sometimes react inappropriately to substances in our internal environment as though they are harmful, foreign, allergenic, inflammatory, or equilibrium disturbing.

For example, progesterone is a natural female hormone. Its blood level rises at ovulation and then falls markedly just before and during menstruation. This often induces severe discomforts.

Progesterone neutralization usually provides startling relief for premenstrual symptoms and menstrual cramps. It also often relieves the pain and nodular swellings of endometriosis; the nausea and vomiting of pregnancy; and intolerance to medications containing progesterone-like substances such as those in contraceptive pills.

Neutralization has been similarly effective in certain other hormonal problems. Estrogen neutralization often can relieve the steady breast pain and lumpiness of chronic cystic mastitis (fibrocystic disease of the breast). Estrone neutralization frequently can relieve some of the discomforts of menopause. Insulin neutralization in diabetics allergic to injected insulin can prevent allergic reactions to insulin.

This suggests the desirability of studying the effects of neutralization with specific extracts in the treatment of imbalances caused by inappropriate bodily responses to a great many other self-produced substances. Such imbalances might include those which cause so-called autoimmune (self-allergic) diseases. One such disease, rheumatoid arthritis, has already been determined to be greatly benefited in some cases by neutralization to foods, inhalants, and chemicals.

VIRUSES

Astoundingly, neutralization with Influenza Virus Vaccine can start providing relief in the majority of patients *within minutes* from both influenza and herpes virus infections. Both of these viruses are globally distributed and have great destructive potential.

Influenza viruses produce annual worldwide epidemics and cause great discomfort, lost worktime, and even death. Influenza is particularly dangerous in the very young, the very old, and persons already weakened by other disorders, particularly of the lungs, heart, liver, and kidneys.

Herpes viruses cause a wide variety of illnesses, such as fever blisters, genital sores, shingles, and postherpetic neuralgia (persistent pain long after shingles sores have healed). They also cause blindness, encephalitis, highly fatal herpes of newborns, chickenpox (varicella), and "mono" (infectious mononucleosis).

As well, they cause a chronic, persistent, disabling disease called Epstein-Barr Virus Syndrome. Herpes viruses probably deal out more human discomfort, severe long-lasting pain, brain damage, and death than any other family of viruses.

Since there has been no really effective antibiotic against viruses, a breakthrough in the treatment of virus infections was badly needed. It is incredible but true that infections caused by two major virus families, the influenza and herpes virus families, usually can be rapidly and successfully treated by neutralization with a single readily available material, Influenza Virus Vaccine.

Successful use of this and other virus vaccines leads me to believe that a great many virus diseases for which no specific treatment is currently available can be similarly helped *during* the disease. This would be done by using *therapeutic* neutralizing doses of vaccines which are already widely used for routine *preventive* immunization against these specific diseases. It is also likely that additional virus diseases will become treatable during the disease with neutralizing doses of new preventive immunizing vaccines as they become available in the future.

HOMEOSTASIS

An impossibly long list? Too wide a variety of different causes and unrelated illnesses? A panacea?

Not at all. The human body has a marvelously complex and comprehensive network of immunologic and biochemical tools for maintaining stability and defending itself from harm by a great many deleterious substances and conditions.

These include foreign materials (allergens); invasive living organisms; body cells that are abnormal, worn out, or cancerous; and fluctuations in blood and tissue levels of hormones and other molecules. These biologic tools maintain organic integrity and balance—*homeostasis*—to protect the internal environment from harmful changes which can be caused by many substances generated both inside and outside the body.

REGAINING AND MAINTAINING HEALTH

When these immunologic and biochemical mechanisms work well, we are in good health, in good equilibrium, in homeostasis. In health we are oblivious to the activities of the harmful substances on the one hand, the unflagging efforts of the protective mechanisms on the other, and the ongoing silent internal battles constantly being waged between these two opposing forces.

When some facet of this protective network changes, biologic and molecular balance or equilibrium reactions in many organs may become altered. Then homeostasis can be lost and multiple symptoms surface.

Neutralization is a new and unique method of quickly regaining and maintaining balance and stability. It reduces or eliminates the symptoms of illnesses caused by many specific substances in the internal and external environment.

In the next chapter, we will turn our attention to how this can work. It is a relatively "heavy" chapter. However, it is important because it answers innumerable questions that patients ask about basic causes of their problems. Hopefully, I have made it interesting and easy to read. I really want you to understand your illness so that you and your physician together can manage it more successfully.

Chapter 3

HOW THE "JUST-RIGHT" TREATMENT CAN MAKE YOU WELL

ALLERGENS CAN CAUSE BOTH LOCAL AND DISTANT REACTIONS

When molecules of potentially allergenic substances such as ragweed pollen or milk enter the body, they may cause *local* reactions in the organ of entry, such as a stuffy nose (for example, ragweed) or diarrhea (for example, milk). Soluble allergenic molecules also may be absorbed into the circulation and be carried in the bloodstream to *distant* organs which may be sensitive to these particular allergens.

The reactions may then be in sites distant from the portal of entry. They may be manifested by such symptoms as hives, headache, hyperactivity, or behavioral changes. So allergenic molecules can reach both local and distant organs, and can therefore cause symptoms in any part of the body.

YOU CANNOT HAVE AN ALLERGIC REACTION UNLESS YOU HAVE A SENSITIVE STRESS ORGAN

Organs sensitive to allergenic molecules are variously termed allergic target organs, shock organs, or stress organs.

Not everyone has organs sensitive to allergens. Allergic people do. That is why they have allergic symptoms.

They inherit the tendency for stress organ sensitivity as well as for allergy. Symptoms may show up at various stages of life, depending partly on genetic programming and partly on environmental stresses encountered along the way.

MAST CELLS AND BASOPHILS RELEASE CHEMICAL MEDIATORS WHICH CAUSE ALLERGIC SYMPTOMS

How do allergenic molecules cause allergic reactions in stress organs? Primarily by reaching two types of cells and attaching to their cell surfaces. This causes the cells to release histamine-containing granules and other potentially harmful chemicals.

The first type of cell is the *mast cell*. The mast cell is filled with bluish granules. It was named by early pioneers in microscopic research because they felt that the granule-containing cell resembled a bag of mast, a term used to describe a pile or container of nuts, seeds, or acorns. Mast cells fix themselves in permanent positions on the *outer* surfaces of capillaries just under the skin or mucous membranes of the respiratory and digestive tracts.

Thus, in an asthma attack, it is usually the mast cells under the mucous membranes of the bronchial tubes that cause the bronchial constriction. And allergic diarrhea is often caused by the mast cells under the mucous membranes of the digestive tract.

The second type of cell is the *basophil*. The name basophil is derived from the fact that the granules in this cell absorb a basic blue dye commonly used in staining blood cells for microscopic examination. The basophil normally resides in the blood stream and therefore circulates constantly throughout the entire body. However, it has the ability to enter tissues when needed to release its granules and other chemical mediators to reinforce the effects of its sister cell, the mast cell (Figure 1).

The granules and molecules released by these two types of cells are called the "chemical mediators" (causes) of allergic reactions. Tissue-fixed mast cells and circulating basophils are the only cells in the body known to contain significant quantities of histamine.

However, many other harmful chemicals are released by these cells. In addition, the chemicals released by mast cells and basophils have the ability to stimulate other types of cells to come to the site of the reaction and release their own potentially harmful chemicals to fight antigens that are more persistent or more difficult to overcome. This double whammy further reinforces and amplifies the overall response to the antigen. When this second flood of chemicals is released destruction of normal tissue may occur, increasing the response from an allergic to an inflammatory reaction.

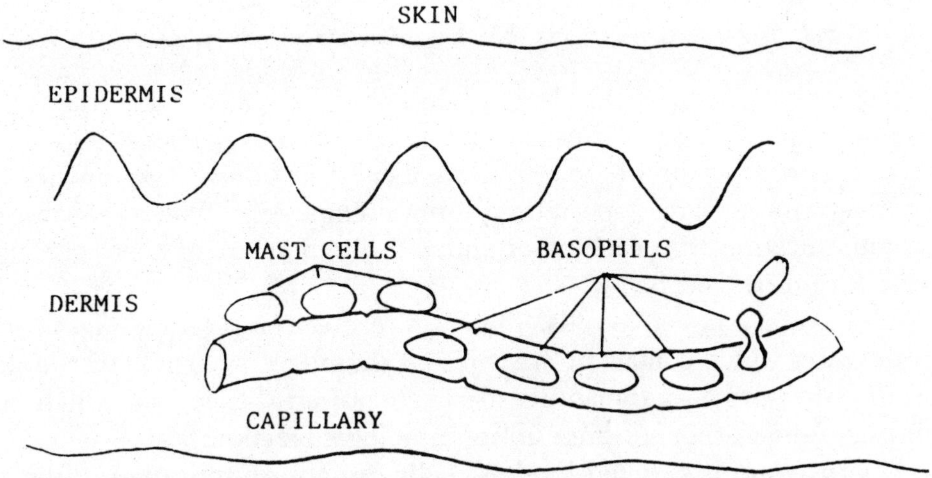

Figure 1. The skin is composed of two layers, the outer epidermis and the inner dermis. The mast cells are attached to the outer surfaces of capillaries, whereas basophils circulate within the capillaries. However, basophils, like other white blood cells, can leave the capillaries when they are needed in the tissues, as shown in the illustration.

THE CHEMICAL MEDIATORS ACT UPON SENSITIVE STRESS ORGANS

Mast cells and basophils are already known to produce many chemical mediators, and undoubtedly more will be discovered. The one we learned about first was histamine.

However, some of the other chemical mediators released by mast cells and basophils can be even more harmful than histamine. You may have already heard about prostaglandins and leucotrienes, two other groups of extremely powerful chemicals released by mast cells and basophils.

The point is that it is really not the allergenic molecules such as ragweed or milk that cause allergic symptoms. Rather, the symptoms are caused by chemical mediator molecules released by mast cells and basophils (such as histamine, prostaglandins, leucotrienes, and the chemicals which attract and activate other types of cells). The way mast cell mediators cause symptoms is by stimulating sensitive stress organs.

Mediator release from mast cells and basophils can be caused not only by allergenic molecules but also by some nonallergenic influences such as virus infections, exercise, chilling, hormonal changes, and other factors.

THE BODY IS A WHOLE FUNCTIONING ORGANISM

Just *below* the superficial layer of the skin and mucous membranes is a dense network of capillaries and fine nerve endings. *Within* the superficial layer of the skin, where intradermal test injections are administered, is a network of highly specialized immunologic cells. These cells are in communication with each other and with the network of nerve endings and capillaries just below.

These are very active cells. They can receive chemical messages from substances which contact or are injected into the superficial layer of the skin. They also have the ability to secrete powerful chemicals which can initiate, amplify, or suppress an immunologic reaction.

The chemicals secreted by these cells can absorb into the capillaries below, just as chemicals in the blood can leave the capillaries moving in the opposite direction to enter the superficial layer of the skin.

Thus the entire skin is a giant immunologic organ. The skin and the whole body are joined as one interacting organism by chemical messenger molecules and cells passing back and forth through the capillaries, as well as by nerve endings which carry messages to and from the brain and other parts of the nervous system.

THE ROLE OF LEAKY PLUMBING IN ALLERGY AND IMMUNOLOGY

The walls of capillaries are only one cell thick. These capillary cells are irregularly shaped but fit tightly together like a three-dimensional tubular jigsaw puzzle to form the capillary tubes.

Mast cells are formed in the bone marrow, circulate through the bloodstream only transiently, and quickly take up permanent stationary positions on the outer surfaces of the capillary cells beneath the skin and mucosa. Mast cells cling to these perimeter capillaries as a great swarm of bees might cling to the branches of a tree.

Each mast cell is like a bee. Allergen injected into the superficial layer of the skin can make a mast cell "sting" the capillary with which it is in contact.

The "venom" in the mast cell's sting consists of the chemical mediators it releases. These mediators force the local capillary cells to contract and become slightly separated from each other, opening tiny crevices or gaps between the capillary cells (Figure 2).

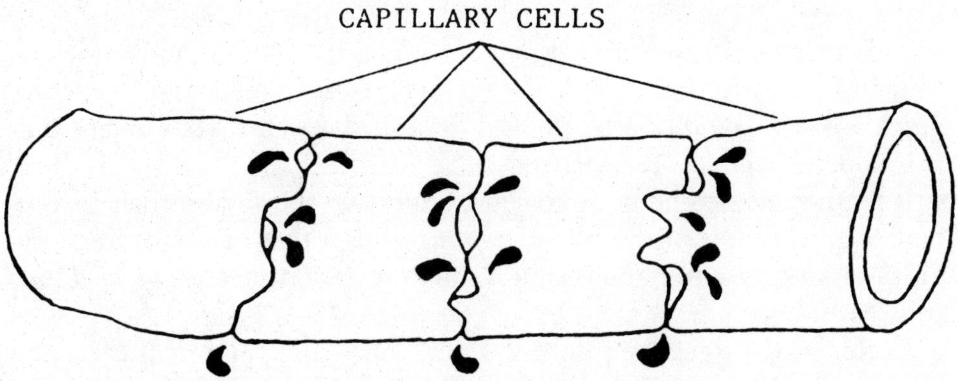

Figure 2. Gaps between capillary cells, with fluid leakage through the gaps.

The gaps let some of the chemical mediators as well as injected antigens enter the bloodstream. They simultaneously allow some of the watery blood serum containing antibodies and other chemicals out of the capillaries into the tissues where the reaction is taking place (Figure 3).

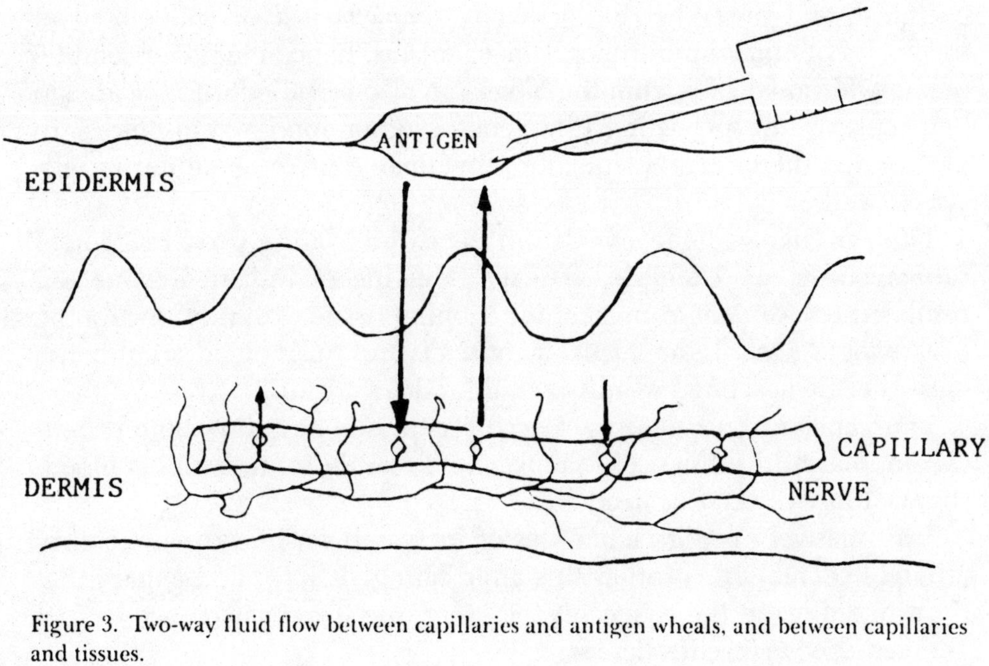

Figure 3. Two-way fluid flow between capillaries and antigen wheals, and between capillaries and tissues.

MEDIATORS ARE GATEKEEPERS

This increased capillary permeability is critical to both allergic and inflammatory reactions. It enables the body to excrete harmful allergens quickly out of the bloodstream and deposit them in tissues where they will hopefully be less threatening.

It further allows the body to send protective substances such as antibodies quickly out of the bloodstream through these gaps. It also provides easier access into the reaction site to certain protective white blood cells.

In this way, protective molecules and cells from the blood can enter into tissues. Here they can exert their defensive function against allergens, microbes, or other harmful substances that may have gained access to the body.

If potentially harmful allergens or foreign substances in the tissues are not quickly neutralized or removed, basophils can move into the area from the bloodstream to secrete additional chemical mediators. This can further widen the capillary gaps.

If still further help is needed, a group of powerful circulating chemicals lumped together under the term "complement" can be called into the reaction. Early investigators did not realize that this was not a single chemical, and they knew only that it *complemented* or cooperated in the action of other immunologic mechanisms, hence the name complement. Additional cells from the blood can also be called into the area to help destroy the persisting allergens or other foreign substances. In performing their cleanup function, they may destroy some normal tissues as well.

This can change the reaction from a reaction of allergy to a reaction of inflammation, for example, arthritis. Healing of inflamed tissue can result in replacement of normal functioning tissue with nonfunctioning scar tissue. As scar tissue heals, it contracts and pulls on adjacent bones and other tissues, often resulting in joint deformities.

Thus, chemical mediators act as gatekeepers. They allow both beneficial and harmful substances to move more readily from tissues to bloodstream and vice versa as needed.

Two relatively benign examples of increased capillary permeability (allergic edema) are swollen lips after eating shrimp, and generalized fluid retention in the tissues of the body due to repeated ingestion of allergenic foods (cyclic edema).

Edema of the brain from an allergenic food may cause headache or brain dysfunctions manifested as impaired memory or thought processes, hyperactivity, or learning and behavior difficulties. Edema of the digestive tract can result in bloating, abdominal pain, diarrhea, constipation, and poor absorption of nutrients. Thus, a variety of ailments can result from allergic edema alone.

VARIETIES OF MANIFESTATIONS OF ALLERGIC ILLNESS

Chemical mediators chiefly cause three types of organ responses: increased capillary permeability, mucus gland stimulation, and smooth muscle spasm. Smooth (nonstriated) muscles are those which are not under conscious control like the striated muscles with which we can deliberately and consciously move various parts of our body. However, the body can also use reflex and conscious efforts through the nervous system, such as hacking, coughing, and vomiting, to quickly get rid of ingested or inhaled irritants and allergens.

In addition to increased capillary permeability, some of the chemical mediators can cause temporary smooth muscle contraction or relaxation. It is well known that bronchial smooth muscle contraction can cause wheezing, and smooth muscle relaxation occurring in arteries can result in dilatation of the arteries, causing lowered blood pressure.

ALLERGY OF THE NOSE

Which organs react to an allergen depends upon which are most sensitive to the particular allergen. For example, if the nose is the stress organ, the thin fluid leakage from nasal capillaries may filter outward from the nasal tissues through the mucosa into the nasal air passages and produce a runny nose. The thin fluid can also drain backward down the throat and produce an irritating cough.

If the fluid liberated from the nasal capillaries is largely held within the tissues of the nose, the tissues swell and cause nasal congestion. Such swelling can result in blockage of the nose and sinus openings, resulting in secondary sinus infections. Allergic nasal swelling can also block the eustachian tubes, which connect the nose to the back side of the ear drum, resulting in recurrent ear problems.

If the mucus-secreting glands rather than the capillaries of the mucosal lining of the nose and sinuses are stimulated by mediators, the mucus formed may be thick, in contrast to the thin watery secretion of capillary leakage. The thick mucus can block the sinus openings or produce a sticky postnasal drip, resulting in such symptoms as sinus pain, headache, throat clearing, sore throat, or cough.

Since mucus is a good breeding nutrient for the viruses and bacteria always present in these areas, this mucus may result in overgrowth of these microorganisms. The overgrowth can overwhelm local defense mechanisms, resulting in tissue invasion and secondary infection.

It is nasal allergy that causes most "sinus trouble" and "ear trouble." And not only allergens but virus infections "caught" from others or initiated by getting chilled can open the defensive gates for bacterial invasion.

Allergic persons seem unduly susceptible to virus infections as well as secondary bacterial infections of the sinuses, eustachian tubes, ears, bronchial tubes, and lungs. Nasal allergy can also eventually result in asthma.

ASTHMA

In asthma, the airways are narrowed and obstructed by three processes: constriction of the muscle coat surrounding the bronchial tubes, swelling of the inner lining of the mucus membranes of the bronchi due to capillary leakage, and thick mucus produced by mucus-secreting cells in the bronchial lining membranes. A fourth problem, hyperactive or "twitchy" airways often present in such patients, can tend to make them wheeze when exposed to nonspecific irritants as well as to specific allergens.

BRAIN ALLERGY

In allergic mental symptoms, the problem apparently is leakage of capillary fluid into various portions of the brain. In migraine, brief constriction followed by prolonged overdilatation of blood vessels occurs in the skull and brain, and also produces fluid leakage from capillaries into these and other tissues.

COLON ALLERGY

In the colon, smooth muscle contraction can cause cramps, diarrhea, or spastic colon. On the other hand, allergic gas formation and smooth muscle dilatation can cause constipation, gas retention, and bloating.

Excessive mucus secretion in the colon can result in mucous colitis. Lack of sufficient mucus can cause dry, hard stools.

Allergic ulceration of the mucosa can cause inflammation and secondary infection. This can cause mouth ulcers. It can also cause chronic ulcerative colitis and ileocolitis (Crohn's disease), with consequent severe diarrhea, rectal bleeding, scarring of the colon, and a tendency to colon cancer.

Thus, in each syndrome, various harmful mechanisms may operate. This accounts for the endless varieties of allergic, allergic-like, inflammatory, infectious, and even malignant manifestations.

NEW KNOWLEDGE

We do not yet know all we need to know to arrive at a complete understanding of allergic, immunologic, and other reactions which affect homeostasis. A great flood of fascinating information from research centers is accumulating now, so we are rapidly learning a great deal more.

THE COMPLEX NETWORK INVOLVED IN MAINTAINING HEALTH

The main thing we are learning is that homeostasis-controlling mechanisms are astoundingly numerous, complex, and interdependent. They include many "turn-on" and "turn-off" switches, and reaction-stimulating and suppressing factors.

The maintenance of optimum health requires exquisitely perfect cooperative interaction of a myriad network of trillions of protective cells and chemicals. These cells and chemicals are analogous to a multitrillion-man military force with a great variety of weapons and tactics, always on the alert, perfectly timed and smoothly coordinated to oppose the thrusts of a constantly probing multitrillion-man army of viruses, bacteria, fungi, yeasts, allergens, toxins, and other threats to health.

THE ROLES OF HEREDITY AND ENVIRONMENT

A second thing we are learning is that many of us have genetic immune "differences," hereditary tendencies to develop flaws in our defense. Some of us have genes that tend to make us prone to develop allergic or other types of illnesses under certain environmental conditions, and for these illnesses to occur in certain organs.

In allergic persons, this altered way of reacting can be triggered by exposure or overexposure to many kinds of substances which are harmless to nonallergic persons. These include pollens, molds, dusts, foods, and other allergens.

THE IMMUNE SYSTEM CAN BE HARMFUL AS WELL AS HELPFUL

A third thing we are learning is that the chief impetus that turns on the protective mechanism is stimulation of the system by the very things that endanger us. This "turn-on" can result in either benefit or harm. For example, it is the invasion of the body by the measles virus that turns on the production of a *beneficial* antibody by certain specialized white blood cells called B lymphocytes. *Lymphocytes* are cells which circulate within lymphatic channels as well as blood vessels.

B lymphocytes only make antibodies. They are so termed because they are derived directly from *bone* marrow cells. T lymphocytes are those which travel from the bone marrow to the *thymus* gland in the lower neck and upper chest. Here they "go to school" and learn several very important lessons, including "helper" and "suppressor" functions.

Helper T lymphocytes are those which have learned to stimulate B lymphocytes to make more antibodies. *Suppressor* T lymphocytes are those which have learned to keep B lymphocytes from making too many antibodies. It is the balance between helper and suppressor T lymphocyte functions that keeps the antibody forming system on an even keel.

When measles viruses invade the body, they are first gobbled up by large cells in the tissues called *macrophages,* which means "big eaters." Macrophages in the circulation are called *monocytes,* named from the prefix "mono" meaning one, because these cells ("cytes") have one large nucleus. Tissue macrophages and circulating monocytes examine the ingested virus and learn its structure.

They send this information to T cells, along with a T-cell stimulating chemical called Interleukin I. Instructed/stimulated T cells then send the structural information to B cells, along with a B-cell controlling chemical called Interleukin II.

B cells respond by growing, multiplying, and manufacturing antibodies against the measles viruses. The quantity of antibodies produced by B cells is kept in balance by helper and suppressor T cells.

These measles antibodies help destroy the measles viruses to cure the illness. Then they continue to be manufactured for years to help protect from future attacks by these viruses.

In fact, future unrecognized exposures to measles viruses can automatically restimulate these specific lymphocytes. These exposures serve as silent boosters of beneficial antibody levels, protecting us from recurrent attacks of measles.

On the other hand, in allergic people with ragweed hay fever, inhaled ragweed pollen can stimulate certain B lymphocytes to produce the *allergic* antibody against ragweed allergen. This does not provide protection, but rather causes chemical mediator release by mast cells or basophils.

This results in symptoms such as occur in hay fever. Each reinhalation of ragweed pollen is likely to stimulate the production of more allergic antibody, causing recurrence of symptoms, not increased immunity.

This paradox of the harmful effect of one part of the immune mechanism is thought to be explained by the fact that it was originally evolved to protect us from worms and other parasites, as well as infecting microorganisms and malignant cells. It just happened that somewhere in our genetic development, the immune mechanisms of some people lost the ability to distinguish between living harmful cells and inert, ordinarily harmless molecules like milk and ragweed.

THE GOOD AND BAD NEWS OF IMMUNOLOGY

So here is the enigma, the contrast of a "good" normal protective immune response with the "bad" altered allergic response. Although several antibodies can be involved, the protecting antibody is usually immunoglobulin G (IgG), and the allergy antibody is usually immunoglobulin E (IgE).

Any substance that stimulates the body to produce any kind of antibodies is called an antigen. All allergens are thus antigens. However, not all antigens are allergens, as some antigens stimulate the production of *beneficial* antibodies such as *IgG.*

However, one antigen can simultaneously stimulate the production of *several* kinds of antibodies. Thus measles virus vaccine is considered an antigen but not an allergen when used in immunization against measles.

But, in a given patient, if the immunizing injection stimulates production of much IgE also, the patient may have an allergic reaction to the measles vaccine injection. In this instance, the measles vaccine is also acting as an allergen.

Whether the antigen is measles virus, ragweed pollen, milk, or another, *it is the antigen that drives the system.* And it often drives *both* of these facets, IgG and IgE, and many other facets as well, simultaneously and in various sequences and proportions. It is the final balance of all these interdependent and highly individualized biochemical and cellular mechanisms, genetic constitution, and environmental exposures that determines whether one is protected from or made sick by the antigen.

IMMUNOTHERAPY INJECTIONS

We have known for a long time that injections of measles vaccine or another virus vaccine can provide immunity against a specific inhaled virus, and that booster injections can increase this immunity. We also successfully use injections of allergenic extracts, for example, ragweed or dust mite extract, to provide protection from these specific allergens. The application of this method to allergens is called immunotherapy.

NOT ALL SENSITIVITIES ARE CAUSED BY IgE

We have used the example of IgE as one cause of chemical mediator release, not because it is the sole cause but because it is the one most investigated, best understood, and most easily described. We already know of at least three other causes of chemical mediator release, but these are too technical to detail in a volume of this sort.

While conventional allergy practice confines the usage of allergy immunotherapy chiefly to IgE mediated reactions, the benefits of neutralizing immunotherapy are much broader in scope. Even certain illnesses in which IgE plays no demonstrable role respond regularly to neutralization therapy.

A PROBLEM AND A SOLUTION IN IMMUNOTHERAPY

One of the greatest problems in immunotherapy has been the difficulty in finding just the right dose of each allergen to provide maximum relief with maximum safety. *What is new and revolutionary about neutralizing testing is that it enables us to find the best treatment dose of each allergen during allergy skin testing.* The benefits of this have far exceeded expectations.

This is true in ragweed allergy, in milk allergy, and in a wide variety of other allergies and nonallergic illnesses. We can now use this homeostasis-restoring dose of the offending substance itself to quickly drive the system back toward normal balance. This levels out the tilted mechanism and relieves the symptoms, *often within minutes.*

By using the "just-right" dose, we seem to be able to turn off the release or harmful effect of histamine and other chemical mediators much more quickly and effectively than ever before. In the next chapter, we will examine the materials and procedures used in achieving these benefits.

Chapter 4

THE NEUTRALIZING SYSTEM: HOW TO FIND THE "GOLDILOCKS DOSE"

Allergy skin testing and immunotherapy employ extracts of potential allergens to help establish the diagnosis and provide treatment for allergic syndromes. The extracts used are sterile solutions of the soluble ingredients of such substances as dusts, dust mites, molds, pollens, feathers, animal danders, foods, and other materials which can cause allergic symptoms in individuals sensitive to them.

THE MATERIALS: ALLERGENIC EXTRACTS

Extracts are manufactured and supplied to practicing physicians by federally licensed laboratories. A full strength extract is termed the stock solution or "concentrate."

In neutralizing testing, the concentrate is serially diluted into nine or more vials, each vial being weaker than the preceding vial. These vials are simply referred to as vials #1, #2, #3, and so on (Figure 4).

The purpose of having several strengths available of each extract is to enable the allergist to test individual patients with weaker or stronger solutions of various allergens as his judgment indicates. Allergists know that not all patients are equally sensitive in general, and that even in the same individual not all allergens are equally allergenic.

So choosing solutions of different strengths to test certain allergens in different patients has been a logical and time-honored practice by many allergists.

THE DIAGNOSTIC PROCEDURE: INTRADERMAL TESTING

Neutralization can be described most simply by breaking it down into its diagnostic and therapeutic features. The diagnostic feature involves administering very shallow intradermal injections of consecutive concen-

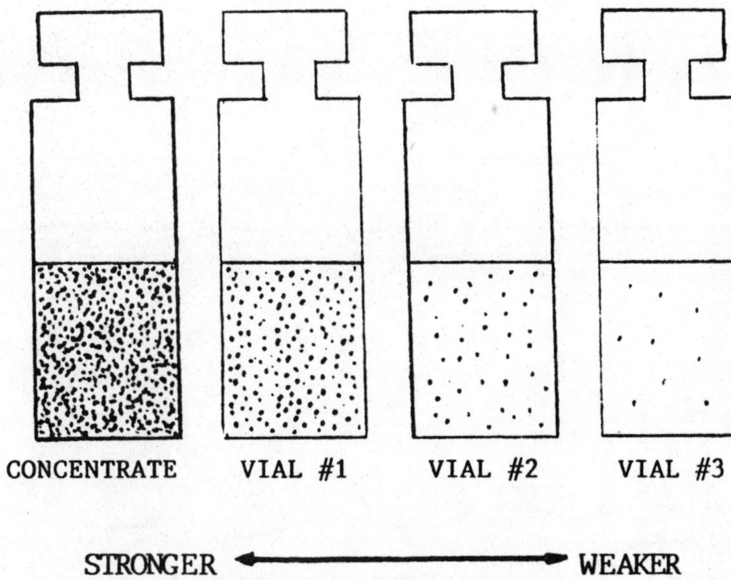

Figure 4. Dilutions of an allergenic extract. The concentrate is the full strength extract, and each consecutive dilution is five times weaker than the preceding dilution.

trations of a potentially allergenic extract such as milk extract, usually at the rate of one test injection per seven to ten minutes (Figure 5).

In a patient allergic to milk, intradermal injections of stronger concentrations of milk extract tend to produce positive skin wheals ("welts"), and injections of weaker concentrations tend to produce negative wheals. About seven to ten minutes are usually required for the skin to form a wheal which can be categorized as either positive or negative.

A positive wheal indicates the occurrence of a local allergic reaction (mast cell mediator release) at the site of the test injection. A negative wheal denotes the absence of such a reaction.

If one injects a relatively strong positive wheal-producing concentration first, and then injects consecutively weaker concentrations at seven to ten minute intervals, the *first* negative wheal concentration encountered while proceeding consecutively weaker is "the strongest negative wheal concentration." This is usually the neutralizing concentration.

For example, if Concentration #2 produces a positive wheal and #3 produces a negative wheal, then #3 is the strongest negative wheal concentration, that is, the most likely neutralizing concentration (Figure 6). All concentrations weaker than this will ordinarily result in negative wheals.

Thus, *the neutralizing concentration is usually the strongest negative-wheal*

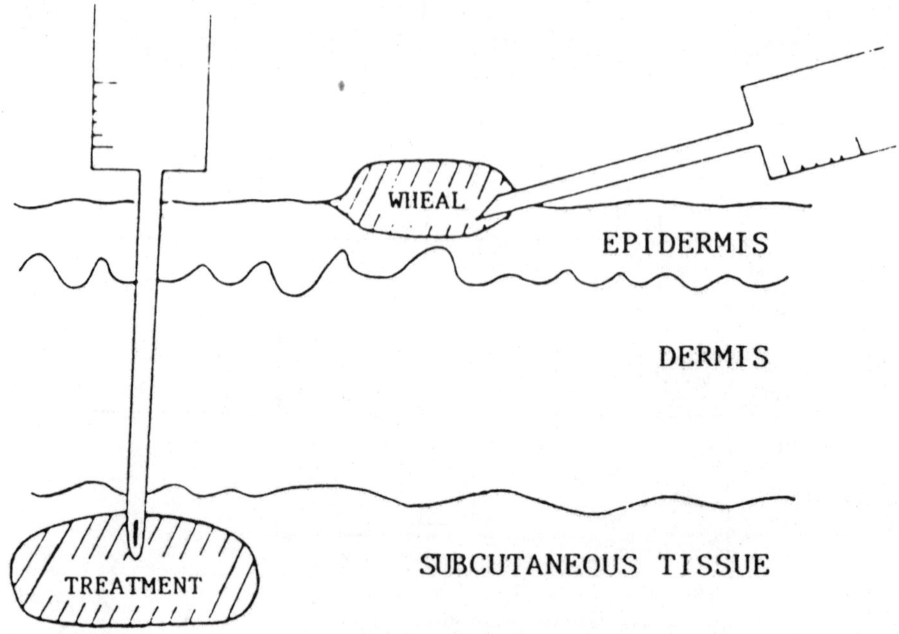

Figure 5. Intradermal and subcutaneous injections.

concentration in the consecutive series. It is just below the strength required to produce a positive local whealing reaction when injected intradermally so is termed *the maximum tolerated intradermal concentration.*

If no symptoms occur during testing, neutralizing doses are determined objectively by whealing alone. However, during testing some patients develop allergic symptoms such as headache, stomachache, congested nose, hives, or hyperactivity. Test-induced symptoms are often,

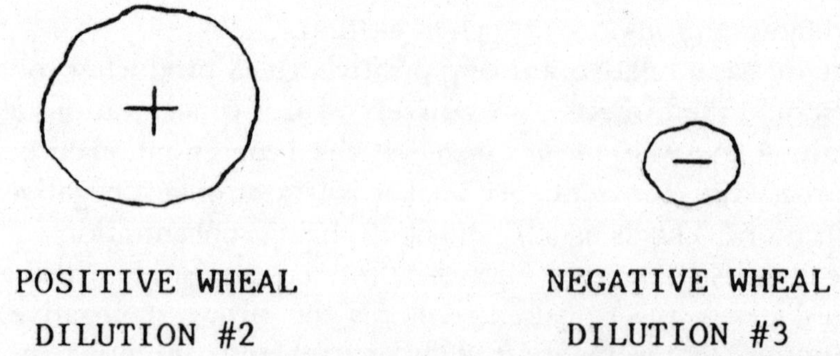

Figure 6. The dilution which produces a positive wheal (dilution #2 in this illustration) is too strong to be a neutralizing dilution. The first negative wheal encountered while proceeding consecutively weaker is usually the neutralizing dilution (dilution #3 in this illustration).

but not always, the same symptoms produced by natural exposure to that particular allergen, although usually much milder.

In some tests, no positive wheals form, but definite symptoms arise. The neutralizing concentration is then the concentration which relieves the symptoms.

Again, the neutralizing concentration always produces a negative wheal. When there is no positive wheal to signal the physician to inject consecutively weaker concentrations, it may be necessary to inject consecutively *stronger* concentrations to find the neutralizing concentration.

For example, if beef produces headache when eaten, an intradermal test injection of beef extract may produce mild headache with or without a positive wheal. When the neutralizing concentration is injected, this symptom usually disappears (neutralizes) within ten minutes.

THE GOLDILOCKS DOSE

This "just-right" dose can be lightly referred to as the "Goldilocks Dose." Like the three bowls of porridge in the home of the three bears, one dose is too strong, another dose is too weak, but this dose is *"just right"* (Figure 7).

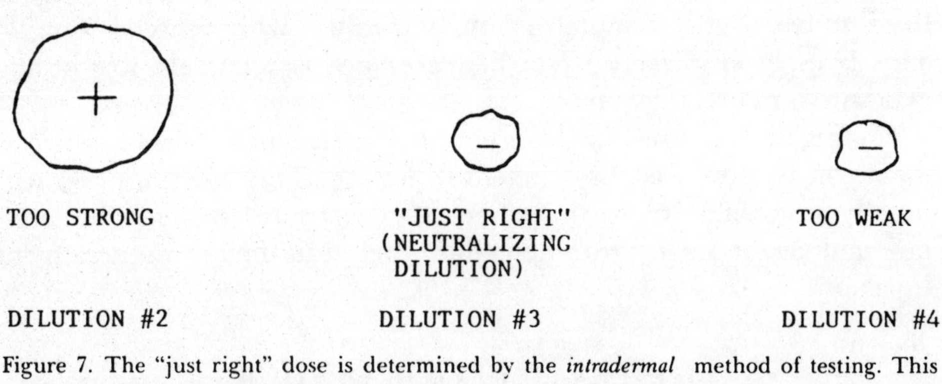

Figure 7. The "just right" dose is determined by the *intradermal* method of testing. This produces a local immunologic response (the wheal) which can be seen, felt, and measured. Subcutaneous injections bury the allergenic extract too deep beneath the skin for precise evaluation by the physician.

It is the golden mean, the homeostasis-restoring dose, the balancing dose, the dose which reinstates stability, the dose that makes the patient *feel* right. It is also the dose that *looks* right to the physician by inspection, measurement, and palpation.

The physician can also observe relief of the *objective* signs of discomfort such as visible hives, nasal congestion, hyperactive behavior, etc. Testing often reveals a remarkable correlation between the patient's desire for subjective relief and the physician's desire for objectively measurable wheal changes and physical signs in the patient.

THE MEANING OF POSITIVE WHEALS AND TEST SYMPTOMS

Asymptomatic Sensitivity. Performing skin tests on a person "off the street" who has never had an allergic illness and who experiences no symptoms from test injections can sometimes result in positive wheals to some injected extracts. However, this person is not sick and needs no treatment.

He is sensitive and the mast cells in his skin are releasing enough mediators at the test site to form positive wheals. This indicates potential future allergic illness. However, he has not yet developed stress-organ sensitivity to these antigens. He is sensitive but not symptomatic.

Symptomatic Sensitivity. On the other hand, in a patient with an allergic syndrome, one or more stress organs is reacting. Therefore, the production of *either* a positive wheal *or* test symptoms from an extract of a substance such as ragweed or milk indicates that this patient is highly likely to experience symptoms from encounters with ragweed or milk. This is especially likely when his resistance is relatively low or the exposure is of great degree.

Finding the neutralizing concentration determines the exact treatment concentration at the moment of testing. This concentration will usually protect and relieve the patient from exposures to these substances, now and also in the future when administered in the form of treatment injections.

THE TREATMENT PROCEDURE: SUBCUTANEOUS INJECTIONS

The treatment feature of neutralization consists in combining the neutralizing concentrations of all the foods to which the patient is sensitive into a single solution and administering injections of this solution subcutaneously at regular intervals (Figure 5). The usual interval is twice weekly.

This generally relieves and protects the patient from whatever symptoms he formerly suffered when he ate these foods. The same treatment system, with certain important procedural modifications, applies to inhalants and many other substances.

RESPONSE

This system of food allergy management allows the majority of patients to continue eating most or all of their allergenic foods without symptoms. This alone is a major breakthrough.

Previous methods of testing with food extracts were usually not very reliable. Treatment consisted only in attempted elimination from the diet of suspected allergenic foods.

Neutralization is also important because it has allowed us to identify many previously puzzling illnesses as being largely or entirely due to foods. It also enables us to provide hitherto unavailable relief through food extract injection therapy.

Whether the patient is sensitive to foods or inhalants, he does not have to wait for many months or years to be built up to a hopefully effective dose and begin improving. The precise effective dose is determined *during* testing.

The first treatment injection contains the full "just-right" effective dose for each substance tested. *No build-up of dosage is necessary.*

Most patients respond remarkably well within one, two, or three weeks. Many note improvement after the first few treatment injections, and some improve *while still undergoing testing.* Of course, patients with complicated problems such as chronic infections, sticky obstructing bronchial mucus, tissue destruction with scarring, and diseases of other organs may show a slower, more limited, or no beneficial response.

IT DOES NOT SEEM POSSIBLE BUT . . .

It does not seem possible that the mere determination of a given dose should be so remarkably effective. It does not seem possible that a single system of therapy can be useful in such a broad range of human ills.

It does not seem possible that the neutralizing phenomenon remained essentially undiscovered or at least not deliberately utilized for most of the three-quarters of a century that the profession of allergy has been in existence. Yet all these points are indisputably true.

AN ADDITIONAL BENEFIT: SAFE SELF-ADMINISTRATION

To repeat, patients with food and inhalant sensitivities usually obtain relief in *ten* minutes when the appropriate neutralizing dose is administered intradermally during testing. This ten-minute relief occurs whether the symptoms were caused by a symptom-inducing test injection or from naturally inhaling or eating the allergen.

The neutralizing dose of each allergen is not only rapidly beneficial, but is proved safe and well tolerated in each patient by office testing under direct observation. Therefore, once the physician is satisfied that the neutralizing doses are correct, the injections are safe and can almost always be self-administered at home.

At home, the injections are given subcutaneously. The subcutaneous injection procedure is readily learned by the patient or a family member through office instruction and supervision. Relief from subcutaneous injections administered at home often occurs within *thirty* minutes.

The patient who develops a stomachache or stuffy nose from excessive exposure to an allergen or from delaying a regularly scheduled treatment injection can usually obtain quick relief simply by giving himself a "booster" or extra injection. He is freed from the necessity of making an appointment and visiting a physician's office for each of his regular treatment injections and always has his relief at hand, whether at night, on weekends, or on out-of-town trips.

The ability of physicians to provide relief-giving injections is not only a great saving of time and money, but also provides a confidence, independence, satisfaction, and improved patient-physician relationship never before known in allergy therapy. In addition, adherence to the injection schedule is much greater than in the patient who must be inconvenienced by having to travel to the doctor's office to receive each of his injections, and can notice no direct benefit from any individual injection.

When recurrence of symptoms clearly follows allergen exposure or delaying treatment injections, and when relief upon resumption of the injections is so rapid, reliable, and convenient, the patient is much more apt to understand and accept the connection between allergy and illness, injections and relief. He is thus more highly motivated to continue his injections on schedule for maximum continuing benefit.

FOR PROFESSIONAL AND NONPROFESSIONAL READERS

The description of neutralizing testing and treatment just presented is a mere outline of principles. Many variations of the basic procedures are required for specific patients, and many modifications of technique are required for testing and treatment with various extracts and vaccines.

I hope that the simple concepts described here are sufficient for the general understanding of the nonprofessional reader. However, it is not intended that physicians read this basic explanation and launch into the procedure.

Experience in management of allergic and environmental illnesses and the development and maintenance of expertise in the fields of allergy, immunology, and neutralization therapy should accompany the use of these procedures. The simplified concepts and procedures described in this book do not constitute a sufficient knowledge base for physician application.

CHAPTER 5

HIDDEN FOOD SENSITIVITY: A CAUSE OF "IDIOPATHIC," "PSYCHOSOMATIC," "HOPELESS," AND "INTRACTABLE" ILLNESSES

Although many additional uses of neutralization have been discovered, the food methodology remains basic. Modifications of technique for inhalants and other allergens are simply variations on the basic theme. It is proper, then, that we first probe deeper into the nature of food allergy and food neutralization procedures before discussing other facets of this subject.

IMMEDIATE (OBVIOUS) FOOD ALLERGY

Allergic food responses are usually classified into two types, immediate (obvious) and delayed (hidden). However, this is very unsatisfactory nomenclature, since many so-called *immediate-type* (obvious) reactions do not occur until hours after exposure, and the food cause of the reaction is not always obvious to the patient.

Similarly, *delayed-type* (hidden) reactions often begin to some degree within minutes after exposure, although the symptoms may not be of the type ordinarily considered "allergic," such as hay fever, asthma, or skin reactions. Furthermore, the food cause of the "hidden" reaction may be discerned by an *aware* patient.

However, this is the way these terms are used at the present time. At any rate, neutralization therapy is usually highly effective for *both* types.

Immediate food allergy is usually relatively easy to diagnose because the symptoms sometimes (not always) occur within a short time after exposure, and are often severe or sudden in onset. It is often recognizable because it is caused by an unusual food or one that is eaten infrequently. The patient may be noticeably sensitive to only one food. The skin test for that food is often positive.

So in immediate food allergy, the causative relationship is often obvious.

A treatment, dietary avoidance of the causative food, is also obvious, although not always easy. Examples of immediate food allergy reactions include the swollen lip that may follow the eating of shrimp; acute hives after eating orange; asthma after drinking milk; or anaphylactic shock after eating egg.

DELAYED (HIDDEN) FOOD ALLERGY

Immediate food allergy was formerly considered to constitute the entire field of food allergy. Delayed food allergy was not believed to really exist. However, we now know that immediate food allergy is just the small, visibly dramatic tip of the iceberg, and that delayed food allergy is far more common.

The subject of food allergy goes far deeper and broader than this. The use of neutralizing testing and treatment has confirmed what pioneers in the food allergy field have been observing and telling us for many decades, namely that some of the most common, chronic, and incapacitating illnesses of mankind are caused by delayed or hidden food allergy.

Patients with hidden food allergy tend to be allergic to many more foods than those with obvious food allergy. Many are allergic in some degree to virtually every food they eat frequently, yet may have no inkling that they are allergic at all.

Allergists themselves have long tended to ignore positive food wheals because they usually differ in appearance from what has been long considered the standard appearance of positive wheals. These differences will be described later.

In any one patient, the symptoms may not emerge noticeably until long after eating the causative foods, and many foods may be causing symptoms simultaneously. Therefore, many such patients suffer puzzling illnesses and are more or less chronically sick. Unfortunately, they are not usually aware that foods have anything to do with their problems, much less able to sort out which specific foods are the culprits.

We now know that hidden food allergy can cause illnesses long called "idiopathic," or self-causing, meaning that we simply did not know their causes. We also know that hidden food allergy can cause illnesses formerly termed "psychosomatic" or "emotional," which are additional wastebasket terms sometimes used when causes are unknown and ordinary examinations and laboratory tests are essentially negative.

This is particularly so when the suffering of the patient appears to be greater than seems justified by the absence of positive physical and laboratory findings. However, this is a common situation in hidden food allergy.

Hidden food allergy is further known to cause illnesses we have long considered "hopeless" or "intractable." This can mean untreatable, resistant to known treatments, or incurable.

We did not know that these idiopathic, psychosomatic, hopeless, and intractable illnesses could be caused by foods. Therefore, we did not know that food allergy treatment could be helpful in such cases. We also did not have the neutralizing system with which to demonstrate the cause-and-effect relationship and provide relief.

If you ask your family physician, "What percentage of your practice consists of functional (psychosomatic) complaints?" he will probably answer, "At least 50 percent." Little does he know that many of these patients are really suffering from allergic illness, particularly hidden food sensitivity.

IgE MECHANISMS OF FOOD ALLERGY

Immediate food allergy has been fairly well studied in the laboratory. However, the existence of hidden food allergy has been denied and its study largely neglected until recently. We are just beginning to learn about the biochemical mechanisms of hidden food reactions.

Immediate food reactions have often been shown to be caused by the same mast cell and basophil released histamine and other chemical mediators which cause the classic inhalant allergy syndromes such as hay fever and asthma. Why do these cells release such harmful chemicals?

The cell surface of each mast cell and basophil is coated as though by barnacles with hundreds of thousands of molecules of the allergy antibody, IgE. An IgE molecule is "Y" shaped, like a lobster, with one tail and two claws. Each IgE molecule firmly attaches its tail end to an IgE receptor in the cell membrane, like an electric plug into a socket, leaving its two active or claw ends to wave about in the surrounding fluid, seeking specific passing allergens (Figure 8).

In immediate allergy, IgE molecules on cell membranes are often the ones that do the dirty work. Like partners in crime, they work in pairs.

Their mode of operation is somewhat like that of two muggers who suddenly emerge from each side of a wooded path to grab each arm of a lone

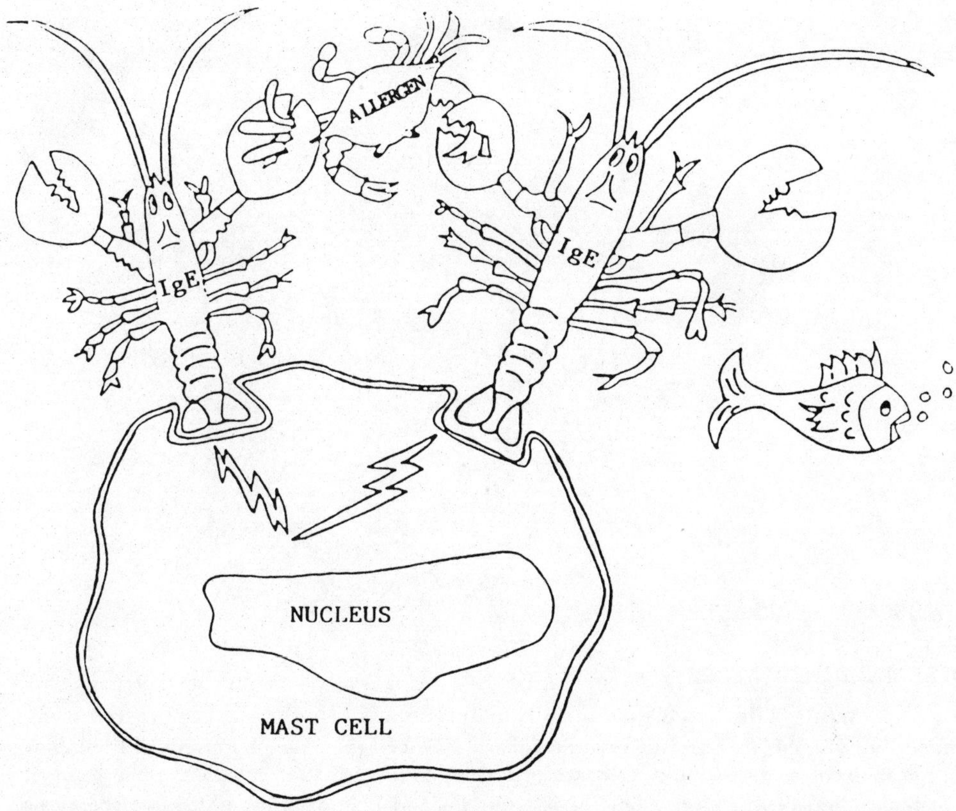

Figure 8. Allergen interaction at the mast cell surface. (The granules have been omitted for greater clarity.) In this illustration, the IgE molecules are sensitive to crab but not to fish. A crab molecule is grasped by two crab-sensitive IgE molecules, causing the mast cell to spew out chemicals and chemical-containing granules that can cause allergic symptoms. This patient is not allergic to fish, and has no fish-sensitive IgE molecules, so can eat fish without suffering allergic symptoms.

passerby. Thus, one claw end of each of two adjacent IgE molecules grabs hold of one allergenic "arm" of a passing allergen molecule (Figure 9).

WHAT GENERATES THE MEDIATOR-RELEASING SIGNAL?

When one allergen molecule is grabbed by two adjacent IgE antibody molecules (this is called an allergen-antibody reaction at the cell surface), a closing or bridging of the gap between the two IgE molecules occurs. The allergen serves as the connector or circuit-closer between the two antibody molecules.

This connection allows the antigen-antibody complex on the cell

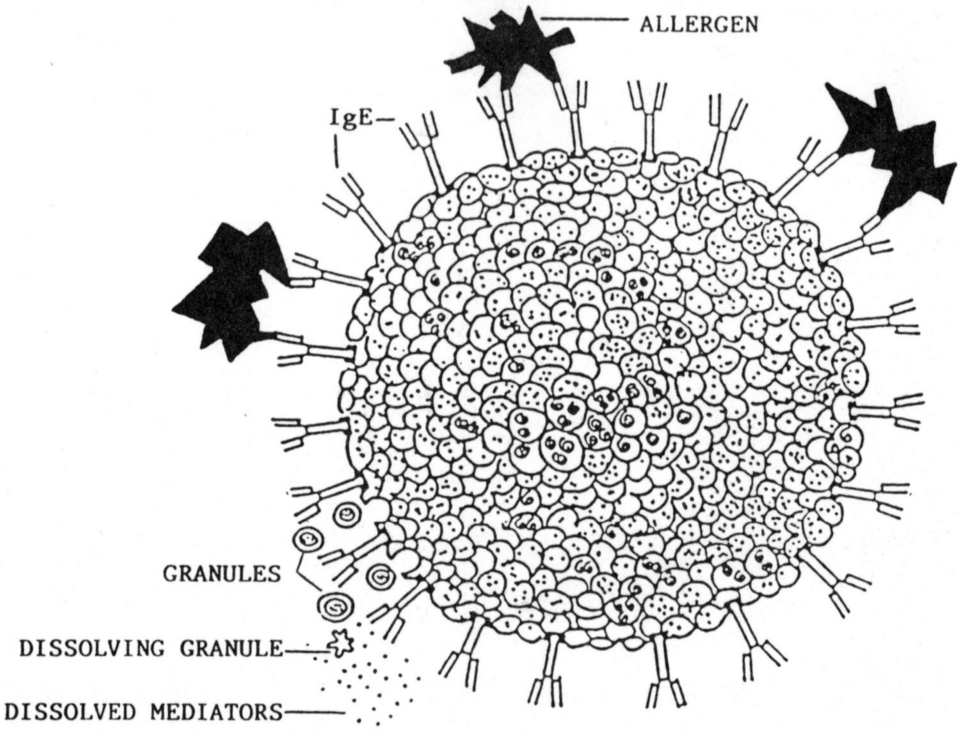

Figure 9. Mast cell discharging granules. A mast cell looks like a plastic bag (the cell membrane) full of seeds or nuts (the granules). Each mast cell may have hundreds of thousands of IgE molecules attached to its cell membrane. When two IgE molecules grasp one allergen molecule, the cell discharges some of its granules and manufactures additional chemicals which can cause allergic symptoms. Granules which have been extruded and are in the process of dissolving and releasing granule-bound chemical mediators are shown in the lower left corner of the illustration.

surface to generate a signal which passes through the tail ends (the electric plugs) of the two IgE molecules through the receptors (the sockets) to the inside of the cell. This is like triggering a panic button, forcing the cell to release its chemical mediators. Presumably this release helps fight the allergen molecules in the body, which the IgE molecules perceive (often falsely) as harmful.

THE SPECIFICITY OF THE REACTION

Since the presence of IgE is often necessary for an immediate allergic reaction to occur, immediate reactions are usually called IgE-mediated reactions. However, just any IgE molecule will not seize just any allergen molecule. If a patient is sensitive only to peanut, this means that he has developed only peanut-specific IgE molecules; they will combine only with peanut allergen molecules.

The claw ends of these IgE molecules are built only for peanut grabbing. Peanut-IgE will not combine with egg, ragweed, or other allergens. The fit is as specific as a key for its lock.

THE SEVERITY OF THE REACTION

The number of IgE molecules the body forms against a given substance like peanut is important. The greater the number, the closer they fit together on the surfaces of the basophils and mast cells, and the more likelihood that two adjacent peanut-sensitive IgE molecules will be able to pair up and grab a passing peanut allergen molecule.

The greater the number of such antigen-IgE combinations the greater the number of mediator-releasing signals sent to the cell, and the greater the amount and rapidity of mediators released. When much free-floating (unbound) allergen in the blood and tissue fluid reaches the IgE molecules on the mast cells or basophils in a short period of time, the release of chemical mediators would be expected to be greater and more rapid, and the symptoms more or less "immediate."

If the number of cell-bound IgE molecules is not great enough, or if the number of arriving allergen molecules is not great enough, there may not be enough chemical mediator release to produce a symptom reaction. The patient may experience no or very mild symptoms.

Or the free mediator concentration in the tissues or blood may not reach the symptom-threshold level (the level required to activate a stress organ) and he may have no symptoms ("asymptomatic sensitivity"). So an allergic patient may have no symptoms on a given exposure because the *allergen* exposure is small, or because his *IgE level* for that allergen is low, or because the quantity of *chemical mediators* released at this time is not adequate to trigger his more or less sensitive *stress organ.*

WHY SYMPTOMS DO NOT OCCUR WITH EVERY MEAL

Thus you may be able to eat such a food in limited amounts or at infrequent intervals without symptoms. However, if you eat the same food in larger amounts or more frequently or at the same time as other allergenic foods, sufficient total chemical mediator release may sum up over a period of time to cause noticeable symptoms. This is one reason why a food will seem allergenic at one time but not at another.

This repeated stepwise release and build-up of mediators over time may be one explanation for episodic, delayed, or hidden food reactions. Another is that some chemical mediators are not quickly released. Some seep out more slowly than others, and some must first be manufactured and released over time by the cell, thus causing symptoms hours later. This is called "the late phase of the immediate reaction."

Reactions mediated by other cells such as lymphocytes, which are finally prodded into action by the chemicals released from mast cells and basophils, may not occur until one or more days later. These are called "delayed reactions."

Alternatively, there may be no symptoms in any case until the overall defense system is overburdened by chilling, fatigue, hormonal changes, infections, metabolic slowing which occurs during sleeping hours, or many other factors. Furthermore, chemical mediator release can be triggered by non-IgE and nonimmunologic factors, the symptom-inducing patterns of which are not all known yet.

THE RAST

A recently evolved laboratory method for determining whether or not a specific IgE (such as peanut-IgE) is present in the blood of a given patient is called the Radio-Allergo-Sorbent Test or RAST. However, the RAST is less sensitive than skin tests, especially for foods, although it is sometimes used to determine the level of IgE in the serum for specific allergens.

Since it is only a test for IgE, the RAST also fails entirely to detect non-IgE causes of allergic symptoms, of which there are several, so is of virtually no value in non-IgE mediated food allergy. The RAST as currently performed is therefore as yet of limited usefulness to the practicing allergist in detecting the presence of hidden food allergies.

The same is true for another laboratory test using enzymes rather than radioactive substances, the ELISA test (Enzyme Linked Immuno-Sorbent Assay). Hopefully this will be remedied by further research.

THE FOOD-ILLNESS CONNECTION

Knowing that foods cause a disease can lead us to the control of the disease. Conversely, learning that we can quickly and effectively control an idiopathic, psychosomatic, hopeless, or intractable illness with food extract injection therapy leads us to the recognition that the illness is really caused by food allergy.

Failure to recognize the food-illness connection has led to untold suffering by millions. It is therefore extremely important for both patients and physicians to understand the depth and breadth of the food-illness connection. Some additional reasons why this connection has been largely overlooked in the past are discussed in the next chapter.

Chapter 6

TEN REASONS WHY YOUR HIDDEN FOOD SENSITIVITIES MAY NOT HAVE BEEN DETECTED

Some foods which cause delayed symptoms are recognized by a few observant patients, particularly if these foods are eaten infrequently. However, for the ten reasons listed below, most delayed type food reactions are not known to the patient.

1. SUMMATION OF FEEDINGS

Absorption of food molecules into the bloodstream begins as soon as the food enters the mouth. Absorption continues at varying rates until the food has been evacuated from the anus.

Food absorption usually occurs for about three or four days. However, it may last up to seven or more days in some instances, particularly in the presence of prolonged constipation.

Many clinical and laboratory observations suggest that the blood level of a food eaten only once seems to reach a maximum at about one and one-half to two hours. It then begins to decline gradually but irregularly.

This level does not seem to finally fall to zero until about four days later. By then the food is usually no longer present in the gastrointestinal tract, and the residual food antigen molecules in the blood and tissues have been completely metabolized.

When a food is eaten daily or several times daily a high food blood level is maintained. Then a reaction to a given food occurs while the patient is still reacting to one or more previous meals of the same food—and may also be reacting to one or more previous meals of other allergenic foods as well.

Symptoms thus tend to be more or less chronic. They seem unrelated to a given meal or a given food.

Anything that causes an increased rate of absorption of a food from the digestive tract is more apt to cause the emergence of symptoms. Increased rate of absorption can occur from intestinal diseases, diarrhea, or taking alcoholic beverages with the food. It can also occur when eating the food on an empty stomach such as when first arising in the morning.

As well, increased food antigen absorption can occur when taken in a liquid form, for example, soup, or when little or no digestion is required before absorption. Absorption of small or undigested molecules can also be increased when there is a deficiency of certain digestive enzymes or of protective antibodies normally present in the digestive system.

Exercising vigorously soon after taking an allergenic food also seems to increase the rate of emergence of symptoms. However, this may be related to increased physical stress more than to an increased rate of absorption.

2. DELAYED AND PROLONGED REACTIONS

One problem that has made delayed food allergy difficult to diagnose in the past is that most of us did not realize that a reaction—even a sudden, severe one—may occur so late and continue for so long a time after a given allergenic food is eaten even once. We did not recognize that such a reaction might not begin or noticeably emerge for many hours and might then last or recur repeatedly for days.

Furthermore, several meals of this food may have been eaten in the past few days so that all these portions of the food are absorbing more or less simultaneously from different segments of the gastrointestinal tract, causing daily or chronic symptoms. Neither did we know that so many other foods eaten in the past few days could also be causing symptoms at the same time.

3. THE GREAT NUMBER OF FOOD INGREDIENTS IN THE SYSTEM

Most people eat three or more meals daily, and each meal usually contains at least five to ten food ingredients. These foods continue absorbing for about three days.

By simple arithmetic 5 to 10 foods per meal times 3 meals per day equals 15 to 30 foods per day. Over a three-day period, forty-five to ninety food portions accumulate in the digestive tract. Thus forty-five to ninety food ingredients are entering the bloodstream simultaneously, potentially impacting on immunologic mechanisms.

This is a conservative figure since many processed foods such as bakery products, packaged cereals, dried or canned mixtures, mayonnaise, salad dressing, etc. may each contain dozens or scores of ingredients. Even a "simple" food such as milk contains a great many potentially allergenic substances.

So a person on an average diet probably has several hundred food ingredients in his gastrointestinal tract and bloodstream at any one time. These are not all necessarily allergenic but the potential is there, increasing the difficulty of detecting individual allergens.

4. PATIENTS MAY BE SENSITIVE TO MANY FOODS

It is not uncommon to see patients with hidden allergies to thirty or more foods who, on initial history, can incriminate only a few foods, such as tomato, oatmeal, and apple. Many patients suffering from recurrent headaches know only that if they eat chocolate today, they will probably awaken tomorrow in the early morning hours with a severe headache.

What they do not realize is that the headaches they have on many days when known allergenic foods are not eaten are due to milk, wheat, corn, soy, egg, beef, coffee, potatoes, tomatoes, lettuce, and possibly other staple foods they eat daily or frequently. This multiplicity of allergens represents a near-impossible tangle which few patients can recognize, much less sort out, without help.

5. REPEATED BURSTS OF ABSORPTION

One interesting observation I have made many times concerning gastrointestinal absorption is that an allergenic food eaten for dinner one evening may cause no symptoms that evening or during sleep. However, when a nonallergenic meal is eaten the next morning, the reawakening of the gastrointestinal tract, which has been dormant during sleep, apparently results in renewed absorption of the allergenic food eaten the day before.

This finally brings forth symptoms. The allergenic food was *eaten* only once, but the increased burst of *absorption* occurred twice, boosting the blood level and producing symptoms in the same manner as though it had been eaten twice.

The patient may even have his headache or stomachache repeatedly, after *several* consecutive nonallergenic meals, from an allergenic food eaten only once but absorbed again in bursts after subsequent meals. He may never be able to pinpoint the causative food because he did not eat it at each of the meals. This is also one reason why some patients who are put on entirely allergen-free diets or total fasts will continue to have symptoms periodically for two, three, or more days before obtaining relief.

6. VARYING THRESHOLDS AND MEDIATOR LEVELS

As discussed, one may have "asymptomatic sensitivity" to some foods. In this instance, the patient may have no symptoms when any one of these foods is eaten once or alone. However, he may have symptoms when eating one allergenic food twice at close intervals, or repeatedly, or when eating several "asymptomatic" allergenic foods together or at close intervals (Figure 10).

This phenomenon suggests that the blood mediator level may be elevated by a single feeding, but not always to the level of the symptom threshold for that food (Figure 11). Eating one allergenic food repeatedly, or eating two or more allergenic foods together or at close intervals, or eating an allergenic food while being exposed to an allergenic inhalant may further elevate the mediator level.

Thus the mediator level finally exceeds the symptom threshold, resulting in illness. This fits clinical observation and is supported in its broad outlines by the research done by Dr. Charles D. May at the National Jewish Hospital in Denver on elevated blood histamine levels and asymptomatic sensitivity in some food-sensitive patients.[24]

7. ADDITIVE EFFECT OF NONFOOD STRESSES

Puzzling symptom fluctuations in the same patient may also be produced at times by *nonfood allergens.* A food-sensitive patient may also be sensitive to inhalant particles, chemicals, or drugs. In a given patient, one particular organ may be the common organ of symptom-expression for both foods and inhalants, and for other allergens as well, just as a wagon's wheels tend always to fall into the same worn ruts in a well-traveled dirt road.

The symptoms may be asthma, headache, diarrhea, itching, muscle/joint pain, or hyperactivity—depending on the patient. Further, the same symptom initiated by allergic stresses may also be precipitated by *non-*

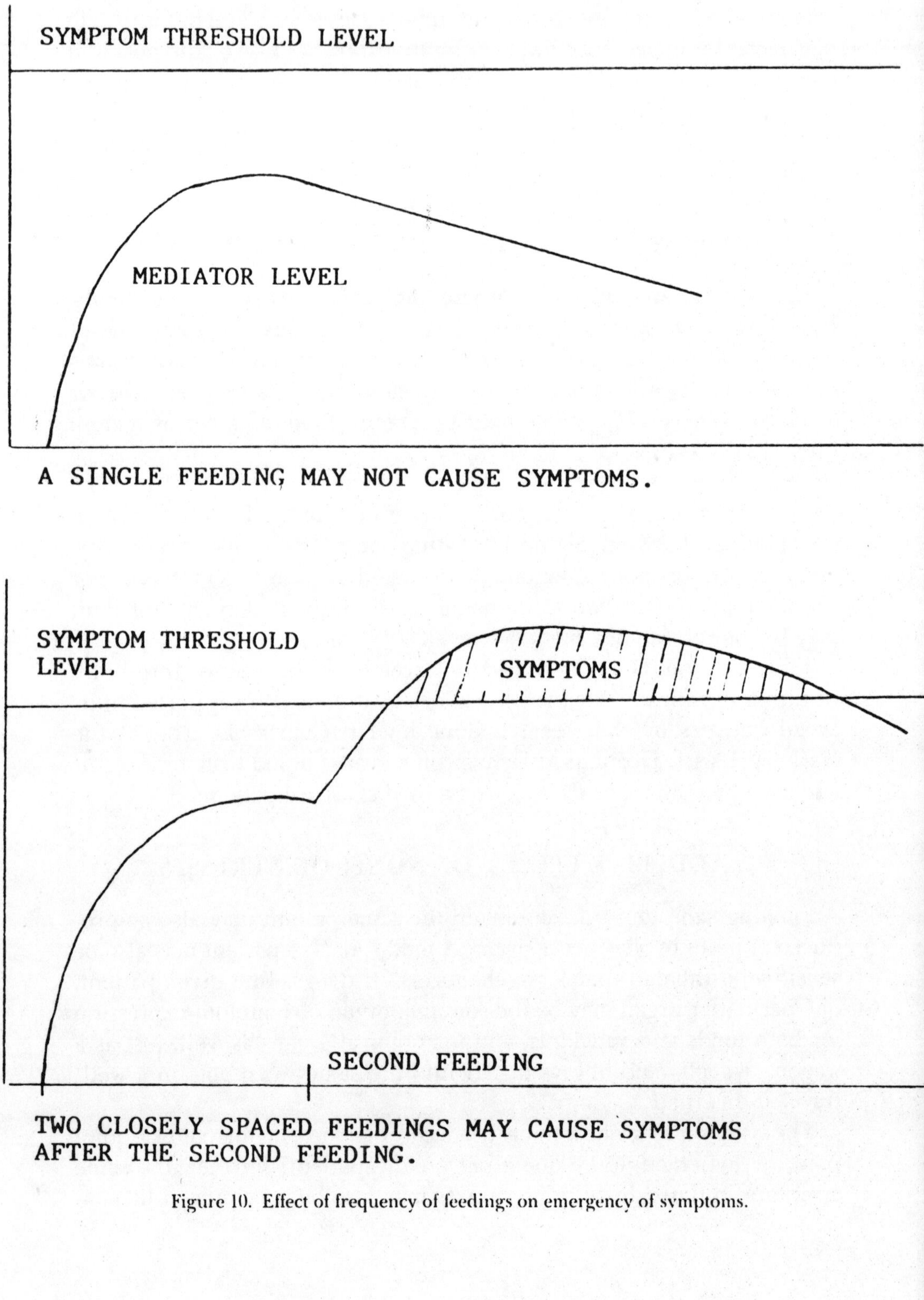

Figure 10. Effect of frequency of feedings on emergency of symptoms.

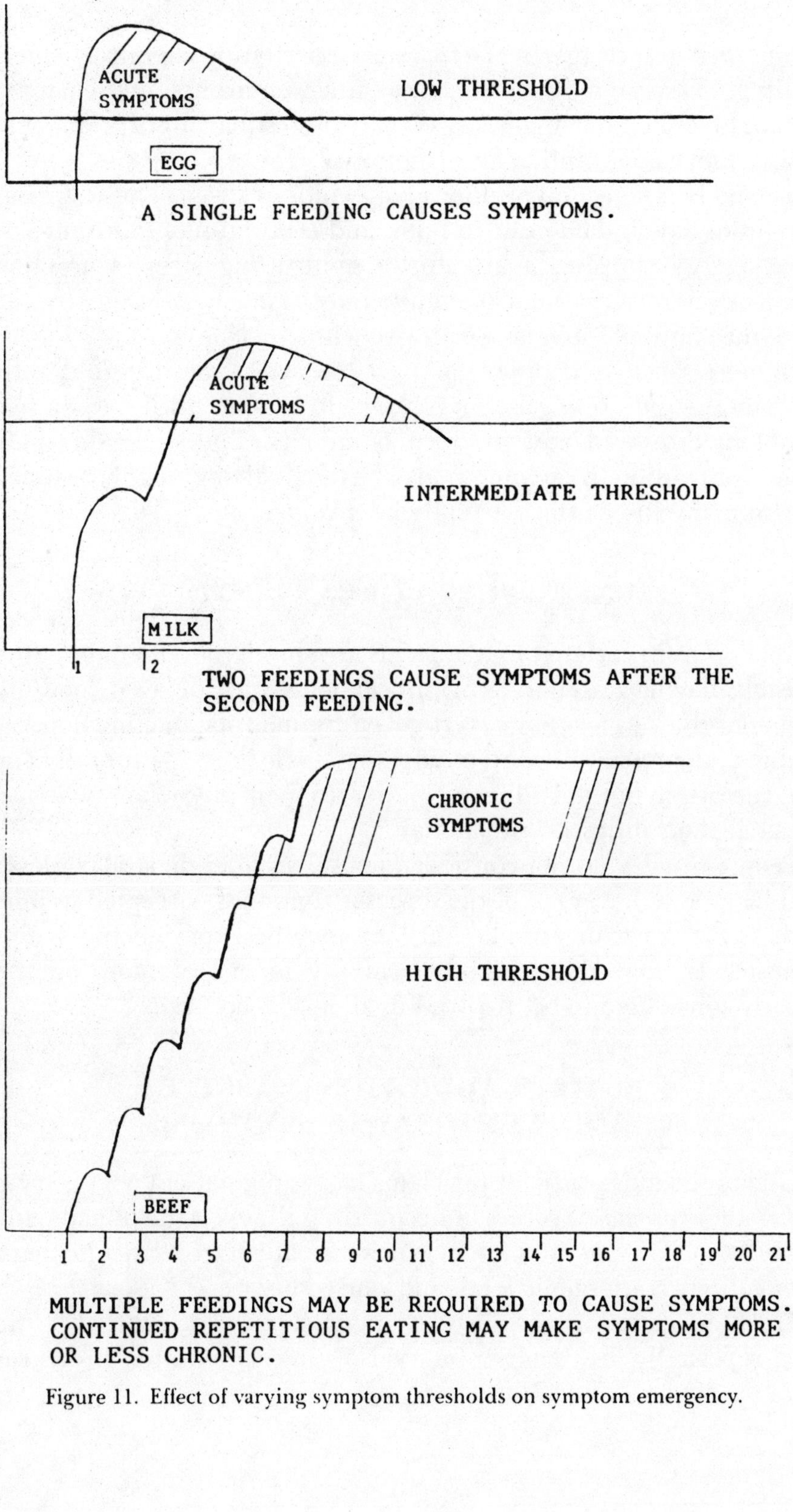

Figure 11. Effect of varying symptom thresholds on symptom emergency.

allergic stresses or triggering factors such as irritating chemicals, infection, chilling, exercise, fatigue, season, weather, environmental changes, the day-night cycle, varying rates of gastrointestinal absorption, menses, postpartum susceptibility, and emotional stresses.

The body is constantly under many kinds of stress. These stresses can vary from day to day, hour to hour, and even minute to minute. Metabolic energy supplies available for controlling stresses are limited. Homeostatic mechanisms can endure only so much. Allergic stresses add on to the "normal" stresses we all live with.

In more sensitive people, who have low symptom thresholds, allergic and nonallergic stresses are more prone to sum up until they exceed the symptom threshold and produce symptoms. The stress that gets the blame for causing the symptom may be the final one, the "last straw," but a great many stresses may actually be involved.

8. UNSUSPECTED ORGANS INVOLVED

Symptoms in certain organ systems are simply not often thought of as possibly having an allergic origin. Patients with delayed food allergy symptoms such as headache, vertigo, gastrointestinal malfunction, mental dullness, depression, hyperactivity, or muscle/joint pain rarely suspect the true origin of their illness. Neither do their physicians, who usually consider their illnesses "functional."

People usually do not consider themselves allergic at all unless they also happen to have one of the diseases commonly accepted as allergic, such as hay fever or asthma. Yet they may be experiencing symptoms almost every day due to food sensitivity in one or more organs not usually considered to be involved in allergic reactions.

9. FOOD ADDICTION (MASKING) AND WITHDRAWAL SYMPTOMS

One of the most difficult problems facing the patient who is trying to fit together the jigsaw pieces of his puzzling illness is the phenomenon of *masking*.[25] This is the situation in which the patient feels *better* immediately after eating an allergenic food, and worse later on.

He often learns—consciously or unconsciously—to eat that particular food repeatedly at whatever interval of time is required in his case to keep him feeling relatively well. *It is primarily when he postpones or misses a meal or snack of this food that he develops symptoms.*

The first sensation produced by eating the masking food is often a pleasant, mild stimulation or relaxation accompanied by a feeling of well-being, extra energy, increased mental acuity, self-confidence, exhilaration, or creativity. If the food is not eaten repeatedly, this may give way to the delayed symptoms, often including central nervous system depression, physical sluggishness, mental dullness, drowsiness, weakness, fatigue, irritability, apartness, depression, or despair.

During the stimulatory phase, he may tend to be energetic, positive, extroverted, gregarious, witty, and friendly; whereas during the depressive phase, he may feel tired, negative, introverted, inadequate, frightened, isolated, lonely, irritable, hostile, or even aggressive. Like Dr. Jekyll and Mr. Hyde, his mood and behavior can change rapidly from supersocial to antisocial.

By eating the masking food often, regularly, and in fairly uniform quantities, the patient maintains the immediate positive effect. This staves off the delayed negative effect. In other words, he masks or overrides his depressive symptoms. He does not consider the food harmful, but rather beneficial. It is a favorite food because he feels so much better when he eats it. Interestingly, he also usually comes to consider it particularly tasty or delicious.

The masking patient does not usually note the immediate stimulation, or at least does not consider it abnormal. In his estimation, this "high" is his normal state.

If he stops the addicting food suddenly and entirely, he may have great central nervous system depression and a physical withdrawal reaction for one or more days, possibly with symptoms such as weakness, trembling, flushing, lethargy, fatigue, headache, imbalance, unsteady gait, joint pains, slurred speech, tingling, or cold sweats. This may possibly cast suspicion on foods eaten on those days but not likely on the one omitted.

Since at any one time several masked foods may be causing either stimulatory or depressive symptoms of various types and degrees simultaneously, the patient is often caught in a maze of conflicting sensations. He may thus exhibit puzzling or volatile mood and behavioral swings which are beyond the understanding of himself and those around him.

10. INCREASED TENDENCY TO LIVE ON "FACTORY FOODS" AND MIXES

An additional difficulty in sorting out food problems has come from the complex, mixed, and chemicalized forms in which these foods are now usually eaten. Factory-processed foods make up an ever larger proportion of the modern diet. They are designed and prepared by chemists in factories rather than by cooks in kitchens. They are often erroneously called "health foods" and are highly touted on television.

Some people live almost entirely on factory-processed foods. These often are mixtures containing a multitude of foods or food-derived ingredients, many of which may not be listed on the labels. Such foods often contain many synthetic and nonsynthetic additives such as artificial colors, flavors, and preservatives, *many of which are not discoverable even by an aware consumer.*

SUMMARY OF THE TEN REASONS WHY YOUR HIDDEN FOOD SENSITIVITIES MAY NOT HAVE BEEN DETECTED

(1) Reactions may require the summation of adverse effects of two or more closely spaced feedings of a single food, or of two or more allergenic foods combined.
(2) Reactions are often delayed and prolonged, so are difficult to connect to the causative foods.
(3) There is a great number of food ingredients in the circulatory system at the same time, all potentially impacting on immune and other mechanisms.
(4) Food allergens are often too numerous for the patient to sort out individually.
(5) The gastrointestinal tract tends to actively absorb nutrients in bursts after subsequent meals which do not contain that food, resulting in several recurrences of symptoms, although the food was eaten only once.
(6) Symptoms may occur only when an elevated mediator blood level surpasses the symptom threshold; thus a food may be tolerated at one time but not at another.
(7) Symptom emergence may require the summation of food allergen and nonfood allergen exposures, physiologic stresses, and immunologic burdens.

(8) Organs may be involved which are not often thought of as expressing symptoms of allergy, so allergy is not considered in seeking causes of the "functional" symptoms.
(9) The masking phenomenon may make one feel better after eating the food (addiction), and worse when failing to eat it (withdrawal symptoms).
(10) There is an increasing tendency to live on processed foods and mixtures containing unidentifiable ingredients manufactured by chemists in factories rather than simple wholesome natural foods containing identifiable ingredients prepared by cooks in kitchens.

THE WAY OUT OF THE TANGLE

Sensitivity reactions do occur to multiple hidden foods, food derivatives, and chemical ingredients of foods. Sorting these out as the causes of symptoms can be very complicated and time-consuming, and total avoidance of them can be very difficult. However, a great deal can usually be accomplished through

(1) *Neutralization therapy* for identifiable allergens,
(2) Eating only *natural, wholesome foods,*
(3) *Avoiding* eating, or repeatedly eating, selected foods which still cause symptoms, especially when eaten too frequently, and
(4) Learning how to avoid *hidden* allergenic food ingredients.

The physician's knowledge and the patient's self-discipline can be critical. The cooperation of food manufacturers could certainly help.

Chapter 7

WHY YOUR SYMPTOMS EMERGE: THE BALANCE BETWEEN TOTAL RESISTANCE LEVEL AND TOTAL STRESS LOAD

Because of all these obscuring phenomena, hidden food allergy has *not* been much accepted or written about until very recently, and is still considered controversial by some. Scientific research in this field is difficult, so there have been very few studies of hidden food allergy. Hopefully, investigators will soon try harder.

On the other hand, for decades psychologic factors in illness have been very much on everyone's mind and tongue. Psychologists and most other people—including us physicians—have been prone to think that most such ailments are due to psychologic stress.

Psychologic stress really can cause many problems. We all have some psychologic stress in our lives on which to blame things. So it is no wonder that although your problem may fit into the food-caused category, you have not known or suspected that your symptoms may be due to hidden food allergy.

If so, it is time to bring it out of the closet and seek relief. This is best achieved by understanding how hidden food allergy interacts with other factors in our lives to make us ill.

STRESSES

We have pointed out that nonfood stresses add on to food stresses. Combinations of several moderately allergenic foods may be tolerated without symptoms until you develop a viral upper respiratory infection, a bacterial sinus or urinary infection, an attack of hay fever or asthma, or an exposure to dust, mold spores, feathers, a fur-bearing animal, a chemical, or a drug.

Your food symptoms may subside or disappear during hot summer weather when chill stress abates, only to worsen or appear again in winter, particularly with the passage of cold fronts and with sharp drops in the nighttime environmental temperature. Symptoms may be worse on humid, foggy mornings; better on dry, cloudless days. Symptoms may emerge chiefly when you exercise, when you are physically fatigued, or when you have had inadequate sleep.

HORMONAL STRESSES

Some food-sensitive women have food allergy symptoms or cravings chiefly before or during menses, and may be relatively or completely free of symptoms at other times. The hormonal stresses and changes of pregnancy and of the postpartum period immediately after pregnancy may also bring out food allergy symptoms.

In some patients, the onset of pregnancy brings welcome relief from allergy symptoms. This is presumably because during pregnancy, the blood levels of cortisol (cortisone), progesterone, adrenalin-type chemicals, and other protective substances are markedly elevated to protect the pregnancy. Shortly after delivery, these blood levels begin declining rapidly, and allergy symptoms tend to return.

Inability to adapt to these rapidly falling blood hormonal levels may result in the occurrence of new allergy syndromes *for the first time.* These are analogous to withdrawal symptoms from long-term drug use, particularly in the instance of cortisone and progesterone. Many women date the *initial* onset of a lifetime of hives, asthma, migraine, depression, or other syndromes from a few weeks or months after a delivery.

THE SUMMING OF MULTIPLE STRESSES

At a given time, individual stresses may be so mild that they remain subclinical, that is, they produce no noticeable symptoms. But multiple subclinical stresses can add on to each other.

Symptoms may be more likely to emerge or be more severe when several foods to which you have asymptomatic sensitivity are eaten on a cold winter day, particularly if you have had inadequate sleep the night before, are exposed to house dust while sweeping, and also happen to be entering the menstrual cycle. Then all these stresses are additive, and symptom causation is multifactorial.

When we speak of exercise-induced asthma, menstrual migraine, or ragweed hay fever, we are emphasizing the triggering factor, the "last straw." However, a large or multiple stress load may underlie some of these reactions. It is the total load which makes the final trigger operational.

Just because in a patient with ragweed hay fever the allergen (ragweed pollen) and the allergic symptom (hay fever) are obvious does not mean that, in the same patient, other allergic stresses (dusts, molds, epidermals, foods, etc.) and nonallergic stresses (fatigue, menses, etc.) are not simultaneously operative and contributing at times to the development and severity of the ragweed hay fever. Of course, in a given patient, *the degree of sensitivity* to one stress factor such as ragweed, peanut, or cold may be so extreme that no other stresses need be operative, particularly if the dose or *degree of exposure* to that individual factor is great.

TIMES OF THE YEAR

We have pointed out that the time of *day* influences the emergence of symptoms, as exemplified by the onset or worsening of symptoms during the early evening, or between midnight and morning. The influence of the time of the *month* in menstruating women has also been discussed.

The times of the *year* are obviously important as concerns pollenation seasons, chilling in winter, and being indoors or outdoors more. The manner of dress also varies with the time of year.

Some people who continue wearing lightweight summer outfits on early fall days, when the sun is shining but the air and earth are cold from the night before, experience "puzzling" fall exacerbations of allergies and infections, especially in the chill or breeze of early morning and late afternoon. The chilling event may take place at any time of day, but the onset of symptoms may not occur until the cool of the evening or between midnight and morning, when the sun has been down the longest, or on arising the next day before the earth has warmed up again.

The same is true of many beautiful sunny spring days which draw people outdoors when the air and earth are still cold from the night before. The manner of dress which is appropriate at noon on such days may provide inadequate insulation at the lower environmental temperatures or windchill in the early morning or late afternoon.

Even summer swimming on hot days is tricky, since the body can be chilled even by a warm breeze on a wet skin. Also, swimming in the cool breezy mornings and evenings of summer days are illness-producing in some chill-sensitive people.

Chill sensitivity is common in allergic patients. Children with mild or moderate nasal allergies tend to have recurrent viral or bacterial infections, particularly middle ear infections, if they take summer swimming lessons in the mornings, especially in outdoor pools.

TIMES OF LIFE

In addition, the strength of our immune and adaptive mechanisms varies with *age.* The infant begins life with a low level of resistance to stress. Increasing resistance accompanies the reaching of maturity and the age of procreation and continuation of the species.

It is well known that immunologic efficiency declines with aging. Allergies, autoimmune diseases, infections, cancers, degenerative disorders, and other health problems increase as we become older. For example, influenza epidemics cause relatively few fatalities in young adults, but can cause a great number of deaths in the elderly as well as in infants.

Disease or dysfunction of a vital organ system may also lower resistance or make one less able to handle life's stresses. This is particularly true in dysfunctions of the cardiovascular system, the lungs, the kidneys, and the liver. These problems are more prevalent with advancing age, and constitute an additional reason that stress exacts a greater toll in the elderly.

One of the questions most frequently asked of allergists is, "Why did I develop my asthma (or other such illness) *now?*" Since allergic illnesses are primarily genetic, and the genes have been present since the moment of conception, why did the asthma begin at age thirty, forty, or fifty?

The declining resistance level with aging is apparently one reason. In addition, over the years the stress level has usually been rising. Eating a food repetitively—or inhaling pollens, dusts, etc.—for forty years impacts the immune mechanism more than exposure for twenty years.

Many illnesses seem to begin when the rising stress level finally exceeds the declining resistance level. In contrast to reports in allergy journals and texts, food allergy is *much* more common with advancing age than in infants, although not nearly as easily noted or identified.

An important part of the protective mechanism of the body is the gene repression system. Although the genes for allergic tendency are present, they may be repressed during health and unable to express themselves as allergic symptoms.

With aging the immune system weakens and the genes tend to escape from repression, that is, they become derepressed. They can then stimulate the production of IgE and other mechanisms which result finally in the onset of illness.

FUNDAMENTAL CONCEPTS

So total allergic load is only a part of the total stress load. However, in a highly allergic patient, allergic stress is a major part of the total stress load.

The concept of *total stress load versus total resistance* is fundamental to the understanding of these disease processes. So also are the concepts of genetically different *general symptom thresholds* among different individuals. Some individuals are very sensitive in general, others moderately sensitive, and still others only slightly sensitive.

There may be different symptom thresholds for different *categories of sensitizing materials* in the same individual; for example, some patients are more sensitive to foods, others to inhalants. There may be variable symptom thresholds in the same individual for different *specific antigens;* for example, one patient may be more sensitive to milk, another to egg.

There may be different thresholds for different kinds of *nonallergic* stress in the same individual, for example, one person may be more susceptible to chilling, another to overheating, another to both chilling and overheating, another to humidity or fatigue, another to exercise or loss of sleep, and another to emotional or hormonal upsets. There may be different *resistance/burden ratios* for the same sensitizing or nonsensitizing stresses at different times of the day, times of the month, times of the year, and times of life.

These factors are closely correlated with symptom emergence and severity, yet largely go unnoticed by the patient. They have been difficult to delineate clinically and even more difficult to study scientifically, so both practicing physicians and scientists have tended to ignore them.

STRESS ORGAN FACTORS—THE OTHER SIDE OF THE COIN

Aside from stress is the presence or absence of susceptible stress organs. If stress levels rise but there are no susceptible stress organs, there will be no symptoms.

It is the presence, degree, and number of stress organ susceptibilities that determine which symptom manifestations will be caused by stress. If mediators are released by mast cells and basophils but there are no stress organs sensitive to these mediators, there will be no symptoms although the blood histamine level may be high (asymptomatic sensitivity) and the skin test may be positive.

Some patients have only a *single* symptom in a single organ, but it is induced by a great many different foods. This is exemplified by a man whose only symptom is asthma, but the asthma is brought on by several different foods as well as by many inhalants; or by his child who becomes hyperactive from each of twenty otherwise wholesome natural foods; or by his wife who has migraine headaches from each of thirty or more sensitizing foods. Another patient may have a fixed *combination* of symptoms, a symptom complex, such as the simultaneous occurrence of blurred vision, imbalance vertigo, a feeling of fullness in the head and ears, and mental dullness, all of which occur from each one of his sensitizing foods.

Still another patient may have *different symptoms from different foods.* For example, in one carefully studied patient, beef causes constipation; chocolate causes eye pain and blurring of vision; milk causes headache; egg causes drowsiness and mental depression; pork causes pain in muscles and joints; orange causes burning nocturnal pains in the knees; rice causes flushes and night sweats; wheat causes forgetfulness and difficulty in concentrating; and corn causes central nervous system stimulation resulting in restlessness, nervousness, and insomnia.

Incidentally, such a patient may tend to be awkward or accident-prone at times because he is pushed too fast by corn stimulation and his perception and reflexes are slowed by wheat and egg. He may learn to avoid injuries and accidents, but must concentrate hard to gauge and control his spatial relationships with the objects and people in his vicinity. The constant effort required for this may itself contribute to his undue fatigue, adding to the fatigue which is common in patients with hidden food allergy due to chronic overspinning of their metabolic energy wheels.

Also, a single food can cause *different symptoms at different times of life.* For example, in one man, milk caused diarrhea in infancy; constipation and extreme gassiness in adolescence; migraine in early middle age; and adult acne and excessive drowsiness in his later years. In this patient, at times, milk has also caused one combination of symptoms minutes or hours after being eaten, and a different set of symptoms the next day.

These variabilities in stress organ responses constitute another reason for the difficulties in diagnosing hidden food allergy.

IT IS TIME TO OBTAIN RELIEF

Closing our eyes to the existence of hidden food allergy has caused untold misery for many people. Many have been afraid to recite their "weird" symptoms for fear of being considered neurotic. It is time for patients and physicians to discuss these symptoms together; to consider the possibility of food causation; to try appropriate challenge feedings, allergy diets, or neutralization treatment; and to obtain relief from hidden food allergy.

—

Chapter 8

HOW YOUR BURDENS COMBINE TO THROW YOUR SYSTEM OFF BALANCE AND MAKE YOU SICK

The hidden connection between a symptom and the causative food is sometimes detected by deliberate observation. It may even virtually leap out at you if you have a prepared mind and a "high index of suspicion."

AN EXAMPLE OF SELF-DIAGNOSIS AND SELF-TREATMENT OF FOOD ALLERGY

A classic example of deliberate discovery followed by accidental confirmation of a hidden food sensitivity was reported by the late Dr. Walter C. Alvarez, eminent chairman emeritus of the Department of Gastroenterology at the Mayo Clinic and a distinguished nationally syndicated newspaper health columnist.[26]

His report concerned his own sensitivity to chicken, a favorite food which he ate often and without apparent harm all his life. However, in later years he suffered "dumb Mondays" (cerebral depression) after eating his usual Sunday dinner of chicken and chicken gravy. In several published descriptions of his reactions, he ascribed his symptoms to chicken gravy and chicken fat as well as chicken itself.

He finally detected this delayed reaction by using a diet diary, that is, keeping a written record of everything he ate and the time that his symptoms occurred. He noted from his diary that he only had dumb Mondays when he ate chicken and chicken gravy on Sundays. He eliminated his problem by reducing his chicken intake and eliminating chicken gravy on Sundays.

Later, while on a two-week camping trip where chicken was not available, he developed an overwhelming craving for it. While returning from the trip, he stopped at a roadside restaurant and voraciously ate an entire broiled chicken.

He was perfectly well that evening; but the next day he developed severe diarrhea, followed by four days of mental dullness and depression and four nights of vivid, colorful hallucinations. When a reaction is long delayed in onset but finally appears suddenly and in greater severity than usual due to having eaten the allergenic food after a period of avoidance of about four to fourteen days, it is called a *hyperacute* reaction.

This example illustrates that you may note no recognizable symptoms from an allergenic food if you eat it in a solid, slowly absorbed form, and in moderate quantity. In fact, you may consider it your favorite and best-tolerated food.

However, if you eat it in large quantity or in a more rapidly absorbed liquid form (such as gravy or soup), you may have a noticeable reaction (for example, a dumb Monday). If you avoid it completely for four days to two weeks, and then eat it in large quantity (for example, a whole chicken) you may experience either a severe immediate reaction or a severe delayed reaction which may last as long as four days. This famous case also illustrates that the brain can be a shock organ in food reactions (dullness, depression, hallucinations).

ELIMINATE BAD DAYS WITH A DIET DIARY

The diet diary, a long-neglected tool in medical diagnosis, can provide you much information about good days and bad. Try keeping a written record of everything you eat, and see what you can learn from it.

But do *not* deliberately challenge your system (as Dr. Alvarez did when he ate a whole chicken after not eating chicken for two weeks) if you have *ever* suffered from severe symptoms in vital organs such as the heart, lungs, or larynx. The symptoms of withdrawal, reintroduction, or challenge feedings can sometimes be quite severe, even when the food is one you have never suspected as causing trouble. And if the food is one you have suspected as causing symptoms in vital organs, dietary changes should not be undertaken without close medical supervision.

If you keep a diet diary, you may find that some food which you eat fairly regularly has been inadvertently eaten in *greater than usual quantity or frequency,* making you feel bad that day, or the next day, or for several days. Or you have inadvertently skipped the food and developed *withdrawal* symptoms. Or you may have skipped it for four or more days, then eaten it at one meal, and suffered an immediate or delayed *hyperacute* reaction. Or you may have skipped it for four or more days, and then eaten it at two or more closely spaced meals, and suffered your immediate or severe reaction after the *second* or a later meal.

THE INFLUENCE OF MASKING SCHEDULES

Some masking patients require a given food at closer intervals than others to maintain masking to that food.[25] Some need an addicting food every two or three days, others once every day, others every six to eight hours, and others every two to four hours. More rapidly absorbed foods are also usually metabolized more rapidly in the tissues and may require closer schedules of ingestion to maintain the addicted state.

This "masking schedule" is one reason why you may note no symptoms during the day, when you are eating the food at two, three, or more meals; but suffer symptoms late at night or on arising. These can be withdrawal symptoms from missing the food during the night's sleep, and are common occurrences in headache patients.

You may have a regular letdown, a headache, or other symptom just before lunch. Or you may note it in the late afternoon as withdrawal effects from a food you ate at breakfast or lunch or both. If you eat the food or beverage again in midmorning or midafternoon or both, you may postpone or prevent the emergence of symptoms.

Perhaps this explains in part the popularity of tea time in Great Britain and the coffee break in the United States. These breaks usually include the ingestion—in addition to caffeine-containing stimulants—of cookies or other snacks containing wheat, corn, sugar, egg, milk, and chocolate. Finally, you may find yourself nibbling your addicting food or sipping your addicting beverage almost constantly to maintain either the "high" or tranquility induced by the allergenic foods, the caffeine, or both.

So the schedule of need for masking differs for different foods in different patients. In a given patient this schedule may determine if and when withdrawal symptoms will occur.

If you are addicted to several foods, each on its own time schedule, your health problems may present an impenetrable maze to yourself, your family, and your physicians.

THE HUMAN EQUATION

Food/symptom correlations such as those made by Dr. Alvarez can be simple and natural once the mind is opened to these phenomena. However, they are often overlooked, ignored, or denied.

Many people, particularly men, are stoics and do not pay much attention to their symptoms. Some consider symptoms as a sign of weakness, or just do not want to be bothered with an analysis of symptoms and their causes.

Even when attention is called to the food/symptom relationship which may have occurred after an inadvertent challenge feeding, a given patient may still deny the correlation. He may say, "I have eaten it thousands of times, it is one of my favorite foods, I have not noted any trouble from it before, and I do not intend to eliminate it or to restrict my diet in any way."

When he resumes eating it *frequently* again, the symptoms quickly become masked or revert to the delayed type. Then the food really does not bother him so far as he can tell.

He thus becomes even more deeply convinced that he is not allergic to it. He continues on with his addictive eating and "idiopathic" symptoms.

INFLUENCE OF THE FORM OF THE FOOD

I have mentioned that a given food may cause different responses at different times in the same patient due to varying amounts, frequencies of ingestion, and physical forms of the food.[27,28] Alcoholic extracts of a food (for example, corn alcohol) are absorbed quickly and seem to cause reactions most rapidly.

Small molecular-weight food derivatives (for example, corn sugar) cause reactions next most rapidly. Larger molecular-weight derivatives (for example, corn starch and corn protein) cause reactions still less rapidly; and slowly-absorbed lipid or fatty fractions (for example, corn oil or corn oil margarine) least rapidly.

A rapidly absorbed form of a food (for example, liquid milk) may produce immediate symptoms, whereas a slowly absorbed form (for example, cheese) may not. In fact, it may be eaten addictively with no symptoms recognized as allergic.

For example, if you eat cheese addictively and have gassiness and three or four stools a day, you may simply consider this your normal bowel pattern. You may not make the "cheese connection."

Another way that allergic masking can be revealed is by taking the food with alcohol or in an alcoholic extract. I have a friend who nibbles raisins—dried grapes—all day and keeps jars of them handy for frequent use. They do not bother him; but rather, satisfy his marked appetite for them.

However, he is puzzled by the fact that whenever he drinks one or two glasses of wine—alcoholic extract of grapes—he develops symptoms. He tolerates most other alcoholic beverages relatively well, but not entirely, because his digestive tract virtually always contains some raisins. Adding alcohol of any type to the digestive tract can increase the rate of absorption of foods already present.

In both instances, increased rapidity of grape antigen absorption is responsible for exceeding his allergic threshold for grape, although it is more noticeable with wine than with most other alcohols. Such a person may never make the "grape connection" unless it is called to his attention.

BLOOD LEVELS, EQUILIBRIUM REACTIONS, AND SYMPTOM THRESHOLDS

The height of the blood level and the rapidity with which it is attained seem to be important factors in determining if the reaction will surface at all. They may also influence the time at which the symptoms will appear.

When a food is eaten, it is not only being absorbed. It is also being simultaneously removed from the bloodstream by being metabolized, bound by antibodies, deposited in tissues, and excreted. The actual blood level at a given time is a *balance* or equilibrium between absorption and elimination rates.

THE STIMULUS

If absorption is slow, the steady elimination of the food antigen from the blood may keep the blood level from reaching the symptom threshold. There may be no noticeable symptoms. If absorption is greater or more rapid, it may exceed the rate of elimination, and the symptom threshold may be reached.

If the threshold is reached very slowly and gradually, the symptoms may be delayed or mild; if the threshold is reached more rapidly and markedly, immediate symptoms may occur and may be severe. Finally there are instances where delayed absorption results in a reaction which is serious because it occurs in a vital organ such as the larynx.

THE ABILITY TO RESPOND

However, there is more to it than absorption rates of the stimulating foods, namely your proneness to respond to these stimuli. Your response may depend on the amount of potential protective energy within your cells as well as the amount of mediators in the cell and IgE attached to the outside of the cell.

High cellular energy *opposes* mediator release. The greater the amount of energy within the cell, the better it can prevent its own release of mediators. It is as though the cell tries not to release its mediators but is forced to by overwhelming outside influences, such as multiple allergen-IgE interactions at the cell surface.

APPLICATION OF GENERAL PRINCIPLES TO SPECIFIC SYNDROMES

These first eight chapters have described the fundamentals and general principles of hidden food allergy. It is now time to apply these to specific syndromes.

Headache is one of the most common syndromes caused by hidden food allergy. How the general principles we have discussed thus far apply to specific syndromes is well illustrated by a consideration of allergic headache, the subject of the next chapter.

Chapter 9

HEADACHE: A COMMON ALLERGIC SYMPTOM

Here we will be discussing allergen-caused headache, not headache due to trauma, tumors, dental problems, eye problems, and other such factors. Allergens can play a causative role in four kinds of headache: migraine headache, sinus headache, tension headache, and cluster headache.

HEADACHE PATTERNS AND RELIEF PATTERNS

Pain is subjective. Objective tests are available for the detection of headache due to brain tumors, abscesses, aneurysms, and other anatomic entities, but the diagnosis as to type of headache in physiologic and immunologic derangements is largely based on your subjective description of your headache.

Each type of headache presents a characteristic pattern. However, some people have atypical pain or more than one kind of headache. The onset, distribution, and other attributes of the pain may not always be characteristic enough to distinguish clearly the type headache involved.

Allergens play a major causative role in several kinds of headache and a lesser role in others. Neutralizing immunotherapy may not only provide relief from your headaches, but can also help us distinguish which type headache you are suffering from.

For example, if you have atypical or mixed headache, you may be relieved of sinus and cluster headaches by inhalant immunotherapy, and migraine headaches by food immunotherapy. This may leave you symptom-free, or with only occasional mild tension headaches.

These may possibly be correlated with situational stress and relieved with aspirin or other minor medications. Since we are interested in obtaining relief, let us focus first on the positive benefits of immunotherapy in specific types of headache.

SOLVING THE MYSTERY OF MIGRAINE

Migraine headache is one of the most prevalent, painful, persistent, and puzzling bedevilments of mankind. It has been estimated that 22 to 44 million Americans suffer from it. Eighty percent of these do not have the typical symptoms that allow it to be readily labelled as migraine.[29]

A distinguished neurologist, Dr. J. R. Saper, stated in an article in the *Journal of The American Medical Association:* "Despite migraine's prevalence and long history in the annals of recorded medicine, this condition has succeeded in defying a firm understanding of its pathogenesis, an objective method of establishing a diagnosis, or a consistently reliable therapy."[30]

Migraine often begins in childhood, adolescence, or early adulthood, and it may then last a lifetime. The pain can be so excruciating and persistent that it can wreck lives, marriages, families, and the ability to earn a living or pursue a career. Many such patients consider committing suicide rather than live with the pain, and some apparently do so.[31]

Migraine has been labelled with all four of the misdiagnoses of hidden allergies: idiopathic, psychosomatic, hopeless, and intractable. Yet most patients with severe persistent migraine can be provided marked relief with allergy management, primarily utilizing neutralization methods described in this book for foods, inhalants, chemicals, and progesterone. Although all the allergic and nonallergic stresses mentioned earlier can initiate attacks, in my experience *allergy is by far the major causative factor in migraine, and the principal allergens are usually foods.*

MIGRAINE AS AN ALLERGIC STRESS DISEASE

I believe that migraine is a stress disease in which the primary stress is usually allergy, just as are hay fever, allergic rhinitis, recurrent laryngeal edema, asthma, eczema, neurodermatitis, adult acne, urticaria, gastrointestinal and cerebral allergies, and certain muscle/joint pains. We do not know all the possible allergens, all the possible mediators, or all the possible nonallergic stresses for *any* of these syndromes, but we are rapidly learning a great many of them.

We also know now that if we neutralize the known allergic stresses and, when necessary, also minimize exposure to the known allergic and nonallergic triggers, we can often provide an astonishing degree of relief in migraine as well as in these other syndromes. When the migraine is caused only by foods, and the number of such foods is small, careful elimination of these foods from the diet may be all that is needed for a lifetime of relief.

Inhalants are the most common allergens in hay fever, allergic rhinitis, asthma, and sinus headache. Foods are the most common allergens in migraine, as well as in recurrent laryngeal edema, eczema, neurodermatitis, adult acne, urticaria, gastrointestinal and cerebral allergies, and allergic muscle/joint pains.

But the reverse is *sometimes* true. Foods can cause upper and lower respiratory-tract symptoms, and inhalants can cause nonrespiratory-tract symptoms. An occasional patient with migraine is helped much more by inhalant than by food immunotherapy. Also, *both* types of allergens play major roles in many patients; in addition, chemicals, drugs, and hormones sometimes enter the etiologic picture.

The basic nonallergic stresses such as fatigue, inadequate sleep, chill, humidity, menses, etc. operate in migraine as well as in allergic asthma and other allergy syndromes. Minimizing or neutralizing one type of stress may be sufficient in one person; but in another, more than one type of stress may need attention.

For example, progesterone neutralization alone may be adequate for some patients with menstrual migraine, but other patients with menstrual migraine require food neutralization as well. Such patients are sensitive to foods but may have no symptoms until the hormonal stress also occurs.

Food addiction, masking, withdrawal symptoms, and hyperacute reactions on deliberate or inadvertent challenge also occur in migraine. Migraine may be precipitated by missing a meal and by religious fast days.

When the total defensive capability is momentarily relatively low, or the total stress burden momentarily relatively high, the resistance/burden ratio is altered unfavorably and an attack may occur. The common occurrence of attacks in the early morning hours seems to be related partially to the abstinence from food during sleep (withdrawal stress) and partially to nocturnal lowering of blood levels of protective substances such as cortisone and adrenalin (lowered defense level).

It may sound strange to hear migraine spoken of as an allergic syndrome. But by my working definition of allergy as a stress disease with an altered resistance/burden ratio in which allergens are usually the major stresses (burdens), it certainly makes sense and fits experience. Most importantly, this concept leads to welcome relief for patients who have not found relief elsewhere.

Many patients with migraine also have other allergic diseases such as asthma, arthritis, depression, adult acne, and chronic ulcerative colitis. Food extract injection therapy for the migraine often provides unexpected health and economic bonuses in the form of great relief of these other conditions as well. Adding inhalant neutralization helps their recurrent nasal, sinus, and ear problems; progesterone neutralization helps relieve their other premenstrual symptoms and menstrual cramps, as well as premenstrual migraine; and influenza virus vaccine neutralization markedly diminishes their fever blister or genital herpes recurrences.

During childhood, many migraine patients had multiple food or inhalant allergies which they "outgrew" and which resurfaced later as migraine and possibly other syndromes. Migraine, like other allergic illnesses, runs in families. Further, the same families have a high incidence of hay fever, asthma, gastrointestinal allergies such as spastic colon and chronic ulcerative colitis, arthritis, cerebral symptoms such as hyperactivity or depression, and hormonal problems such as premenstrual or menstrual symptoms.

These syndromes all seem to be expressions of the same hereditary tendency, the tendency to inadequately control some facet of the defense system, usually resulting in inadequate suppression of the release of chemical mediators. The symptom manifestations seem to depend on which mediators are most operative and which stress organs are most sensitive in a given patient at a given time.

THE ALLERGIC BASIS OF MIGRAINE

The stress organ in migraine seems to be the arterial system that supplies blood to the head and brain. It is apparently the arteries and their subdivisions which are affected by the chemical mediators.

The blood supply to the head comes chiefly from the internal and external carotid arteries, coming up to the head along each side of the neck. The internal carotid artery serves the brain, the eyes and eyelids, and part of the inner lining of the nose; the external carotid artery serves the skull, skin, muscles, and other tissues of the head.

Not this entire arterial system, but sometimes only one arterial branch, is sensitive to circulating chemical mediators in a given patient. For our purpose, what matters is that we prevent or relieve the suffering, regardless of which arteries or mediators are involved. Research discovery frequently lags far behind clinical discovery.

In most patients, we can provide relief now. We can find out why later, when laboratory science catches up with clinical science. We do not yet have enough information in many aspects of medicine to satisfy us intellectually, but in many instances we do have enough to take effective action in patient care.

TYPES OF MIGRAINE

There are two main types of migraine, classic migraine and common migraine. Each classic migraine attack consists of three sequential stages.

The first stage is arterial constriction. This is followed by the second stage, an overdilatation of the previously constricted arteries, causing pounding headache. The third stage consists of increased capillary permeability in the subdivisions of the arteries, resulting in swelling of surrounding tissues including the brain. In common migraine, on the other hand, headache may be the only symptom.

THE THREE STAGES OF CLASSIC MIGRAINE

Constriction: The first stage, arterial constriction, occurs in arteries that supply the visual part of the brain and usually lasts only a few seconds or minutes. During this brief time, the patient with classic migraine suddenly notices visual changes such as dancing or jiggling lines in his field of vision (scintillating scotomata), bright spots like blips on a radar screen, or blurred vision. If the allergenic or nonallergenic stress is mild, this may be all that happens; if it is greater, the painful second stage follows. Nausea and sometimes vomiting may also occur, hence the common name of "sick" headache.

Dilatation: The second stage, arterial dilatation, brings severe throbbing pain due to the pulsation of the increased flow of blood with each heart beat through the now distended arteries. The arterial involvement and the pain are often on only one side of the head, which accounts for the origin of the term migraine (hemicrania).

However, the pain may alternate sides, and both sides may be involved in some instances. The pain may last a few hours, all day, and even two to three days. If you are constipated or if the allergenic foods are eaten repeatedly, the pain can last much longer or be continuous. This can occur even in hospitalized patients if the hospital meals contain the allergenic foods.

Fortunately many people lose their appetite with each attack, or vomit up the food, or have diarrhea, and these help the attack to subside more quickly. Some perceptive patients have learned to shorten their attacks by inducing vomiting, or using laxatives and enemas. This may also be one explanation for the persistent survival of the practice of the "high colonic irrigation" as a therapeutic procedure for these and other patients with hidden food allergies. They ascribe their relief to the emptying of "poisons" from their colons, when the relief may actually be due to getting rid of allergens.

Edema: Edema of various tissues supplied by the involved arterial branches brings additional symptoms. The nostril on the side of the pain may become congested and runny, the eye on that side may become bloodshot and teary, and that side of the face may flush and sweat.

Edema of one side of the brain may cause tingling or other disturbances of sensation in one half of the body in some patients, and some are temporarily paralyzed on one side. When this occurs, the condition is called *complicated* migraine. The brain swelling may also cause fatigue, lethargy, sleepiness, depression, confusion, and behavior changes. The fatigue may be due to edema of the brain or to general exhaustion.

A Total Body Reaction: The nervous system is very sensitive to changes in its supply of oxygen and nutrients. In migraine, one gets the impression that the brain does not allow its blood supply to be restricted very long. It seems to cancel out constriction of brain arteries quickly by inducing compensatory overdilatation.

But constrictive mediators seem to continue to circulate and to cause reduced blood supply to other areas of the body. During the painful dilatation phase in the cranial arteries, continuing constriction in other arteries may make you continue to feel chilled, often with cold blue hands and feet. You may also be pale, dizzy, and trembly. You may have muscle spasm pains in the abdomen, chest, pelvis, hands, and feet. The mouth may be dry, and the heart beat may be rapid and pounding.

The increased capillary permeability and other effects of multiple circulating mediators can produce symptoms in many areas of the body. There may be swelling of the face, hands, and feet, or generalized body swelling (cyclic edema). Constipation, diarrhea, irritability, glare sensitivity, and noise sensitivity are common. As mentioned, asthma, spastic colon, chronic ulcerative colitis, arthritis, and other allergic syndromes may occur or alternate with migraine attacks.

Patients with migraine customarily seek out dark, quiet, isolated rooms for the duration of the attack. They often lie down and place cold cloths or pillows over their eyes to shut out all light. Blocking out light may be an automatic protective adaptation to minimize the signals reaching an overstimulated brain, particularly the occipital lobe which is the visual center in the back of the brain.

The coldness of the cloth and the weight of the cloth or pillows on the closed eyes and head may also serve to reduce local edema about the eyes and head. This could dampen the overexuberant cranial circulation, thereby decreasing swelling and pain in the eyes and head. Squeezing the lids together, rubbing the lids, or applying pressure to areas around the lids or beside the eyes or temples sometimes seems to help. Some combat the general chilliness by using extra layers of clothing, a blanket, or a long soak in a hot tub.

When the attack is over, the patient is usually left extremely weak, fatigued, drained of energy, and "all washed out." This sense of fatigue is common in several other allergy syndromes but is particularly pronounced in migraine.

Only 20 percent of patients with migraine have visual or gastrointestinal features as described (classic migraine). The other 80 percent (common migraine) have vague or no noticeable preliminary visual symptoms, no nausea, and more prolonged pain. As there is as yet no objective method or laboratory test for diagnosing migraine, and the diagnosis rests chiefly with the patient's description of his subjective symptoms, these 80 percent are particularly difficult to diagnose and may be erroneously placed in the category of "psychosomatic."

HOW IMPORTANT ARE EMOTIONAL FACTORS?

Thus there are some who say that many of these are emotional headaches rather than migraine, or that migraine itself is emotional in origin. In my experience, emotionally induced headaches are usually of the tension (muscle contraction) type, not migraine. Migraine is most often caused by allergens and further aggravated or triggered by the same nonspecific stresses that trigger other allergic syndromes.

One of these nonspecific stresses is the emotions. However, the emotional factor in instigating migraine attacks is relatively minor or infrequent, and attacks of emotionally triggered migraine are usually mild and brief. It is natural for anyone not familiar with the hidden allergy factors to erroneously blame all these mysterious attacks on emotions.

However, the *secondary* emotional impact of sudden, unpredictable, and unrelenting attacks of severe, pounding, recurrent head pain over years or decades can be considerable. Control of the head pain by allergic management usually greatly relieves the secondary emotional facet, but some patients never forget their old dread of being suddenly struck with fierce pain. Some come to look upon it as punishment from heaven for some imagined wrongdoing, when it is actually wholesome foods that they have innocently eaten.

HORMONAL FACTORS

Hormones often play an important role in migraine, as in other allergies. Migraine attacks can begin at any age but often begin with puberty, and may be worsened by or occur only before or during menstruation.

They may be aggravated by using oral contraceptive tablets. These tablets usually contain two types of hormones, estrogens and progestogens. Progestogens are compounds similar to, but not identical with, natural progesterone. They can be given by mouth, whereas progesterone cannot because it is destroyed in the stomach.

In these patients, the body's response to progesterone and progestogen levels seems to make the difference. Classic migraine may become more severe in pregnancy when progesterone levels are high, and might diminish or disappear completely at menopause when progesterone levels are low—as though *low* levels of progesterone are more beneficial than higher levels in classic migraine patients.

On the other hand, common migraine usually becomes better or disappears completely during pregnancy, returns after delivery, and worsens at menopause—as though *high* levels of progesterone are desirable in common migraine patients. So it appears that the difference may be in the body's response to the progesterone *level,* not to the progesterone as such. It is as though the wrong level of progesterone for a given individual triggers the release of mediators, and the right level turns off the release of mediators.

MIGRAINE VARIANTS AND EQUIVALENTS

When migraine headache is regularly accompanied by other symptoms such as abdominal pain, the syndrome is called a migraine *variant.* When no headache occurs, but recurrent symptoms such as eye pain or vomiting and abdominal pain occur, this is called a migraine *equivalent* (for example, "ophthalmic migraine" or "abdominal migraine").

Abdominal migraine and other migraine equivalents without visual involvement or headache seem to me to be simply allergic reactions in the gastrointestinal tract and other organs. They respond to neutralization in the same manner as other types of allergic reaction including migraine itself.

So migraine is a good syndrome to consider as a model of hidden allergy and of the interactions of various allergic and nonallergic stresses. That is the subject of the next chapter. Migraine patients will be particularly interested in delving deeper into their problems. If you do not have migraine, but have some other resistance/burden syndrome, you should still benefit from the understanding of how various factors affect migraine and other such syndromes, perhaps including your own.

Chapter 10

MIGRAINE AS A MODEL ALLERGIC/STRESS DISEASE

Migraine is almost a perfect model of the interplay of the various stress factors we have been discussing. Most migraine patients are unaware of the fact that they are allergic to most of the foods they eat very frequently and even to some they eat infrequently.

In some people, a specific symptom threshold may be extremely low, and the quantity of that specific food required to precipitate an attack may be very small, almost molecular. In others, migraine appears only on repetitive eating of large amounts of one or several allergenic foods. These two extremes represent both ends of a bell-shaped curve.

If people are aware of any of the foods to which they are allergic, it is usually chiefly the infrequently eaten ones. Some know that they have attacks when they eat or overeat only chocolate and possibly a few other foods, when actually they may be sensitive to ten, twenty, thirty, or more. Some have two kinds of allergy and experience immediate IgE-type reactions (urticaria, vomiting, diarrhea, or others) without headache from one infrequently eaten food such as shrimp, and migraine from many of the frequently eaten foods in their diet.

In some people with migraine, no one of their food allergies is necessarily of a major degree, but all together they tend to place an unbearable burden on homeostatic mechanisms. The total stress load hovers close to the total symptom threshold much of the time, and the final straw that precipitates headache may be either an extra stress-elevating factor or an extra threshold-lowering factor. When the stress level temporarily exceeds the symptom threshold, an attack may occur.

EXPLANATIONS FOR MYSTERIES OF MIGRAINE

Many mysteries of migraine become clear once you perceive the allergen/stress connection and understand the concept of allergic addiction. They explain why one person can obtain relief of headache by taking a laxative or enema and eating lightly or fasting a day or two, while another develops headache on religious fast days due to withdrawal of addicting foods. They explain why some obtain relief by entering a hospital, thereby getting away from the allergen-filled air and the snack-filled refrigerators in their homes.

They also explain why some may obtain relief by taking no nourishment except intravenous glucose; while highly corn-sensitive patients may be made worse by glucose, the commercial form of which is made from corn. Some report that they dare not touch alcoholic beverages, never realizing that alcoholic beverages are rapidly absorbed extracts of foods. Foods that contain such nonallergenic headache precipitants as tyramine, nitrites, bisulfites, or monosodium glutamate may also be causing migraine through their content of allergenic foods or chemical ingredients.

The basic burden is usually a multitude of hidden food allergies, on top of which there may also be inhalant, chemical, and hormonal sensitivities. Then one of the foods may be eaten in greater quantity or in greater frequency than usual, or an extra inhalant exposure may occur, finally triggering a migraine attack.

Chemicals may enter the picture in the form of perfume or other chemical odor or a chemical additive to food or water. One allergenic culprit may even be a medication such as a migraine "reliever," a vitamin or iron preparation, a pain pill, or an injection taken in hope of obtaining relief. Factors in cigarette smoke, caffeine-containing beverages, and contraceptive tablets may also be causative.

The total allergic burden may also be tolerated adequately until a nonallergic burden adds on in the form of a humid, foggy, or rainy day; a cold night; exposure to winter wind; passage of a cold front; or change of season or climate. Overwork, exercise, fatigue, lack of rest, loss of sleep, or another physical stress may be the final burden triggering an attack of migraine.

The final burden may be hormonal (progesterone). Migraine attacks occasionally tend to occur at ovulation when an egg departs from an ovary and heads for the uterus. The ovary then immediately starts secreting progesterone to help the egg embed in the soft thick inner lining of the uterus.

This causes progesterone blood levels to begin rising. If the egg is fertilized, progesterone levels remain high to protect the pregnancy. If the egg is not fertilized, progesterone levels rise for only one week, and then rapidly subside for another week, at which time menstruation occurs.

Migraine attacks in some patients tend to occur during the entire two weeks before menses when progesterone levels are unstable, rising to a peak one week and then falling to baseline the next. More commonly, migraine attacks tend to occur just before onset of menses when progesterone levels are falling most rapidly and reaching the lowest level of the cycle. In this instance, it may be progesterone withdrawal or a diminishing progesterone/estrogen ratio that triggers the attack.

Just as in some patients with asthma, some migraine patients have their attacks at almost the same hour every morning, commonly 3:00 to 4:00 A.M., whether they ate the allergenic food at breakfast, lunch, or dinner the day before. Others have their attacks regularly at about midnight, or on arising in the morning.

This suggests that the schedule of the food addiction/withdrawal phenomenon is modified in these instances by factors operative in the cool early morning hours, such as chill, low cortisol blood levels, low adrenalin blood levels, and low metabolic rate. Whether the patient is a light or heavy sleeper may affect the time that he awakens and perceives the pain.

Migraine patients are often compulsive workers and high achievers. Some have less headache on work days, more on weekends.

Weekend headache is usually described as a letdown phenomenon. Is work really a needed stress, withdrawal from which induces headache? Is the weekend decrease in work tension accompanied by a fall in levels of protective substances such as adrenalin? Or is it that these patients have learned to eat carefully during the week so as to be able to maintain their high-level work outputs; and on weekends relax their guards, reward themselves, give in to the temptation of chocolate binges, spicy foods, restaurant meals, or alcoholic beverages?

As in asthma, an infection can also be the final precipitant of a migraine attack. This is true whether it is a viral upper respiratory infection or a bacterial infection of the sinuses, urinary tract, or other areas.

Whatever the final triggering stress, the food allergy burden is basic in the majority of patients, and controlling the food allergies can provide remarkable relief in such instances. On the other hand, inhalants, chemicals, or hormones can be primary burdens in a minority of patients.

When no clues are available as to what the primary problem is, you can be tested and treated for foods for the best chance of providing relief. Degree of response to food extract injection therapy or diet or both then indicates whether or not to test inhalants. On the other hand, if you have chronic nose and sinus congestion as well as recurrent migraine, you may be benefited by testing and treating selected inhalants before beginning food testing.

A history of sensitivities to chemicals and drugs or a failure to respond completely to food and inhalant treatment indicates the need for careful attention to chemicals. You may require coverage for all these types of allergens, and in some instances, for progesterone as well.

IMPLICATIONS OF THE ALLERGIC BASIS OF MIGRAINE

In all fields of medicine, treatment depends upon diagnosis. What makes a good specialist is the ability to recognize, diagnose, label, and classify—not necessarily relieve—all or most of the syndromes in his field of specialization. In a given specialty, each patient's illness must fit somewhere into the classification of diseases within that specialty. When no objective means of diagnosis is available for a given symptom or syndrome, modern medical philosophy and training usually dictate a descriptive label or a psychiatric diagnosis.

Since the vast majority of people with severe migraine do not even have typical symptoms before an attack or any other specific diagnostic marker which enables them to be categorized definitively as migraine, they may have to live with the general diagnostic classification of "headache"—and possibly of "neurosis" as well. In these common migraine patients, the allergens are usually the same as in classical migraine, and similar relief frequently follows management of the allergenic and nonallergenic stress factors.

WHAT IS SO NEW ABOUT FOODS CAUSING MIGRAINE?

Since antiquity, it has been known that some people with migraine develop attacks when they eat certain foods. However, this was previously considered an isolated or unusual phenomenon. More recently such reactions have been connected with tyramine, nitrites, bisulfites, monosodium glutamate, and other substances in certain foods, but not often with an *allergic* response to the foods themselves.

What is new is the knowledge that hidden food allergies are by far the major cause of migraine attacks, and that food extract injection therapy or meticulous diets or both can usually offer great relief. Later chapters will describe neutralizing responses to inhalants, chemicals, and hormones for patients with migraine and other syndromes.

NEUTRALIZATION CAN PROVIDE BOTH DIAGNOSIS AND RELIEF

In the preceding chapter, I quoted the words of a distinguished neurologist: "Despite migraine's prevalence and long history in the annals of recorded medicine, this condition has succeeded in defying a firm understanding of its pathogenesis, an objective method of establishing a diagnosis, or a consistently reliable therapy."[30] Although there is much yet to learn, neutralization makes much of this statement obsolete.

With neutralization testing, we can often induce headache with one concentration of an allergen and relieve it with another concentration of the same allergen, usually within ten minutes. A subcutaneous food treatment injection in a patient who feels a headache beginning can often relieve or abort the attack. Regular treatment injections with food extracts usually provide marked or complete prevention of further attacks.

Relief and prevention make the diagnosis. Thus neutralization often provides both diagnosis and relief, and indicates the role of allergy in causation.

Chapter 11

DOUBLE-BLIND STUDIES IN MIGRAINE

I am well aware that it is a major heresy to state that food allergy is the most common cause of migraine, and that food extract injection therapy can offer much relief. These facts will be accepted by scientists only if proved by rigidly controlled double-blind studies.

In this kind of study, courses of active food extract treatment injections must be alternated with courses of placebo (blank) injections containing no food extracts. To keep psychological factors from influencing the outcome, neither the physician nor the patient can know which of the two types of injections are given at any time. Case reports of four migraine patients I have studied in this manner are presented here.[8,20]

METHOD

These patients were first tested to enough of their staple foods so that they could live for the duration of an eighty-day study on only the foods covered by their food extract injections. The neutralizing doses of all these foods were combined into a single solution, unique for each patient, and self-administered subcutaneously each day for each twenty-day active extract course. Four courses alternating twenty-day active and twenty-day placebo injections comprised the eighty-day study.

A placebo or blank injection was prepared containing only the inactive diluting solution, tinted to prevent recognition. The patients could not detect any difference in appearance between active and placebo extracts.

The first extract chosen for instituting the study was determined by the flip of a coin by a third party and neither the patient nor I was aware which extract was employed. The four alternating consecutive twenty-day courses were designated courses A, B, C, and D. Thus depending on the flip of the coin, one patient's active extract courses might be A and C, another's B and D. This provided an unusually clear and repeated comparison between responses to active extract and placebo.

A careful symptom survey was made when the study was begun, and symptom changes were recorded during and at the end of each of the four 20-day courses of therapy. Each patient was carefully instructed and repeatedly reminded to eat only foods whose neutralizing doses were included in the active treatment injections. Their adherence to this diet and their responses were followed by carefully analyzed diet, symptom, and medication diaries. Some slips did occur, but were noted and taken into account, as will be described. As the following examples indicate, the active extract proved to be far superior to placebo in every case.

Case Number 1

B.L.: A twenty-nine-year-old white female with recurrent severe migraine headaches since early childhood, becoming progressively worse in recent years. In the preceding six months the headaches had awakened her in the early morning hours *every day.*

She reported that headaches had followed the ingestion of coffee, chocolate, beef, pork, and ice cream. She had been taking combinations of pain medications regularly for nine years. She also often required injections of Demerol®. Additional symptoms which accompanied the migraine attacks included recurrent vertigo, tinnitus (ear-ringing), nausea, abdominal cramps, and depression.

The first series of injections administered was of Active extract. *After the third daily injection,* she required no further medications, and was completely free of headache, vertigo, tinnitus, and depression for the remainder of the twenty days. She stated that this was the longest she had ever gone without a headache since early childhood. The nausea and abdominal cramps were also markedly improved.

On the second series (Placebo), headache returned on the fourth day. For the balance of the twenty-day period the headache was as severe and frequent as before therapy. Her pain medications were of no benefit, and she came to the office with a wet cloth over her forehead and eyes, crying in pain. The vertigo, nausea, and depression had also returned in full force, with a moderate recurrence of tinnitus.

On the third series (Active), she noted improvement by the second day and almost total clearing of headache *by the third day.* From the fourth day on, she remained free of headache and all other symptoms except mild occasional abdominal cramps for the balance of this twenty-day period.

On the fourth series (Placebo), her headaches returned to a slight degree but not as severely as on the preceding series of placebo. However, her nausea and abdominal cramps worsened, and her depression returned in full force.

This case illustrates a typical response to food injection therapy in a patient with severe, prolonged, intractable migraine and several additional food-caused symptoms. It demonstrates a clear and marked difference between placebo and active food extract injections. It also indicates the rapid response of lifelong symptoms to food extract injection therapy, with marked improvement in just three to four days.

The partial holdover (hyposensitization) benefit noted on the second placebo series occurs commonly in this system of therapy, particularly when the injections are administered daily for a while. This is further evidence of its effectiveness in building steadily greater and longer-lasting resistance to the untoward effects of allergenic foods.

This holdover benefit is similar to the prolonged benefit inhalant-sensitive patients obtain on prolonged inhalant injection therapy. Many may discontinue inhalant injections and yet remain free of inhalant-caused symptoms for a period of time, often for weeks, months, or years.

Case Number 2

M.H.: A fifty-seven-year-old white female with recurrent, severe, left temporal migraine headaches accompanied by nausea and vomiting since early childhood and progressively worsening. In the seven months prior to the study she had been awakened by severe headache *every day,* usually at about 4:00 A.M. About three times a week the pain became so severe that she required multiple injections of Vistaril® and Demerol for relief.

Every three weeks or so, even these failed to provide relief, and she had to be hospitalized and heavily sedated for three to seven days. Hospitalization had been necessary nine times during the past seven months. She also had glare sensitivity and adult-onset acne accompanying the migraine and becoming progressively worse as the migraine became more frequent and more severe.

She had been thoroughly and repeatedly worked up by her family physician as well as by the chairman of the neurology department at a medical school. Although the diagnosis of migraine was made, no etiologic foods were sought or found.

Her only clues as to precipitating factors were that one headache seemed to follow the ingestion of a chocolate brownie, and that some headaches were preceded by the ingestion of alcoholic beverages. However, she felt certain that foods and alcohol were not related to the present headaches because she had been careful not to ingest chocolate products or alcoholic beverages during the preceding seven months, yet the headaches continued and even worsened.

The first series of injections (Placebo) did not affect the severity or frequency of the symptoms. On the second series (Active), the headaches became noticeably less severe *after the third injection* and the glare sensitivity and acne became markedly better. She required no hospitalizations, and had only one mild migraine headache during this twenty-day period.

On the third series (Placebo) she went rapidly downhill. By the fifth day her migraine had returned to its original severity and frequency (every day) and her nausea and vomiting had become uncontrollable despite medication. By the sixth day, when Demerol and Vistaril were no longer able to relieve the headache, she had to be admitted to the hospital for five days. Despite heavy medication, some headache continued to be experienced daily for the balance of the twenty days.

On the fourth series (Active) she noted improvement again *on the fifth day.* She had no migraine or nausea for the balance of the twenty-day period.

This second case of severe, lifelong, intractable migraine illustrates again the marked and rapid relief obtained from food extract injections, and the rapid and severe return of symptoms when placebos were substituted.

Case Number 3

C.B.: A fifty-two-year-old white female with severe migraine headaches for the past twenty-five years. The headaches were always accompanied by nausea and usually lasted two to three days. She had been regularly taking Cafergot®, Darvocet-N 100®, and Phenaphen #3®. The only known food reaction was shrimp, which caused hives and laryngeal edema but not headache. Symptoms which accompanied her migraine included recurrent vertigo, fainting spells, laryngeal edema, nausea, flatulence, diarrhea, eczema, and urticaria.

On the first series (Active), her headache and all other symptoms completely cleared *after the third injection* and she was free of all symptoms for the remainder of the twenty days. On the second series (Placebo), headache and flatulence returned after the seventh injection and progressively worsened to their original intensity. On the third series (Active), the headache and flatulence cleared *after the first injection* and all symptoms remained clear for the balance of the twenty days. On the fourth series (Placebo) all symptoms continued to remain clear.

This is the third case of severe, prolonged, intractable migraine, with a typical galaxy of accompanying severe allergy symptoms, all responding in the same rapid and dramatic pattern as in the cases previously described. There was also a similar holdover protective benefit when the fourth course was placebo, as in Case #1.

Case Number 4

D.H.: A thirty-six-year-old white female with a history of severe migraine headaches since early childhood. During the preceding six years the headaches increased progressively in frequency and severity. For the preceding eight months severe pain occurred *daily* and was virtually constant. An acute headache awakened her between midnight and 5:00 A.M. every morning. She also complained of recurrent vertigo. The only known food allergy was catfish, which caused vomiting but not headache or vertigo.

She had been scratch-tested by another allergist ten years before, revealing positive tests to several inhalants and seventeen foods. She received inhalant injections for two years and reduced the intake of the seventeen foods as instructed with no benefit. She was carefully studied repeatedly by her family physician and twice by neurologists, the second of whom referred her to me after exhaustive neurologic testing.

On the first series (Placebo), the basic pattern of daily headache remained. On the second series (Active) she was *better the first day and clear the second day.* She had only one headache during the remainder of the twenty days, which followed the ingestion of chocolate. Although the neutralizing dose for chocolate was included in her treatment injections, it did not provide complete protection from chocolate ingestion, as determined by repeated challenges and attempts to provide protection after the study was completed. (In such instances, elimination of the nonresponding food—chocolate in this instance—from the diet, combined with the use of neutralizing injections for the responding foods is required for complete relief of migraine.)

On the third series of injections (Placebo) her severe daily headaches returned on the third day and they continued daily for the remainder of the twenty-day period. On the fourth series of injections (Active) she noted complete relief of headache *by the third day,* and had only three headaches during the entire twenty days.

The first of these three headaches occurred when she inadvertently ate oats, for which she had not been tested. The second occurred after repetitive eating of wheat, from which she was protected except from too-frequent ingestion as determined by repeated wheat challenges after the study was completed.

The third followed bottled lemon juice, which was not supposed to have been included in her diet. Lemon allergy extract was in her food injections, and freshly squeezed lemon juice did not bother her, but bottled lemon juice repeatedly caused headaches on later challenges.

A preservative or additive in the bottled lemon juice was assumed to be the culprit. The bottled lemon juice contained water, lemon juice concentrate, lemon oil, sodium benzoate, and sodium bisulfite.

This is the fourth case of severe, prolonged, intractable migraine responding markedly and rapidly to food injection therapy. Her experiences with chocolate, oats, wheat, and chemical additives in factory-processed lemon juice indicate some of the problems encountered in therapy.

Most such problems are readily managed by either testing, retesting, limiting frequency of ingestion, or total avoidance of individual incriminated food items and additives. This patient remained free of migraine by continuing her injections twice a week, eating only foods covered by her injections, eating wheat only at one meal each four days, and avoiding chocolate and chemical additives.

SUMMARY

As is suggested from these four reports, most patients with severe lifelong, intractable migraine receive marked relief after only a few days of food extract injection therapy, and they often relapse within a few days or a week after discontinuing the injections. Some may still have an occasional attack caused by eating a food not covered by their injections; if so, this food can be tested and added to the treatment set.

Others may have an attack after eating too much or too frequently a food which is in the treatment extract; this can be relieved by an immediate booster injection of food extract, or by retesting this food to see if the body's dosage need for it has changed, or by reducing the quantity or frequency of that food in the diet. An occasional food cannot be covered completely by treatment and must be totally eliminated from the diet. This is particularly true of chemical additives.

Many drugs are used for migraine, but all have limitations and side effects, some very serious. Some people do not respond adequately to any drugs currently available. The unique value of controlling the allergic *causes* of migraine is that it usually provides far greater relief than treatment of symptoms, and usually does so *without drugs.*

RELIEF IS REAL, NOT DUE TO PLACEBO EFFECT

It is obvious to any physician with long experience in neutralizing testing and treatment that the marked benefits of food extract injection therapy are real, not hypnotic. Under direct observation it is clear that some test doses make the headache worse, some cause no change, and only the neutralizing dose relieves the symptoms induced by a provoking dose. How would a "hypnotized" patient know which dose to "neutralize himself" on? And if he could turn his headache off by his own volition, why does he seek help from a physician?

The characteristic wheal pattern of a positive wheal on the overstrength dose and a negative wheal on the neutralizing dose is objective, not under the control of the physician or the patient. Worsening and relief of headache during testing almost always comes before the wheal is fully developed. The patient has no way of knowing what the wheal pattern will be even if he were to try to modify his symptom responses to correlate with the wheals.

When a patient on treatment injections delays or skips his injections for a while, his symptoms tend to return. If he then resumes his injections, relief often comes within thirty minutes after the first injection. When a patient is taking his treatment injections regularly, and they suddenly fail to help or they even cause some symptoms, retesting reveals that some doses have changed, and resumption of treatment with the newly determined doses provides quick relief again.

The placebo hypothesis is also denied by responses of infants. Infants in the first few months of life with severe symptoms such as eczema, diarrhea, or asthma respond to test doses just as described for adults. Infants also respond remarkably well to treatment injections. Their terrible itching, frequent stools, wheezes, or other symptoms often begin improving after the first few treatment doses. The same is true of children with migraine.

If suggestion were the primary relieving factor, how could the benefit last so long? Hypnosis usually wears off very quickly, as anyone can testify who has ever tried hypnosis for control of obesity, smoking, or migraine. The benefits of neutralization continue.

One could argue that each self-administered treatment injection is a sort of hypnotic reprogramming. This is absurd since the benefits are so specific. Protection is obtained only from the allergenic foods contained in the treatment solutions, and many patients do not long remember exactly which foods are in their injections.

When a patient is allergic to virtually every food, he usually has no symptoms so long as he eats only foods covered by his food extract injections. When he unknowingly eats one noncovered food, he may have a migraine attack.

When this noncovered food is then tested and the proper dose added to the treatment vial, ingestion of the food no longer induces migraine. When I have deliberately omitted a given allergenic food from a treatment extract with the patient's concurrence to see if the patient could detect which food was omitted, he has almost always been able to correctly identify the omitted food.

When a patient is well protected for a long time by his injections but notes that he again begins to have migraine whenever he eats one specific food such as wheat in his treatment solution, retesting wheat alone may be all that is needed. This will usually reveal that the wheat neutralizing dose has changed, and a new treatment extract containing the new wheat dose again eliminates the migraine.

When an effective food treatment solution loses its effectiveness after a long period of usage, and the patient is unable to identify which foods are now inducing symptoms, retesting all the foods usually determines that the body's neutralizing dose needs have changed for many foods. Treatment with injections containing the newly determined neutralizing doses again quickly provides relief.

No suggestion is made to the patient undergoing testing that he will either have symptoms or obtain relief on any given dose. No leading questions are asked or directive statements made. The physician himself does not know in advance which dose will produce symptoms or which will relieve them.

Many patients entering my office have already been to many other physicians, prestigious clinics, pain centers, and medical school hospitals. They have had every opportunity to respond to the unconscious suggestive effect of great expectations, impressive medical centers, white-coated father-figures, multiple diagnostic manipulations, and therapeutic medications and procedures. They have often been subjected to acupuncture, biofeedback therapy, nutritional therapy, and even attempts to provide relief by skilled hypnotists and psychiatrists. Why did these supersuggestive placebos totally fail, and food injections succeed?

Much remains to be learned, not only about allergic reactions in general, but also about chemical mediators, how they act, and how they interact with the brain and other organs. This may take decades to unravel. Meanwhile, the ability to provide much relief is in our hands *now.*

Chapter 12

HEADACHE FROM YOUR SINUSES AND EARS

The respiratory sinuses are like air pockets in the bones of the skull. One of their functions is to lighten the weight of the skull, which would otherwise be solid bone. A second function is to help warm and humidify incoming inhaled air. A third is to manufacture protective mucus.

HOW THE SINUSES WORK

The sinuses are lined by a membrane made up of two kinds of cells, goblet cells and ciliated cells. The purpose of the goblet cells is to constantly secrete a thick, clear, lubricating mucus. The mucus drains from each sinus through a tiny hair-sized canal into the nasal cavity or upper part of the throat behind the nose.

Each sinus membrane is covered by a blanket of this mucus. The mucus blanket is constantly in motion, moving along slowly and steadily around the inner lining of the sinus, out through the tiny canal into the nose and nasopharynx, and then on down into the throat.

Here it is met by a similar mucus blanket moving upward from the trachea and bronchial tubes. The mucus converging in the throat from both upper and lower airways is reflexly and subconsciously swallowed into the stomach.

The sinus mucus blanket is pushed along its path by the ciliated cells in the lining membrane of the sinuses, nose, and throat. These are specialized cells with little cilia or hair-like projections like whips that all beat together in rhythmic waves.

Under a microscope, ciliary action would look like a wheat field repeatedly and regularly rustled by sharp gusts of wind, with the wheat stalks swaying together. The cilia actively beat in such waves under the blanket of mucus, moving the overlying mucus along.

The sinus mucus blanket protects, insulates, and lubricates the underlying membranes of the nose and throat. It also catches and traps bacteria, viruses, mold spores, dusts, pollens, and other inhaled particles that land on the mucus blanket, and moves them on into the throat and stomach. The stomach is the "garbage disposal unit," digesting and destroying the mucus and its trapped particles and organisms.

HOW BLOCKED SINUSES CAN CAUSE HEADACHE

The sinus entrances must remain open not only for mucus to get out, but also to allow air to move into and out of the sinuses. If air cannot move in both directions through the sinus openings, the air pressure in the sinuses cannot be kept the same as the atmospheric air pressure.

Sinus blockage can result in the air within the sinuses being absorbed through the sinus membranes into the bloodstream, and not being replaced by air from the atmosphere. This results in a *negative* pressure or vacuum in the sinuses. Such a vacuum can cause a sinus headache.

Of course, sinus blockage can also obstruct the exit of mucus from the sinuses. The goblet cells in the sinus membranes continue secreting mucus, and the sinuses become overfilled, resulting in a *positive* pressure. This too can cause sinus headache.

Sinus blockage is often caused by *allergic* edema of the membranes of the sinuses and their openings. In allergic patients, when allergenic particles such as pollens deposit on the nasal and sinus membranes, the allergen molecules diffuse into the membranes and combine with IgE molecules bound to mast cells lining the capillaries just below the membranes.

This causes local mediator release from the mast cells, leading to allergic edema of the nasal and sinus membranes. As sinus canals are surrounded by bone, the membranes can only swell *inward* against themselves, thus sealing off the passageway.

When sinus *infection* occurs due to viruses or bacteria, it is an inflammatory edema that swells the membranes and blocks the sinuses. Mucus formation continues and the pressure and pain thus become increased.

The addition of microbes, plus the white blood cells, antibodies, and other protective substances sent in to fight the microbes, makes the mucus still more copious and usually turns it yellow or green. Infection causes irritation of the sinus lining, so can also produce oozing of blood. In this case, the mucus may at times appear blood-streaked.

So either allergy or infection can cause sinus blockage and headache. In infection the mucus is often yellow, green, or blood-streaked.

"SINUS TROUBLE": HOW HEALTHY SINUSES CAN BE BLOCKED BY A SICK NOSE

Even when the sinus membranes themselves are not swollen, the sinuses can be obstructed by swelling of the lining membrane of the nose. As in the sinuses, nasal tissue swelling is usually caused by edema from allergically increased capillary permeability or from inflammatory edema of the nasal tissue due to infection.

The color of the membrane of the nose is attributable to the red blood cell-filled capillaries just below the membrane. The healthy nasal membrane is the same pink color as the mucus membrane of the mouth. Allergic edema of the nose from capillary leakage results in pale, moist, boggy, waterlogged nasal membranes.

This edema impairs the circulation in the membranes. In severe cases, the circulation is so poor that the membranes look pale or blue. The membrane cells receive less oxygen and nutrients, and cannot as readily dispose of their waste products. Under these circumstances, the membranes are like six-cylinder engines working on only three cylinders. Their protective function is diminished, and they are more susceptible to infection.

The infection need not be caused only by viruses or bacteria "caught" from other people. The viruses and bacteria normally present on everyone's respiratory membranes, but ordinarily stalemated by mucosal and body defenses, can invade when either local or general defenses are diminished. Both local and general defenses can be weakened, diverted, or dissipated by allergy.

Thus, much infection is secondary to allergy. This is why control of allergy is so often effective in reducing the incidence of recurrent upper respiratory infections, sinus infections, ear infections, bronchial infections, and pneumonia.

It is simply amazing how patients with repeated infections of these types usually quit having them soon after the institution of allergy controls. These controls may be simple, such as educated avoidance of chilling, getting a pet out of the house, or removing a carpet from the bedroom; or they may require instituting neutralization therapy for inhalants as well, and sometimes also for foods.

CHILLING, INFECTION, AND ANTIBIOTICS

I cannot leave the subject of sinus infection without a word about antibiotics. Many people can overcome their colds and sinus infections without antibiotics. Some obtain complete relief from just five or ten days of antibiotics. Whatever microorganisms are not eliminated by a short course of antibiotics can be finished off by the patient's own natural defenses.

However, many allergic patients do not have a sufficiently strong defense mechanism to "finish off" the infection. They come in with a history of ten or more severe respiratory infections, often complicated by repeated asthma attacks or pneumonia each winter.

In actuality, they are usually having *one* infection in the early winter treated repeatedly with too-short courses of antibiotics, with nine *recurrences* of the original infection. They can be saved much suffering and repeated antibiotic therapy by being treated thoroughly for the first infection, thus preventing the nine relapses.

Thorough treatment may require two, three, or more weeks of antibiotic therapy for the first attack. However, this is far better than ten courses of antibiotic therapy and ten asthma attacks, pneumonias, or other complications of upper respiratory infections treated with inadequate antibiotic therapy.

Another important point about antibiotics is that many upper respiratory infections and asthma attacks are triggered by viruses. Viruses cannot be killed by any of the antibiotics available today.

But *allergic* people who contract viral respiratory infections or asthma often quickly develop secondary *bacterial* infections. The viruses may disappear spontaneously in a few days, but the bacteria often persist and cause progressive worsening of the illness. These bacterial complications can be severe, frequent, and life-threatening, especially in allergic and asthmatic patients.

Bacteria *do* respond to antibiotics. Allergic and asthmatic patients with a history of repeated severe winter attacks should start taking an antibiotic *as early as possible* in each attack. They should also continue the antibiotic *until thoroughly well* to prevent repeated relapses. This may require taking the antibiotic an additional three days or so after the disappearance of all noticeable symptoms.

In addition, I would like to note here that chilling, infection, and antibiotic therapy are all related. Chilling lowers resistance in many allergic people, leading to "colds," sinus infections, ear infections, asthma attacks, pneumonias, and other allergic and infectious problems.

If you develop a sinus infection from becoming chilled, and you then proceed to get chilled again before the sinus infection is well, the second chilling further lowers resistance. This allows the established infection to drive deeper into the tissues.

This increases the severity and duration of the illness, and prolongs the need for an antibiotic. So learning to protect yourself from chilling, being careful not to become chilled again when you already have an infection, and taking an antibiotic early enough and long enough are all part of the overall protection you may need.

SEROUS OTITIS: HOW HEALTHY EARS CAN BE BLOCKED BY A SICK NOSE

Another condition, serous otitis, has similar allergic causes and similar responses to therapy. The outer ear canal comes to a dead end at the ear drum; the drum completely seals off and separates the outer ear canal from the middle ear cavity. The middle ear cavity connects to the nasopharynx through a narrow tube called the Eustachian tube. Blockage of the nasal end of the Eustachian tube by either allergic or inflammatory swelling of the nose results in inability of air to move from the nose through this tube to the middle ear cavity behind the drum.

Air pressure on both sides of the drum must be equal in order for the drum to maintain its normal position and tension and to be able to vibrate properly. Eustachian blockage results in the absorption into the circulation of the air in the middle ear. Then the pressure in the middle ear becomes less than the atmospheric pressure in the external ear canal, producing a vacuum in the middle ear.

The vacuum pulls the drum inward, producing an inward bulging or retraction of the drum toward the middle ear. This reduces its ability to vibrate. The result is difficulty in hearing, particularly the finer, high-pitched sounds. The increased tension on the drum can cause pain in the ear or on the entire side of the head.

If the vacuum lasts long enough, it pulls thin serous fluid out of the capillaries in the membrane into the middle ear cavity, where it puddles. The patient may feel the fluid trapped in the middle ear, especially when he tilts his head. This sequence can usually be prevented and relieved by allergy management.

In some patients, the thin serous fluid becomes drier and thicker due to reabsorption of the watery portion of the fluid. The remaining proteinaceous material may then become so thick that it forms a sticky glue-like plug ("glue ear"), which can only be removed surgically through an incision in the drum. Then allergy treatment can be instituted to decrease the tendency for this condition to recur.

DISTINGUISHING FEATURES OF SINUS HEADACHE

Now that we have described the anatomic and physiologic fundamentals, let us return to our discussion of headache. Sinus headache is usually easily distinguished from migraine headache.

If sinus infection is present, there may be a history of exposure to someone with a "virus cold," or to an inhaled allergen, or simply to a chilling event that lowered body resistance and allowed ever-present viruses and bacteria to invade the sinuses. When infected, the inner lining of the nose usually looks red and congested, whereas in the uninfected state it may have been either pale from allergy or just normally pink. The mucus is thick and yellow, green, or blood-streaked, and can often be seen draining down the back of the throat.

Fever, sore throat, cough, and elevated white-cell count may also be present, although not necessarily so. Sinus x-rays may show swollen sinus membranes and sometimes the presence of accumulated fluid or mucus in the sinuses. If the sinus blockage is caused by allergy, and no secondary infection is present, the membranes of the nose look pale, boggy, and moist; any drainage is clear or milky, not yellow, green, or blood-streaked.

A microscopic examination of a stained smear of nasal or sinus mucus can sometimes help differentiate between allergy and infection. In allergy and in some nonallergic conditions, the smear often reveals the presence of many eosinophils, specialized white blood cells that tend to move into areas of allergic inflammation to "clean up" allergic debris, to remove damaged cells and molecules, and to neutralize harmful mediators. Their function is to help return the tissues to a normal state. In infection, the cells which predominate are more often the neutrophils, the white blood cells which are most highly specialized for destroying microorganisms. They are called "neutrophils" because they do not take up either red or blue stains well, and so look neutral-colored under the microscope.

The location of the pain is dependent on which sinuses are blocked.

The pain can be virtually anywhere about the head, but most commonly is in the face just below the cheek bones, or in the forehead, or in the back of the head. In the case of serous otitis, the pain is chiefly in the area of the ears and temples.

The face or forehead may be swollen and tender to touch. The pain is dull and steady, not sharp and throbbing as in migraine, and there is usually no nausea or vomiting. The pain may be temporarily worsened by changing head position, and temporarily helped by decongestant nose drops which may open the sinuses for a while for better drainage.

The pain may last for weeks, months, or years until the underlying allergic and infectious factors are controlled. When long lasting, the repeated prolonged use of nose drops may itself irritate, swell, and eventually atrophy the membranes, causing an inflammatory condition called rhinitis medicamentosa.

When a recurrent or chronic smoldering, low-grade sinus infection persists, it may sap your strength; make you feel listless, tired, and unmotivated; and lead to job failure, social failure, and depression. I have seen many lives turned around simply by adequate management of the infection plus allergy treatment to decrease the tendency to future recurrent infections.

INHALANTS VERSUS FOODS IN SINUS HEADACHE

Even in the absence of infection, there is no question but that inhalant allergens are common causes of nose, sinus, and Eustachian blockage and pain. Inhalant management alone usually provides rapid and continuing relief.

But the patient who fails to improve adequately or clear completely on management of inhalant allergy, infection, and anatomic abnormalities should be considered for possible food investigation. Food allergens absorbed from the gastrointestinal tract can traverse the bloodstream and combine with food-sensitive IgE molecules on the mast cells just below the membranes in the nose, sinuses, and Eustachian tubes.

Chemical mediators released by basophils or by mast cells from other areas of the body can also reach these tissues and cause allergic reactions. So foods, although less commonly than inhalants, can cause increased capillary permeability in the sinuses and Eustachian tubes just as in the lip, larynx, and other areas.

Chapter 13

TENSION HEADACHE: A CHARLEY HORSE OF HEAD MUSCLES

When most people speak of tension headache, they refer to headache caused by *emotional* tension. However, headache specialists use the term to mean *skeletal muscle* tension.

Tension headache is caused by painful contraction of the skeletal muscles of the face, head, and neck. It is like a "charley horse" of the head.

Specialists do generally feel that emotional factors cause most muscle contraction headaches. The chief emotional factors incriminated are anxiety and depression.

Anxious patients are described as tense, apprehensive, easily embarrassed, and sensitive to the opinions of others. They are constantly worried. They may have insomnia, restlessness, irritability, fits of aggression, weeping, and psychosomatic symptoms referable to many organs.

According to certain psychologists, chronic anxiety may be the result of forbidden aggressive, hostile, and unacceptable sexual strivings which threaten to break through the repressing influence of social and moral taboos. The head pain is considered an anxiety-reducing protective behavior pattern which develops when the patient is in an anxiety-producing situation. Such a situation may be related to sex, marriage, family, job, social setting, or personal habit.

Depressed patients are said to think little of themselves, and to dwell on their mistakes and inadequacies. They often complain of poor memory and impairment of concentration.

There is no question that many people experience at times the characteristic feelings of anxiety and depression as well as headache. But there is also no question that many of these same symptoms may also be caused by food allergy.

Allergy frequently coexists with anxiety or depression. One of the most gratifying events in medical practice is the sudden lifting of the pall of chronic anxiety or depression experienced by some patients when they carefully follow allergy diets or are given food extract injection therapy.

Painful muscle contraction headache can be caused by a variety of disorders such as tumors, infections, and diseases of the eye, ear, nose, teeth, and jaw-joints. Some tension headaches accompany sinus headaches. Some are associated with migraine headaches, apparently secondary to the irritation of the muscles by the throbbing dilated arteries passing through them, and by edema of the muscles from the allergically increased capillary permeability of migraine.

These secondary types of tension headache are best managed by correcting the primary problem. Treating the food allergy, removing the tumor, clearing the infection, correcting the diseases of the eye, ear, nose, teeth, and jaw-joints, and treating the sinus problem and the migraine usually relieve such secondary tension headaches.

Physicians interested in food allergy are very familiar with the ability of foods to cause muscle spasms and joint pain in various parts of the body. We frequently see food-allergic patients suffering from muscle and joint pains of the chest, back, abdomen, arms, legs, or the back of the neck.

We sometimes produce and relieve these pains during testing and can then prevent recurrence of pain by allergy treatment, particularly for foods. We are not at all surprised to see some patients with muscle pains of the head respond similarly to testing and treatment with allergy extracts.

HOW IS TENSION HEADACHE RECOGNIZED?

Since tension headache is due to muscle contraction, the pain is steady, not throbbing. The patient usually describes it as a feeling of tightness, using such terms as "band-like," "vise-like," or "cramp-like." The muscles are often tender to touch or pressure, and it may hurt to comb the hair or wear a hat. Even the weight of the hair can make a difference, and keeping the hair cut short to reduce the drag of long hair can reduce the pain somewhat in some patients.

Chilling drafts often increase muscle contraction and pain in the head area as in other areas. In tension headache as in migraine, the pain is often worsened by exercise, fatigue, weather changes, menses, and even weekends, holidays, and vacations. Some patients note that eating certain foods—or not eating them—is followed by increased pain. Thus, many of the same allergic and nonallergic stresses that cause other syndromes we have discussed operate here also.

My purpose is not to state that all tension headaches are due to or aggravated by allergy but that some of them undoubtedly are. When tumors and other diseases are ruled out, allergic factors should be investigated.

When psychiatric help is needed, it should be sought. But psychiatric help, even when successful, may require many years to reduce the pain, or to teach the patient how to bear up under it or live with his problem. On the other hand, a patient can usually be markedly helped in a few weeks with allergy management if his headache is basically or even partially allergic.

Constant or recurrent pain distracts the mind, turns the patient's attention inward on his bewildering symptoms, and reduces his concentration and perception of what is going on in the world around him. All of these reduce his ability to learn from experience or from teaching. Recurrent pain focuses his attention on the pain itself, or on when the next pain will strike, or on how he can alter his day-to-day behavior to minimize the chances of being struck again by pain.

Many psychiatric problems diminish, or at least are much more readily coped with, if the patient is no longer burdened by the suffering and introversion that accompany allergy-caused symptoms such as headache. When the pain is controlled, the mind is freed.

These patients can return to being productive, interacting members of the family, the classroom, and society. Their achievements increase, and their self-confidence and feeling of worthiness naturally improve. If tutoring or counseling is still needed, it should then be sought for the situational or character problem or for the secondarily altered protective thought and behavior patterns.

Chapter 14

CLUSTER HEADACHE: SURPRISING RELATIONSHIPS TO ALLERGY

Cluster headache, like migraine, is a vascular headache. Just as in migraine, the carotid arteries are the shock organs and the pain is caused by dilatation and leakage of these arteries and their branches. Interestingly, cluster headache occurs much more often in males, whereas migraine occurs more often in females.

Cluster headache is also called histamine headache or Horton's headache because in 1956, a Canadian physician, Dr. B.T. Horton, popularized the idea that it was caused by histamine. Although attacks in susceptible people can sometimes be precipitated by injections of histamine, other agents that widen blood vessels, such as nitroglycerine and alcohol, can have the same effect. Antihistamines are of little or no help, and histamine desensitization has not been a reliable method of treatment.

Cluster headache differs from migraine primarily in its unusual pain pattern. There are many sharp head pains in rapid succession, each pain lasting only seconds or a few minutes, occurring in clusters or groups that last usually from thirty to ninety minutes. There is complete freedom from discomfort between pains and between clusters of pains. These clusters may occur two or three or more times a day, often at the same time each day.

This time pattern can be likened to the effects of a gusty windstorm on ocean waves. Each wave is analogous to one pain. Each sharp gust of wind causes a cluster of great waves to come crashing against the shore in rapid succession. Between gusts, the waves quickly subside. Between waves and between gusts, the shore is quiet.

Cluster headaches are even more prone than migraine to be on one side of the head. The pain comes without warning and there is no visual or gastrointestinal prodrome.

It may begin suddenly in one eye; or it may begin high in one nostril, spreading quickly to the eye and then to the forehead and temple on that side. The nostril on that side becomes congested and watery, the eye becomes bloodshot and teary, the face on that side may become red and sweaty, the eyelid on that side may droop, and the pupil constrict.

The pain is pulsating or throbbing, that is, more severe with each heart beat. The arteries on that side of the temple may be so dilated that they can be visualized and palpated. The pain is so severe that many patients have considered suicide.

These patients do not seek a dark, isolated room where they can rest and be quiet. Nor do they put a pillow or cold cloth over their heads. Rather, they pace the floor and are totally unable to sleep or rest.

When the cluster attack is over, it subsides rapidly. The patient is energetic and is quick to resume his usual activities. By contrast, the subsidence of migraine usually leaves the patient tired, somnolent, and lethargic.

Cluster headaches tend to arouse a patient from sleep even more than migraine. They are prone to occur during sleep, naps, or relaxation. The onset of pain can be so sudden and severe that the patient jumps out of bed before he is fully awake.

POSSIBLE ALLERGIC FACTORS IN CLUSTER HEADACHES

I have been impressed by the occasional similarity in the time periods of cluster headache attacks and allergic asthma attacks. Cluster headache attacks sometimes appear during each spring tree-pollinating season; each fall weed-pollinating season; each winter chill, dust, and mold season; or, less frequently, each warm midsummer grass season.

Some attacks last only as long as the specific pollen season. Like asthmatics with multiple sensitivities, attacks can occur at two or more separate seasons, and can even continue for several consecutive seasons.

Also, just as in asthma and other allergic syndromes, seasonal inhalant exposures comprise only one of the stresses that seem to bring about the attack. It is well known that attacks can be brought on by alcoholic beverages, with the pain usually appearing fifteen to thirty minutes after ingestion of the alcohol. Eating hot dogs has also been found to be a precipitating factor.

In both instances the widening effect on the blood vessels of alcohol and the nitrites used as preservatives in hot dogs have been assumed to be the culprits. To my knowledge, no one has seriously studied the possibility of allergic causation due to the food origin of alcohol; the increased absorption rate of foods eaten at the same time as the alcohol; and the well-known sensitivity responses to food additives, chemical dyes, flavorings, and preservatives in alcoholic beverages, hot dogs, and other such factory foods.

It is also well known that changing the cluster headache patient's environment, hospitalizing him, or removing him from "stressful" situations may relieve and even abolish an attack of cluster headache. These have been interpreted to indicate the importance of emotional stress situations. From an allergy viewpoint they may well indicate the fact that the patient has been removed from the cold or pollen-filled outdoor air; the dusty, moldy, or chemicalized environment of his home; his indoor pet or carpet; and his snack-filled refrigerator.

The various nonspecific triggers of allergic reactions, such as chill, fatigue, emotional events, and others, seem also to trigger cluster headaches. Most cluster headaches occur in males, but when they occur in females, menstruation can act as another nonspecific trigger of cluster headache attacks.

From the seasonal incidence of some cluster headache attacks, one would expect that if any allergy treatment was helpful, it would be inhalant immunotherapy. That is exactly what my experience has been. Many such cluster headache patients have obtained marked relief if treated with inhalant neutralizing injections begun well in advance of the season. Relief can be obtained in some cases even if treatment is begun during the season; but a preseason start improves chances for benefit.

Foods must also be treated in some people, and the nonspecific triggers of allergic reactions often require attention as well. By individualizing the care to suit the needs of the patient, overall allergy management can be very helpful to many patients with cluster headache.

My first recognition of the relationship of asthma and other allergic syndromes to cluster headaches was a chance occurrence. The first patient who came to me for cluster headache had never had asthma. He developed mild headache when I tested him with intradermal injections of some inhalant antigens, particularly pollen. He also developed mild *asthma* spells when tested for molds.

Both the headache and the wheezing cleared when I administered the neutralizing test doses of the antigens that had caused them. Since then, I have noted allergic factors in many cluster headache patients, and have provided much relief by treating these factors.

Many people with cluster headaches also have nasal, sinus, bronchial, gastrointestinal, or other allergic problems, for which they may be seeing multiple specialists. The same allergens are causing symptoms in multiple organs.

Relieving their cluster headaches also usually relieves many of these other symptoms as well. Again, cost-effectiveness is added to relief-effectiveness.

Chapter 15

HIDDEN DIGESTIVE ALLERGY: A CAUSE OF MOUTH ULCERS, IRRITABLE BOWEL/SPASTIC COLON, CHRONIC ULCERATIVE COLITIS, AND CROHN'S DISEASE

Food allergy can cause symptoms and illnesses in all portions of the G-I tract, from the mouth to the anus. These range in severity from minor annoyances to life-endangering conditions.

FOOD CANKER SORES VERSUS HERPES COLD SORES

In the past, we tended to ascribe most recurrent sores in and around the mouth to herpes virus infection. We rarely, if ever, suspected food allergy as an important causative factor.

Now that rapidly effective therapy is available for both food allergy and herpes virus infection, a clear distinction is important in order to choose which treatment to use. Usually, this distinction can now be readily made.

Canker sores are almost always on mucosal surfaces, *inside* the mouth. Cold sores (fever blisters) are almost always on a skin (cutaneous) surface, usually on the skin around the lip or on the vermilion border (the lipstick area). Canker sores are usually scattered about on different sites within the oral cavity with different attacks, while cold sores often recur in precisely the same skin site in every attack.

The shape of canker sores is usually irregular and amoeboid; they are relatively large in diameter; and they are flat, depressed below the mucosal surface, and punched out in appearance. Cold sores are often first pink, pinpoint in size, and elevated above the skin surface.

They may first appear as tiny papules (pimples) which grow and change to blisters, with redness and swelling (inflammatory edema) of the underlying and surrounding skin. The blisters then join together, ulcerate, ooze, and crust. Canker sores do not crust.

FOODS AS CAUSES OF CANKER SORES

Canker sores are almost always due to food allergy. They respond rapidly and reliably to dietary avoidance or food extract injection therapy for the causative foods. Canker sores can often be made to recur for the purpose of diagnosis by meticulously avoiding the suspected food and all its derivatives for four days and then eating it in large quantity at two or more consecutive meals on the fifth day.

If no foods are suspected, a diet diary should indicate which foods have been eaten, possibly repeatedly, at the last meals before the sores appear. If ulceration has been frequent, you should suspect the five or ten most frequently eaten foods or beverages in your diet, and all foods eaten in binges or with great relish. Citrus fruits and tomatoes are common offenders.

All these foods can be avoided simultaneously until the ulcers heal, and can then be re-added one by one in challenge fashion to pick out the causative foods. When the causative foods cannot be determined by these procedures, diagnosis and relief can still usually be provided by neutralizing testing and treatment.

HERPES AS THE CAUSE OF COLD SORES

Cold sores, on the other hand, are due to recurrent herpes virus infections, and almost always respond rapidly and reliably to neutralizing injections of Influenza Virus Vaccine. They are only rarely affected by dietary changes.

During intradermal testing with consecutive concentrations of Influenza Virus Vaccine, the pain of the cold sore usually subsides markedly or completely within thirty minutes after administering the neutralizing concentration. This provides the diagnosis through relief.

This is not a placebo effect as other test concentrations of Influenza Virus Vaccine do not provide relief, the neutralizing dose of Influenza Virus Vaccine does not relieve the pain of canker sores, and food extract injections do not relieve cold sores. The same characteristic, objective wheal pattern seen in intradermal food testing is produced by intradermal tests with Influenza Virus Vaccine.

Future recurrences of herpes attacks can often be aborted at the outset of the attack by just one or two self-administered subcutaneous injections of the neutralizing concentration, usually with relief of pain in thirty minutes and rapid disappearance of the lesions, often within hours. Usually recurrent attacks quickly become much milder, briefer, and less frequent. *After treatment for one or two attacks, it is common for recurrent attacks to change from weeks apart to many months or even years apart.*

This remarkable rate of decrease in recurrence does not require regular weekly preventive injections. Injections are not usually needed at all between attacks. All that is needed in most cases is the few injections required therapeutically to relieve the attacks themselves.

TRUE HERPES ULCERS WITHIN THE MOUTH

In rare instances, crops of ulcers within the mouth *can* be caused by recurrent herpes virus infection. In these instances the ulceration is usually far more severe, extensive, prolonged, and debilitating than when caused by foods.

This condition causes incredible suffering. Eating, drinking, swallowing, and speaking can be excruciatingly painful. Brushing the teeth is out of the question. In the past it was notoriously difficult to treat, but great relief now usually accompanies neutralization with Influenza Virus Vaccine.

Also, a rare patient will have true herpes-caused cutaneous cold sore recurrences whenever he eats a specific allergenic food which triggers reactivation of the herpes virus. In rare instances, a severe cold sore on the skin surface of the lip can penetrate to the mucosal surface of the lip, producing a through-and-through lesion involving both the skin and mucosal surfaces.

OTHER CAUSES OF MOUTH ULCERS

Of course, the acute generalized herpetic mouth ulcers of young children are caused by the herpes virus, but this is not recurrent; it occurs only once in a lifetime. The pain from multiple severe mucosal ulcerations of the mouth and throat is often so great that the child is unwilling to eat or drink for ten to fourteen days or longer and may become dehydrated. This may require hospitalization for intravenous fluid therapy. I have never had an opportunity to use Influenza Virus Vaccine neutralization therapy in acute herpetic gingivostomatitis, but it does offer the possibility of reducing much suffering and expense.

Once this condition heals, the virus retreats and takes up permanent refuge in nerve cells. However, the virus is prone to travel back down the nerve fibers to the skin to cause fever blisters years later when the skin is traumatized or the body's immune defenses are temporarily too weak to hold the virus in check.

A wide spectrum of other conditions is capable of producing mouth ulcers. This includes a skin disorder called erythema multiforme; infections; drug reactions; vitamin and iron deficiencies; autoimmune diseases such as lupus and Reiter's Disease; and immunodeficiency states such as Behcet's Syndrome, Crohn's Disease, and reactions to toxins such as gluten, a constituent of some grains. They also include blood disorders, malignancies, and many others. In some cases, no cause can be found.

Despite the length of this list and the need to be aware of serious conditions, many are obvious and others are rare diseases. Most recurrent oral mucosal ulcerations of "unknown cause" are due to food allergy, and most recurrent cutaneous sores about the lips are due to herpes. Both usually respond well and quickly to specific therapy, as described.

DR. ALVAREZ AND CHOCOLATE-CAUSED CANKER SORES

I would like to conclude this discussion of canker sores and cold sores with another quotation from Dr. Walter Alvarez, the eminent Mayo Clinic physician I quoted earlier with "dumb Mondays" from chicken:[26]

> "When I was a boy of 12, I decided I'd never again go into an ice cream parlor because I had noticed that often after eating ice cream or partaking of some soft drink, I felt miserable for the rest of the day and my mouth was sore. Years later I learned that chocolate was another enemy of mine. When I said goodbye to chocolate, that was the end of my discomfort and canker sores in my mouth."

FOOD AS CAUSES OF STOMACH, INTESTINE, AND BOWEL SYNDROMES

Allergic disorders of the gastrointestinal tract can produce many symptoms including difficulty in swallowing, nausea, vomiting, indigestion, "heartburn," gassiness, bloating, abdominal pain, constipation, diarrhea, and bloody stools. These syndromes may occur in various combinations as manifestations of many diagnostic entities labelled as pharyngeal edema, esophageal spasm, gastritis, nervous stomach, irritable bowel, spastic colon, mucous colitis, chronic ulcerative colitis, and Crohn's disease.

Such conditions are generally considered functional or due to nerves and emotional stress. Yet many are easily demonstrated to be caused chiefly by food allergy, and these patients usually obtain marked relief from food extract injection therapy.

Infants and small children with many serious and even life-threatening gastrointestinal conditions are often benefited by this treatment. These conditions include recurrent and chronic vomiting, stomachaches, colicky pain, and chronic diarrhea.

Infants as young as one or two months of age can be readily tested and successfully treated by the neutralizing method. Their response is usually remarkably rapid and provides further evidence that neutralization responses are not dependent on a hypnotic or placebo effect.

When people experience chronic or recurrent gastrointestinal symptoms, they usually have no idea that food sensitivity may be the cause of their troubles. They may blame the symptoms on constitutional weakness; or on other factors such as spiciness, greasiness, roughness, acidity, inadequate dietary fiber, vitamin or mineral deficiencies; or digestive enzyme deficiencies. Often, they feel that emotional stress is their problem.

While all these factors do need consideration, food allergy needs consideration also, and is usually overlooked. I believe it is a more common cause than all the other factors combined.

PROBLEMS WITH SYMPTOMATIC RATHER THAN SPECIFIC TREATMENT

Patients with obscure bowel symptoms tend to take antacids, analgesics, bowel relaxers, or tranquilizers. They also ingest more milk products, or eat more bran (wheat), or take megadoses of vitamin C (which is usually made from corn).

They may use capsules, tablets, or liquids containing starch (corn, wheat, potato), milk sugar (lactose) or other sugars (cane, beet, corn), chemicals, and other sensitizing agents. Although the drugs may dampen the patient's symptoms or his ability to perceive them, some of these medications may be allergenic and add to or perpetuate the allergy problem.

Many of these drugs can also cause nonallergic side effects such as drowsiness, nervousness, nausea, headache, stomachache, or diarrhea and further complicate the symptom picture. For example, one of my patients was for decades repeatedly thrown into several days of nausea and depression by a great many foods. About the third day of her depression, she usually developed diarrhea, and would quickly evacuate the etiologic foods, clearing spontaneously by the fourth day. But during the first two depressive days she tended to take stimulants, antidepressants, antianxiety drugs, and antinauseants; and during the third and fourth days she would add drugs to combat the diarrhea, thus delaying bowel evacuation.

Once on these drugs, she was reluctant to stop them for fear of recurrent symptoms. So she was in a nearly constant drugged state, with confusing and debilitating side effects of multiple medications, perpetuating her own illness. Her brain and other organs were driven back and forth by drugs which not only were unneeded but worsened her physical and mental condition; delayed return to normal; and led toward drug dependence, habituation, and a feeling of physical and emotional weakness.

Since her depression was accompanied by great physical lethargy, she took to bed with each attack, and her bed rest was further prolonged by the lethargy occurring as a side effect of some of her medications. She thus spent an inordinate amount of her life in bed, putting great strains on her family and great limitations on her ability to function, achieve, and enjoy life.

It is important to treat such people early, before years or decades of drug usage, faulty thought patterns, counterproductive habits, and inappropriate interpersonal relationships have become entrenched. However, even late institution of therapy can often relieve much symptomatology.

When an x-ray examination shows spastic colon, or when a patient receives a descriptive diagnosis of nervous stomach, irritable colon, chronic diarrhea, chronic ulcerative colitis, or ileocolitis (Crohn's disease), this says nothing about causative factors. It in no way negates the fact that this patient's syndrome may be caused by food allergy and may be relieved by food extract injection therapy.

RELIEF AND COST-EFFECTIVENESS IN LIFE-THREATENING ILLNESSES

The ulceration of chronic ulcerative colitis and Crohn's Disease are analogous to the ulceration of aphthous stomatitis. In my experience, all are usually caused primarily by food allergy, and all usually respond quickly to food extract injection therapy.

Chronic ulcerative colitis and Crohn's disease are often treated by lifelong cortisone therapy and sometimes by surgical removal of the colon and/or part of the ileum which may necessitate living with a colostomy or ileostomy. Persistent ulcerative colitis can eventually lead to carcinoma of the colon. So these can be severe life-limiting and even life-threatening illnesses.

I have therefore observed these patients particularly closely. I have been gratified to note that most of them have become greatly improved or virtually free of their problems after the early institution of food neutralization treatment, combined in a few instances with meticulous avoidance of one or a few problem foods.

They also have usually been freed of the need for prolonged cortisone therapy with its many potential complications, as well as the need for expensive hospitalizations and operations. In these as in so many other syndromes, neutralization is usually both highly relief-effective and cost-effective.

INFANTS AND CHILDREN

When allergy produces chronic diarrhea or chronic edema of the gastrointestinal mucosa in a child, food absorption is diminished, the child becomes undernourished and lethargic, and a descriptive label of "failure to thrive" may be applied. This sometimes life-threatening syndrome usually responds exceptionally well to early institution of food extract injection therapy, and again saves much suffering and expense.

Infants typically respond rapidly if treated early, and *no infant is too young to be tested and treated.* In fact, delaying institution of treatment too long may result in inability to regain catch-up growth.

Although the stomachaches, gassiness, diarrhea, and other allergic symptoms are often controlled even by late treatment, the child may never attain his full potential height. So parental awareness and early investigation are very important, and nutritional as well as allergy therapy may be needed.

CHRONIC CONSTIPATION CAUSED BY FOOD ALLERGY

There have been many patients in my practice who have been constipated by foods. The effect is often subtle and difficult to recognize.

For example, one man has a regular, dependable, quick, easy, and painless bowel evacuation each morning. But if he eats pork one day, the next morning his evacuation is delayed; the stool is harder and drier than usual; some straining is required; and there may be slight pain. The movement may also be incomplete, and a second urge may come later in the day to finally complete the evacuation. If he is busy and ignores the second urge, he tends to be uncomfortable that day and even more constipated the next day.

If he eats pork on two consecutive days, he may have no urge and no evacuation at all the third day. If he continues to eat pork, he has to regularly use stool softeners or lubricants, laxatives, or enemas for relief. So he has learned never to eat pork closer than at intervals of four or more days.

I am not singling out pork as a frequent culprit in constipation. Any food can do it. Usually it is a frequently eaten food when the constipation is chronic. But I have seen acute constipation from such unlikely foods as asparagus, broccoli, spinach, and other ordinarily healthful and beneficial foods. I have often wondered if some patients who require surgery repeatedly for intestinal obstruction could be suffering unknowingly from food-induced constipation caused by repeatedly eating one or several constipating foods.

CHRONIC CONSTIPATION CAUSED BY INHALANT ALLERGY

I have learned much about allergic symptoms by recording and scoring the degree (0, 1+, 2+, 3+, or 4+) of every symptom that can be extracted from the patient by detailed questioning, whether due to allergy or not.

I then rescore each symptom at each subsequent visit and note which symptoms improve after which treatments. One of my most surprising findings has been the frequent relief of severe chronic constipation when patients receive *inhalant* allergy neutralization therapy!

In other words, when a patient with an inhalant allergy syndrome also gives a history of chronic constipation, the constipation is often noted to improve markedly or disappear when inhalant neutralization therapy is administered. Although I have long noted that individual foods could cause constipation, and food avoidance or food neutralization could be helpful, I was quite surprised to discover that there could also be an inhalant-constipation connection. It is because of this observed correlation that I speculate that the mediators released into the bloodstream by inhalant allergens can sometimes alter bowel function and lead to chronic constipation.

Chapter 16

HOW BRAIN ALLERGY CAN CAUSE ATTENTION DEFICIT DISORDER, HYPERACTIVITY, LEARNING DISABILITY, BEHAVIOR PROBLEMS, IMPAIRED MENTAL FUNCTION, DYSLEXIA, AND OTHER BRAIN DYSFUNCTIONS

It is conservatively estimated that about 5 to 15 percent of the children in the United States alone are afflicted with the hypersensitivity/learning disability syndrome. Some suggest that as many as 9 million children have some degree of this disorder.[32,34]

Children with behavior and learning problems are the largest group of children referred to psychiatric clinics. As many as 60–70 percent of the clientele at child guidance clinics are referred by teachers and parents because of such symptoms.[34]

However, the incidence may be much higher. Many do not come to the attention of physicians. Others are taken only to a specialist to evaluate their vision, hearing, reading, writing, speech, poor scholastic achievement, "bad" behavior, lethargy, incoordination in sports, or other specific problems that do not always get them included in this category.

Neither does it often get them to an allergist who might resolve the underlying cause. Further, the full scope of the problem can only be appreciated when one realizes that this must be virtually a worldwide situation, affecting adults as well as children.

SYMPTOMS AND CONSEQUENCES

The symptoms are sometimes confusing, "soft," or highly variable. This makes diagnosis that much more difficult and the consequences of long-delayed diagnosis that much more severe.

Some hyperactive children are considered as just unusually energetic or not well-disciplined. They may be simply unable to sit through a meal, complete an assigned task, listen to the end of a story, or wait for another person to finish speaking before impulsively interrupting with thoughts of their own on an entirely different subject.

Others are in constant physical motion, moving, running, jumping, fidgeting, or wriggling. Some are awkward, clumsy, bump into people and objects, knock furniture over, or have repeated accidental injuries. Some cannot accept directions, discipline, or authority, no matter how skillfully or persistently applied.

Some just seem to be sensitive or bad tempered and aggressive. Others are hypoactive, limp, lethargic, drowsy, cry easily, or are depressed. Some do not realize that they cannot see letters or objects as others do.

Some cannot spell accurately or write legibly or evenly. Some cannot properly sort out what is being said to them. They may misunderstand or forget instructions almost as soon as they are given.

Such children cannot understand why they are considered by their siblings, parents, peers, and teachers as difficult, strange, incorrigible, lazy, or "out of it." They gradually find themselves criticized or punished beyond tolerance, leading to friendlessness or isolation.

They may start out life as potentially loving, intelligent, and talented. However, they may still tend to become academic and social failures as children, difficult juveniles as teenagers, and maladjusted loners as adults.

On the other hand, other conditions can cause these and similar problems and need to be considered. Possible causes include anemia and other blood cell disorders; chronic nose, sinus, or ear allergies; occult smoldering infections; autoimmune diseases; hypothyroidism or other endocrine problems; lead or other poisonings; intestinal parasites; visual problems; hearing problems; neurological or psychiatric illness; birth injury; psychologically damaging homes or parents; hereditary abnormalities; and many others.[34,35] Just because a child behaves "differently," we cannot *assume* it is due to food allergy.

CAN HYPERACTIVITY/LEARNING DISABILITY BE CAUSED BY FOODS?

Since ancient times, it has been known that some people are seriously affected both physically and mentally by foods that do not bother most other people.[36,37] One of the earliest recorded references to the cerebral benefits of elimination diets was in the first chapter of the Book of Daniel.[38] Physicians have been publishing books and articles over at least the past century describing cerebral symptoms or unusual behavior brought on by food reactions.

However, as in migraine, the food connection was long overlooked or considered to be a rare phenomenon by both allergists and the medical profession in general. Until attention was focused on this relationship, and particularly until food neutralization became available, there was no way to know how common this problem is and how often it can be helped. We now know that many of these patients behave the way they do because they have hidden sensitivity to some of the ordinary foods in their diet, and sometimes to other substances as well.

THE BRAIN AS A STRESS ORGAN

Food reactions which cause increased capillary permeability or other sensitivity effects in the brain seem to make the brain cells work too rapidly, too slowly, or in abnormal patterns. *So cerebral responses to allergenic foods usually take the form of stimulation, depression, or inappropriate behavior.* In fact, all three may be occurring simultaneously in some patients from individual or multiple food, inhalant, and chemical sensitivities.

One of the foremost leaders in the recognition of cerebral allergy was Dr. Frederick Speer, Clinical Professor of Pediatrics at the University of Kansas. In 1970 he edited a remarkably comprehensive book on this subject (*Allergy of the Nervous System*).[39] The eminent contributing authors included a neurologist, a pediatrician, and five nationally recognized allergists. Each chapter is followed by a list of bibliographic references. You can learn a great deal about the subject by reading this book and its references.

The foreword to Dr. Speer's book was written by Dr. Walter C. Alvarez, the Mayo Clinic physician I quoted earlier with "dumb Mondays" from chicken and canker sores from chocolate. At the risk of some repetition, here is Dr. Alvarez' entire foreword to Dr. Speer's book:[26]

> I rejoice to see this book 1) because I know it is much needed and it can do great good, 2) because it is full of facts and data on the history of the subject, and 3) because of my long interest in food allergy. Back around 1930 I was one of the small group of men who were studying food allergy and had learned that it can produce a dulled brain.
>
> For years before I knew I was highly sensitive to chicken fat, I suffered from what I called "*dumb Monday,*" when I was too dull to do

much constructive work like writing. Finally I discovered that the bad Mondays were due to the Alvarez family's habit of having chicken for Sunday dinner. When I stopped eating chicken, that was the end of my troubles on Monday.

Then one day, when I happened to tell my dear friend, Dr. Clifford Sweet, an able pediatrician, of my dumb Mondays, he said, "That gives me an idea; among my young patients I have many with 'dumb Monday'; I must inquire now to see if they have what you had." Months later, when I saw Cliff, he told me that a study had soon shown that the dumb Monday children were suffering from food allergy, and it came most often on Monday because on Sunday the child usually ate something not eaten during the rest of the week. Cliff said, "I now have a big 'Dumb Monday' club."

My most remarkable personal experience with brain dulling due to food allergy came many years ago when, on a Friday evening, coming down from a mountain trip, very hungry, I ate a whole broiled chicken. Next day I had a severe diarrhea, and with this I became so dulled I could not read with comfort. And that night I had hallucinations of sight, such as I had never had before and haven't had since. In the evenings when I would close my eyes, I would seem to go into a strange new world with many colors. These visions came every night until Tuesday when again I was well.

The most remarkable case of brain injury due to allergy that I ever saw was that of a lad of twenty or so, whom I saw in consultation. The doctor in charge asked me, "Could this fellow's indigestion and abdominal pain be due to food allergy?" I said, "Perhaps. But, as you say, his main trouble is that last year, while in his sophomore year in college, he had some brain damage so severe that he could no longer study and had to go home. Before that, he was a grade A student, as were his four brothers when they were in college." However, I said that he could try the elimination diet.

Two days later, when I met the doctor, he said "Quick, come with me; I want to show you a miracle; that lad whom you saw, when put on the diet, not only lost his indigestion and abdominal pain, but he became bright." I went to the room, and sure enough, the lad was bright; his face was wide awake; his speech was quick and clear; and he said, "I am going right back to college." Then when a few tests showed that he was markedly sensitive to eggs, he told me that he had fallen ill when his mother had started giving him, each morning, an omelet made of five eggs.

Similar to this lad's case was that of a man of thirty who came to consult me because of indigestion. When my examinations failed to show anything wrong, I put him on my usual elimination diet of nothing but oatmeal, lamb, rice, butter, sugar, and canned pears. The next day he came to say, "Look, doctor; a miracle has happened, and I feel bright again. Some years ago my father died, leaving me a big factory, but I never could do anything with it because I felt so dumb; I was too dull to work, so I got an able manager to run the business for me, and I spent my days browsing in my club. Now I feel so well that I am ready to go back home and get to work." A little study then showed that his trouble was due to the eating of a certain type of fish which he loved so much that he had been eating a serving of it every day.

As we all know, food allergy can sometimes bring on a spell of migraine. However, there are usually other causes. My large experience at the Mayo Clinic with hundreds of women with migraine left me with the strong impression that even when a migrainous woman finds that she is allergic to, let us say, chocolate, and she stops taking chocolate in any form, she will still have some attacks of migraine.

What impresses me is that still, with all of my forty years of study of food allergy, in some cases I fail to think of this disease when I should, and some brother physician has to make the diagnosis for me. This suggests that many physicians who have never been interested in food allergy must often be failing to make this diagnosis when they should do so.

DIETARY DIAGNOSIS

In case you wish to follow Dr. Alvarez' suggestion of an elimination diet, I would prefer you omit oatmeal (a cereal grain, and usually eaten with milk and sugar), butter (a milk derivative), sugar, and canned pears (which are now usually sweetened with sugar or corn sweetener). You could substitute less-frequently eaten foods such as lamb, duckling, turkey, and several species of scale fish (simply broiled in a covered Pyrex® dish or aluminum foil to maintain the moisture and tenderness), and a careful selection of raw and lightly cooked fresh vegetables (in simple form) not previously eaten very frequently.

Safflower or other infrequently used oil can be used for salads and cooking. Sea salt should be the only seasoning. Some of the vegetables and some salt can be broiled with the protein foods to add flavor.

This is a nutritious diet, but you must always be aware of the nutritional safety that comes from eating as wide a variety of wholesome foods as possible. Additional individual natural foods should be added experimentally one at a time every few days after the first week or so. By this time marked improvement should have been noted.

Additional protein foods, vegetables, and fruits should be added first. The last foods tried, if at all, should be milk, eggs, chocolate, individual cereal grains, citrus, coffee, tea, beef, pork, chicken, sweets, and other foods you have most frequently eaten in the past.

Factory-made foods or complex mixtures should not be used. Vitamins and other food supplements usually should be avoided until the *full* safe diet is established. If vitamins are then desired, they should be tried individually on an experimental basis to see if they cause symptoms, which many do if they contain allergenic fillers or are made from allergenic sources.

MIGRAINE IS NOT CAUSED BY CHOCOLATE ALONE

In regard to migraine, Dr. Alvarez referred to great improvement but not total elimination of migraine by avoiding one food such as chocolate. The reason for this incomplete clearing is now apparent to you, namely that migraine is usually caused by sensitivity to *many* foods and often to some nonfood antigens and nonallergic triggers as well. Total relief is not usually achieved by eliminating one food.

THE DAWNING RECOGNITION OF CEREBRAL ALLERGY

Dr. Speer's book contains chapters on inhalants, drugs, and nonallergic factors, as well as foods as causes of cerebral reactions. I would also like to quote Dr. Speer's own words from his preface:[39]

> No source of nervous complaints is more commonly overlooked than allergy. This depends on the striking similarity of many allergic manifestations to psychogenic illness. Physical evidence of allergy is often meager or absent, and symptoms may be numerous and vague. The patient himself is often painfully aware that his symptoms seem to have the earmarks of a neurosis. As a result he may complain very little. The whole story may not come out until he is assured that allergic symptoms are inclined to be multiple, diffuse, and bizarre. One may speak of such an individual as a "pseudoneurotic."
>
> That allergy may cause disorders of the nervous system is not a new discovery. Even before the term allergy was coined, physicians were aware that things that "disagree" with people may cause irritability,

fatigue, headache, and even convulsions. When allergy emerged as a distinct specialty, phenomena of this type were promptly recognized as true allergic states. An extensive literature on neurologic allergy has since accumulated.

HYPERACTIVITY, LEARNING DISABILITY, BEHAVIOR PROBLEMS

Cerebral sensitivity reactions in a child may affect different parts of the brain and result in a bewildering variety of symptoms and diagnostic labels such as attention deficit disorder, hyperactivity, hyperkinesis, learning disability, dyslexia, minimal brain dysfunction, allergic tension-fatigue syndrome, sleep disorder, impulsivity, sluggishness, childhood depression, incorrigibility, or behavior problem. Many (not all) children with such labels are really suffering from food and other sensitivities.

Moderate degrees of cerebral allergy in both children and adults may go unrecognized and unlabelled but are nevertheless negative factors in the achievement of the individual and in his enjoyment of life. Taken together, the many people who suffer poor cerebral function or cerebral malfunction make for less productive individuals, communities, and nations. Greater degrees of cerebral allergy can cause great misery and economic loss to the individual, to the family, and to society.

For simplification, we will refer in this book to all these cerebral manifestations as Attention Deficit Disorder (A.D.D.) since this is the officially chosen nomenclature of the moment. A.D.D. is not always due to sensitivity reactions, but it commonly is.

Many A.D.D. children and adults respond well to allergy-type management, especially to *food extract therapy, elimination or rotation of incriminated foods,* and *chemical avoidance.* Even *inhalant extract therapy* alone provides surprising relief in some patients with cerebral symptoms. Neutralization treatment is so rapidly effective that, in most cases, a few weeks' trial is sufficient to determine whether it is going to be fruitful or not.

This is in marked contrast to the long years of medical therapy, job retraining, and even institutional care currently required when these problems are approached entirely from the psychological or neurological point of view. The cost effectiveness achieved by simply avoiding allergenic foods or utilizing neutralization therapy can be enormous. The long-term use of Ritalin® and other palliative-stimulating drugs, with all their inadequacies, side effects, drug dependence, abuse, and cost[40] should rarely if ever be necessary when the problem is attacked from the standpoint of eliminating or neutralizing the causes.

It would be a pity for anyone who needs and can benefit from this help not to avail himself of it. If he does not, he may be doomed, possibly for life, to continue to achieve below his potential, or to remain a burden on his family and society. The earlier the treatment the better, since long-established harmful or antisocial habit patterns may be difficult or impossible to modify later, even when the allergic problems have been controlled.

It is also extremely difficult to catch up scholastically, socially, and morally when one's brain has been blocked, distracted, or distorted for years. Such a brain is unable to perceive the signals and sort out the lessons of life that should be a part of normal growth and development, and a part of the memory bank from which we later draw to make prudent judgments.

So even after successful allergy care has been achieved, a certain amount of one-on-one tutoring, social training, special schooling, and psychiatric or psychologic support may be required for a while. Too long a delay in instituting appropriate allergy care can lead to irreparable damage and much additional rehabilitational expense.

This subject is vast and cannot be covered here in complete detail. Many practical, simple, and informative books have been published on this subject.[8,41–77]

I highly recommend starting with *Allergies and the Hyperactive Child* by Dr. Doris J. Rapp (published by Sovereign Books, Simon and Schuster Building, 1230 Avenue of the Americas, New York, New York 10020, 1979) and *Can Your Child Read? Is He Hyperactive?* by Dr. William G. Crook (published by Professional Books, P.O. Box 3494, Jackson, Tennessee 38301, 1977).

I further recommend Chapter 6, "Food Allergies, Behavior and Criminality" in Dr. Alexander Schauss' book *Diet, Crime, and Delinquency* (published by Parker House, 2340 Parker Street, Berkeley, California 94704, 1980).

I have already mentioned Dr. Speer's book, *Allergy of the Nervous System* (published by Charles C Thomas, Springfield, Illinois, 1970).

The recent book by Dr. Albert Rowe, *Food Allergy: Its Manifestations and Control and the Elimination Diets* (published by Charles C Thomas, Springfield, Illinois, 1972), is an expansion of an early classic which emphasizes the value of elimination diets.

The book *Food Allergy* by Drs. Rinkel, Randolph, and Zeller (published by Charles C Thomas, Springfield, Illinois, 1951) is also a classic, and emphasizes the value of rotary diets.

The book *An Alternative Approach to Allergies* by Drs. Randolph and Moss (published by Lippincott and Crowell, New York, 1980) goes deeply into the role of chemicals as well as foods in cerebral sensitivities.

A book has recently been released entitled *Adverse Reactions to Foods* sponsored by The American Academy of Allergy and Immunology and The National Institute of Allergy and Infectious Diseases (published by The National Institute of Health, No. 84-2442, July, 1984). All of these books have additional lists of references for those who wish to dig deeper.

A DOUBLE-BLIND STUDY

The following double-blind case study illustrates the value of food extract injection therapy in a child with hyperactivity, learning disability, and behavior problems. A four-year-old white boy was presented with marked hyperactivity, restlessness, crying spells, short attention span, and insomnia.

He was a disciplinary problem in nursery school and at home, described as "nervous, cannot sit still, unusually aggressive, fighting other boys, and unable to accept normal discipline." When corrected, he flew into a rage and beat on the floor with his fists or ran out of the room screaming. He slept poorly and wandered around the house at night.

He had marked allergic shiners, frequency of urination, nightly enuresis and daily incontinence, wetting his pants frequently through the day and appearing surprised and embarrassed at doing so. In the office he was cooperative but serious, distant, and completely uncommunicative.

His hyperactivity was reportedly worsened after chicken, Kool-Aid®, and Tang®. His grandmother, father, and sister all were known to have food reactions, and his father was reportedly hyperactive also.

On his first series of twenty daily injections (Placebo) his symptom picture was unchanged.

On the second series (Active) he had complete clearing of his urinary frequency, enuresis and daytime incontinence, and his hyperactivity and shiners gradually but definitely improved.

On the third series (Placebo) his behavior deteriorated rapidly, and by the tenth day he was "as bad as ever."

On the fourth series (Active) there was moderate to marked improvement in all symptoms, particularly the hyperactivity; and he was a smiling, communicative boy at school, in the home, and in the office.

This case illustrates the effectiveness of food extract injection therapy versus placebo in the hyperactivity, learning disability, behavioral aberrations, sleep problems, and urinary dysfunctions of some food-sensitive children.

UNDUE FOCUS ON ADDITIVES HAS RETARDED PROGRESS

Excellent pediatricians, psychologists, and nutritionists have studied hyperactivity and concluded that it bears little or no correlation with the diet. However, their studies have been confined almost exclusively to the behavioral effect of artificial colors, artificial flavors, preservatives, and natural salicylates in the diet.

Additives do sometimes play a significant role, but *hyperactivity is chiefly caused by cerebral reactions to natural wholesome foods* such as milk, wheat, corn, egg, chocolate, beef, potato, chicken, soy, and peanut. Commonly eaten sweets are often troublesome. It is a shame that many eminent researchers have been focusing virtually all of their efforts and time on additives, and have essentially ignored the foods themselves.

If you give children a typical diverse and chemicalized American diet plus cookies made from wheat, milk, egg, and corn syrup, and add a small amount of artificial color or flavor to the cookies eaten by only half the children, you are not likely to see a statistically significant difference between behavior of the additive group and the nonadditive group of children. They are all eating wheat, milk, egg, and corn syrup, and possibly many other allergenic foods and chemicals as well. The extra degree of hyperactivity which might be caused in some instances by the chemical additives in the cookies eaten by half the children would get lost in the evaluation of subjective changes and in the statistical analysis of the data.

In addition, inhalant particles and inhalant chemicals play roles also, and these have not been controlled in any studies done thus far. Further, there are thousands of chemicals, as well as colors, flavors, preservatives, and natural salicylates in foods. In my experience, *natural* salicylates such as those in foods are different from aspirin (acetylsalicyclic acid) and rarely cause problems; it is the foods themselves that produce the symptoms.

The actual researchers have usually been careful to conclude that the specific additives studied and the conditions of the study simply revealed no significant behavioral differences between the study and control groups. However, some of those who quote the research articles tend to broaden this conclusion erroneously and state that "these studies show that hyperactivity is not caused by additives or by allergy."

What a surprise observers would be in for if they visited offices which employ precise neutralization testing. There they could see infants and children be made fussy, hyperactive, groggy, noisy, abusive, or intolerable with one test dose of a food or inhalant extract, and a little gentleman or lady who lies quietly or sits and looks at pictures in a magazine on a neutralizing dose of that same food or inhalant extract.

What gratification they could experience if they listened to the mothers in the examining rooms, describing how Johnnie's grades, behavior, and social adaptability have improved markedly within weeks after starting his allergy injections; and how happy his teachers, neighbors, and playmates are with his new pleasant personality.

Chapter 17

MULTI-SYSTEM DISEASE: HOW ALLERGIES CAN MAKE YOU SICK ALL OVER

Allergic reactions can produce a multitude of very puzzling symptom combinations and organ dysfunctions. Chemical mediators can be released by allergens circulating through several organs simultaneously.

Even when chemical mediators are released only locally by mast cells, they may enter the bloodstream and act at many distant shock organs as well as locally. Mediators released by basophils in the blood can reach all organs within fifteen seconds.

Mediators entering or released in the brain can indirectly affect a variety of organs, since the brain controls the entire body. So the symptoms of allergic illness can be extremely complex.

Some unfortunate patients have symptoms in one or several organ systems from hidden food and chemical sensitivities. But they have no typical "allergic" syndromes, such as hay fever, and so are not recognized as allergic patients. History, physical examination, laboratory tests, and x-rays usually fail to show the allergic causes of the symptoms.

Therefore, such patients are often considered hypochondriacs, neurotics, or weak-willed people who easily succumb to the minor emotional stresses of daily living. If such patients never get to a physician interested in hidden food allergy, they may never obtain relief.

Food allergic patients constitute many, though not all, of the so-called "functional" cases seen daily by practitioners of every specialty. They include the baggy-eyed, bloated, gassy, crampy patient. They include the anxious or frightened patient with heart palpitations, skipped heart beats, mysterious flushing sensations, and tingling which may involve only limited areas, such as the fingers or toes, or come in great waves over the entire body. They include the aching patient with muscle spasms, joint pains, finger stiffness, leg cramps, and chest pains without chest disease.

In addition, there is the tired patient who is groggy and sluggish in the mornings, falls asleep in meetings or classes, or feels compelled to take naps after lunch or supper. There is the stuffy-nosed patient with episodes of faintness, imbalance, floating sensations, or feelings of "fullness of the head."

There is also the persistent bed wetter with emotional instability or aggressiveness. There is the hyperactive child in constant motion, with accident-proneness, a tendency to break things, short attention span, inability to concentrate, learning disability, and behavior problems. Such a child may be doomed to suffer the "difficult-child syndrome," or may be allowed excessive permissiveness because despairing parents have given up trying to control him with normal love and discipline. There may be stubborn disobedience, ego-destroying criticism, child battering, rebelliousness, truancy, vandalism, increasing punishments, efforts to find escape through alcohol or drugs, and even criminality.

There is also the dreamy "out-of-it" child whose brain seems curtained off from the normal maturing sensory stimuli of childhood, who is unable to comprehend needs for or methods of appropriate social interaction, cannot adapt to his peer group, becomes cruelly teased and ridiculed, and then withdraws to a safer distance and becomes a loner. There is the child who has periodic spells of bizarre behavior, or of wandering about the house or neighborhood at night, or of banging his head against the bed or wall for hours, or of staring into space for long periods, or of inappropriately picking fights with much larger children.

There is also the constant nibbler who likes to have chocolate, hard candy, jelly beans, peanuts, citrus fruits, coffee, tea, milk, sugar, corn, wheat, or other specific foods at frequent intervals all day. There is the food addict who is considered hypoglycemic, may develop obesity, or be sick or inordinately hungry each morning until he takes his first masking "fix." There is the alcoholic who begins with an allergic addiction to whole-grain corn and gradually progresses through more rapidly absorbed, better-masking corn products until his tolerance diminishes to the point that he can no longer tolerate corn products at all, and he has to limit his drinking to wine.

There is the insomniac with restless legs who finally falls asleep and then awakens in the night with his pillow or pajama collar drenched with perspiration. There is the patient whose night itchings disturb his sleep or cause him to scratch and claw at his skin in his sleep. There is the patient who loses sleep because he must get up frequently to urinate, partly due to gas pressure from the colon on his bladder, and partly because of allergic fluid retained in his tissues from the foods eaten the previous day and finally being absorbed and excreted during the night.

These are the "weak," "psychosomatic," "hypochondriacal," "functional," or "polysymptomatic" patients. Many of them are living on vitamins, food supplements, hormones, stimulants, tranquilizers, analgesics, hypnotics, cortisones, and other medications, some of which are themselves producing or masking allergy symptoms as well as causing nonallergic side effects.

Such people may not be basically neurotic, but may simply be less able to cope with daily situations because of their allergy symptoms. These symptoms sap their energy, distract them, and keep their attention turned inward on their discomforts and puzzling sensations rather than on the world around them.

Some may become secondarily neurotic, for they note that they are "different," and cannot figure out why. They come to suspect that they are simply inadequate, and they live in constant bewilderment and fear of what kind of people they are and what is happening to them.

As they shop for relief among physicians and clinics, their self-esteem is further diminished and their anxieties magnified by the absence of a specific organic diagnosis, and by the sympathetic explanation that their symptoms are "only due to nerves." They get caught up in pharmacologic confusion by the multiplicity of medications which never end, which produce their own side effects, and which add to their feelings of weakness and dependence. They feel diminished by the unspoken signals that they are somehow less than normal people.

These unfortunates exist on symptomatic and supportive care, rather than specific therapy. They usually have descriptive, rather than etiologic, diagnoses.

Many of those who are not primarily depressed by specific cerebral sensitivity reactions or by their medications become secondarily depressed from the feeling of being hopelessly trapped. They may end up with multiple medications, surgical procedures, electroshock therapy, or prolonged psychotherapy, most of which turn out to be blind alleys since their allergy problems remain.

They may become alcoholics or drug addicts; or they may be divorced or incarcerated in mental institutions by their noncomprehending, despairing or exhausted spouses. Thoughts of suicide are readily admitted, and undoubtedly sometimes carried out.

To the physician who deals primarily with typical allergic disease—"atopic disease"—this list of "allergic" symptoms may seem strange and unfamiliar. By the current popular definition of allergy as a disease that can be demonstrated to be caused by IgE or another immunologic factor (despite the fact that our tests for such factors are extremely limited and inadequate), the type of sensitivity which produces these symptoms may not yet properly be called allergy.

But we are interested here in people, rather than semantics. The sensitivity to foods and other substances which make certain patients ill in these strange ways has been attested to for decades by many observant allergists. Some of these physicians or their loved ones were themselves sensitive in some of these ways and suffered many of the symptoms, illnesses, and feelings just described.

So we can just call them hypersensitivities, sensitivities, adverse reactions, or intolerances if we wish. The reality is simply that they exist and can usually be successfully diagnosed and treated using methods described here. These methods fit well the training, experience, expertise, equipment, personnel, and techniques of allergists and other physicians who specialize in environmental medicine.

COST EFFECTIVENESS OF NEUTRALIZATION THERAPY

It is in these patients with multisystem disease that neutralization therapy can save the greatest patient expenses. Many of these unfortunates have been requiring the services of several specialists, undergoing repeated hospitalizations, diagnostic and surgical procedures, and regular visits to psychiatrists.

Some children have had repeated psychological, neurological, vision, and hearing tests, and have had to be sent to special schools or utilize individual tutors. Lawyers' fees and judicial proceedings have been required for adolescents and adults involving vandalism, wife battering, child battering, divorce proceedings, and various criminal charges. Cerebral symptoms can result in diminished career goals, institutionalizations, and multiple other societal expenses.

Of course, all of society's ills are not related to allergy, immunology, or an altered resistance/burden ratio. But there is no doubt that some certainly are, and these can usually be prevented or greatly helped by comprehensive resistance/burden management including neutralization therapy.

Chapter 18

METHODS OF DETECTING HIDDEN FOOD SENSITIVITY:

I. THE MEDICAL HISTORY, PHYSICAL EXAMINATION, LABORATORY TESTS, AND DOUBLE-BLIND STUDIES

THE WEAKNESS OF THE HISTORY

It is sad but true that the diagnostic methods upon which most allergists depend are of little value in detecting *hidden* food allergy. The medical history may help place the patient into a descriptive diagnostic category, for example, migraine, hyperactivity, depression, aphthous stomatitis, irritable bowel syndrome, cyclic edema, adult acne, neurodermatitis, or multisystem disease. However, an *allergic* cause of these diseases is rarely suspected.

Even when certain more classic allergic diagnoses are entertained, for example, chronic urticaria or atopic eczema, standard history-taking methods are virtually helpless in delineating the specific causative allergens. Physicians do not often ask questions concerning food allergens, and if they did, few patients could give them accurate answers.

Instead, most such illnesses are considered "functional," usually meaning emotional or stress-related. Many physicians will tell you, "Fifty percent of my practice consists of functional diseases." What they do not know is that the majority of these patients are probably suffering from allergy-caused symptoms. The "stress" is often allergic stress.

Practical allergy training is sadly neglected in many medical schools and residency training programs. Many well-trained physicians are unaware of the existence and importance of hidden food allergy.

Since hidden food allergy is not often considered in diagnosis, and there are as yet no reliable laboratory tests for hidden food allergy anyway, many fine specialists tend to overlook this diagnosis. Since they recognize it so rarely, they feel it is unimportant or virtually nonexistent.

Here I would like to remind you again of the words of Dr. Walter Alvarez:[26]

> What impresses me is that still, with all of my forty years of study of food allergy, in some cases I fail to think of this disease when I should, and some brother physician has to make the diagnosis for me. This suggests that many physicians who have never been interested in food allergy must often be failing to make this diagnosis when they should do so.

THE WEAKNESS OF THE PHYSICAL EXAMINATION

The physical examination is also of little or no help in making the diagnosis of hidden food allergy. Food allergy patients often have no observable physical signs whatever, or none that would be considered significant by most physicians.

Physical signs that do sometimes occur, such as facial pallor in children, lower eyelid edema, and "shiners" (reddish or grayish discoloration of the inner angle of the lower lids near the bridge of the nose), can occur in other conditions and are not often noted as useful clues to allergic disease. Even when there is a syndrome present that is very frequently due to food allergy, such as migraine, atopic dermatitis, urticaria, irritable bowel syndrome, or hyperactivity, the physical exam offers little or no help in directing the attention of the specialist to food allergy in general or to specific causative foods.

THE WEAKNESS OF THE MEDICAL LABORATORY

The food-allergic patient can be tested by every laboratory procedure available in a fine hospital or large medical center, to no avail. I must repeat that *there are yet no reliable laboratory tests available for hidden food allergy.* So a "thorough hospital workup" is of little or no help in making this diagnosis.

However, the medical history, physical examination, and laboratory workup can exclude other diseases, and is often important for this purpose. Furthermore, the diagnosis *can* be made and relief provided by the growing number of physicians who are becoming aware of the importance of hidden food allergy and effective procedures for its management.

THE DESCRIPTIVE DIAGNOSIS SUGGESTS THE LIKELY CAUSE

How can you get some idea as to whether or not you have a food allergy problem? First, as pointed out by Drs. Bock and May and others at National Jewish Hospital in Denver, your syndromes, your descriptive diagnoses, offer clues.[78] *The name of the syndrome can tell you the probably cause of the syndrome.*

The most commonly encountered syndromes caused by food allergy have been reviewed repeatedly in this and earlier chapters (migraine, irritable bowel syndrome, and so on). If you have one of these syndromes and have been unable to find relief, you would do well to consider food allergy as a possible cause.

However, virtually all of these syndromes can also be caused by other types of stresses and other diseases, some quite serious. For example, you could have a tumor of the brain, the bowel, or other organ. If these have not already been ruled out, you should consider seeing your personal physician or appropriate specialist to do so.

CERTAIN SPECIFIC SYMPTOMS SHOULD AROUSE SUSPICION

In addition to these general *syndromes,* a second clue to the possible presence of hidden food allergy is your specific *symptoms.* Are your symptoms (or your child's) the type that one would expect to see in food allergic patients from what you have read so far in this book? Is there a complete absence of pertinent physical and laboratory findings to account for the symptoms otherwise?

One source of information concerning this is the list of symptoms enumerated by patients entering our office, induced in our office during testing with food extract injections, successfully neutralized under our observation, and then brought under control by our food extract neutralization treatment.

Some examples are headache, vertigo, or ear ringing; itching, rashes, hives, generalized swelling, or localized swellings which come and go; canker sores, throat or esophageal spasms, nausea, vomiting, abdominal pain, diarrhea, excessive gassiness or bloating; short attention span and hyperactivity; sluggishness, drowsiness, foggy-brain spells, feelings of fullness in the head and ears, depression; bizarre behavior or sudden periodic personality changes; unexplained muscle or joint pains; or allergic rhinitis or asthma that have not responded to inhalant extract immunotherapy and inhalant avoidance measures.

Most of these symptoms are simply clues. They are not necessarily caused by hidden food allergy, but should suggest allergy investigation if other causes have not been found.

KNOWN ALLERGY TO A FEW FOODS SUGGESTS HIDDEN ALLERGY TO OTHERS

Third, ask yourself what you already suspect or know about specific foods bothering you now or in the past. Did you have problems with infant formulas, cow's milk, eggs, chocolate, or other foods as a child? If you are aware that your symptoms sometimes have been induced by one or two specific foods, you may well have the tendency to hidden food allergy. In this case you could be allergic to a great many more foods which you simply have been unable to pinpoint.

You would do well to question your parents about what kind of symptoms you might have had as a small child. If you had feeding problems, breathing problems, repeated throat or ear infections, food intolerances, diarrhea, or rashes and then "outgrew" these symptoms, the same foods that gave you symptoms then may well be those which are bothering you now. They may now be causing such hidden or delayed symptoms as headache, vertigo, or depression, and there are likely to be many additional foods involved now as well.

FOOD BINGES, ADDICTIONS, OR UNUSUAL EATING HABITS

Fourth, unusual eating habits may be a clue. If you consider a food or beverage particularly delicious and eat it in occasional great binges, or alternatively eat it almost constantly and addictively, you may well be allergic to it.

If a particular food makes you feel better, or if not having it makes you feel worse in some way, you are likely to have an allergic addiction to it. You may also be addicted if you feel dependent on it, or feel that you can't live without it.

Do not exempt any food from suspicion; the ones you are sure you tolerate best may be the very ones causing the most trouble. Do not be reluctant to mention it on the assumption that you would have to give it up; neutralization can probably allow you to continue to eat it without suffering the unpleasant consequences.

PHYSICAL APPEARANCE

Fifth, take a good hard look at yourself in the mirror. Many allergic patients have chronic subnormal absorption of food nutrients from childhood, and grow up sallow, thin, or short. On the other hand, addictive eaters tend to be obese.

Patients with hidden food allergy may be bothered to an unusual degree with adolescent acne, or may experience adult acne. Many have dark lower lids (shiners), deep-set eyes, long silky lashes, bags under their eyes, allergic reddening of the inner angles of the lower lids, or fan-shaped wrinkling of the lower lids (Dennie's lines). There may be a permanent crease in the skin just above the tip of the nose from repeatedly and unconsciously rubbing or wiping it.

Are you a mouth breather? Do you have a dental overbite ("buck-teeth")? Both can be caused by chronic allergic obstruction of the nasal passages. Early allergy therapy can prevent heavy orthodontic expenses later.

Incidentally, I have noted a higher than expected incidence of severe chronic nasal obstruction, present since infancy, in patients with certain neurologic disorders, particularly multiple sclerosis. Since the carotid arteries supply the nasal tissues as well as the brain, some as-yet unknown correlation may exist between allergically leaky vessels and nasal and cerebral syndromes.

As mentioned, some patients are bloated or obese from addictive eating. Others are swollen and puffy from generalized allergic edema. Stomach rumblings or excessive gassiness may be a clue, as also may be fluctuations in weight due to eating water-retaining allergic foods. Do you look bad and feel bad all over without known cause after thorough medical investigation?

These signs are "soft," nonspecific. None of them are absolutely diagnostic of allergy, and the absence of these signs is not proof that allergy is not present. They are simply examples of clues that may be useful in increasing the suspicion that hidden food allergy may be a problem when no other answers have been forthcoming.

THINK OF WHAT LEAKY PLUMBING CAN DO

As discussed, allergic signs and symptoms are often vascular phenomena. Allergic mediators can cause constriction, dilatation, or leakage of blood vessels anywhere in the body.

Many of the diagnostic signs in the area of the eyes, nose, and face seem to reflect vascular changes in branches of the internal carotid artery, which comes up into the brain and gives off branches to the eyes and nose. The eye and nose areas are readily observable to the physician, so these signs are easily recognized.

When the vascular changes occur only in more hidden branches such as those to specific brain areas, or in the blood supply to other internal organs, there may be no visible localizing diagnostic signs whatsoever. Instead there may be behavioral, respiratory, gastrointestinal, or other symptoms, often of a nonspecific nature.

THERAPEUTIC TRIAL SUPPLIES THE FINAL ANSWER

Allergists, like other specialists, strive to be totally objective and scientific. However, this is not yet achievable in any specialty. In the field of hidden food allergy, we seek diagnostic clues assiduously, but they are only clues nevertheless. *In practice, the final answer is in your response to a therapeutic trial of neutralizing treatment, diet diaries, or meticulously performed challenge feedings, elimination diets, and rotary diets.*

Chapter 19

METHODS OF DETECTING HIDDEN FOOD SENSITIVITY: II. CONVENTIONAL SKIN TESTS AND FEEDING TESTS

It is difficult to write of a "conventional" methodology, because different conventional allergists use different methods. Even allergists who have been trained in major allergy/immunology centers do not all think or practice alike.

One training center focuses more on practical clinical allergy procedures, another on research concepts and laboratory techniques. One places great stress on asthma and allergic rhinitis; and another on immunologic disorders such as lupus, rheumatoid arthritis, immune nephritis, immuno-deficiency diseases, transplantation immunology, and tumor immunology.

Milk allergy is recognized and much discussed in a few centers, but few concern themselves much with food allergy in general. I do not know of any that recognize the broad importance or teach an effective treatment of *hidden* food allergy.

Even among those which emphasize practical clinical allergy procedures, the methodologies employed for reaching a diagnosis and carrying out therapy are variable. So the following discussion will describe long-used procedures which are considered conventional but are not necessarily used in all centers.

ENDERMAL TESTS

Although several laboratory procedures for allergy diagnosis are now under study and in clinical use, none has yet fulfilled its promise in clinical practice. Skin testing is still of major importance in establishing allergy diagnosis.

Skin tests are divided into two main categories, endermal and intradermal. Endermal procedures are more superficial. They consist of scratch, puncture, and prick tests, usually using the point of a needle or other sharp instrument to scratch, puncture, or prick the *outermost* surface of the skin.

The *scratch* test is usually performed by making a quarter-inch scratch on the surface of the skin, deep enough to break the superficial layer of epidermis but not deep enough to reach the capillaries and draw blood. The *puncture* test is performed by thrusting the point of the needle directly down like a spear at a right angle through the superficial layer of epidermis.

The *prick* test is performed with a needle puncture much like a puncture test but with the needle inclined at an angle, so that an upward flipping or pricking action as the needle is being withdrawn can unroof a bit of epidermis. This creates a slightly larger crevice than is obtained with the puncture test.

Ideally, the scratch, puncture, or prick is made through the drop of allergenic extract on the skin so that a tiny bit of the extract can be introduced into the superficial epidermis. The volume of extract introduced has been estimated as approximately a millionth of a millileter—but this could vary greatly with the method employed.

The scratch test was the first skin test method used for either inhalants or foods. Interestingly, the first physician to report the successful use of scratch tests for food allergy and to correlate a positive scratch test with food-caused symptoms was Dr. Oscar Schloss in 1912;[79] and Dr. Schloss was the teacher of my teacher, Dr. Bret Ratner.

INTERPRETATION OF ENDERMAL WHEALS

Allergists interpret endermal whealing in a variety of ways. Most base interpretation of allergen wheals on the comparison of endermally placed wheals produced by saline (the negative control) and histamine (the positive control).

One generally accepted concept is that, in order to be significantly positive, an allergen wheal must be larger than the saline control wheal and at least as large as the histamine control wheal. In other words, to be positive, an allergen must cause the release by local mast cells in the skin of at least as much histamine as is introduced by the histamine control.

Not all allergists or immunologists agree with this interpretation. Some have stated that, considering the tiny amount of allergen introduced so superficially, an allergen wheal of any size whatsoever should be considered positive, even if it is only one millimeter in diameter. Actually, a negative wheal does not rule out allergy; there are many technical and immunologic variables that can account for a negative wheal in the presence of a true allergy to the antigen being tested.

INTRADERMAL TESTS

Intradermal testing consists of producing a wheal by injecting a known volume of allergenic extract *underneath* the most superficial layer of epidermal cells with a hypodermic syringe. Interpretation is usually based on comparison of the antigen-produced wheal with a saline-produced wheal.

POSITIVE WHEALS ARE DUE TO CAPILLARY LEAKAGE

The cause of positive whealing is the fluid that flows out of the opened pores of underlying capillaries (increased capillary permeability) and forces its way up to the site of allergen deposition. The outward fluid flow from capillaries is caused by chemical mediators such as histamine, released locally by mast cells. This mediator release is due to the reaction of the injected allergen with the IgE molecules bound to mast cells lying along the capillaries beneath the test site.

IgE has been aptly described as a gatekeeper, causing the release of mediators which open the capillary gates (pores between capillary cells) to allow clear fluid laden with protective antibodies from the blood to be carried to the allergen molecules introduced into the skin. Thus the antibodies can combine with the allergen molecules and prevent them from doing harm.

VARIABILITY IN PROCEDURES

Scratch testing is the oldest of all the methods, and is still used by many practicing allergists and researchers. Recently, more have been adopting prick tests.

Some allergists use only an endermal procedure and never do intradermal tests. Some allergists and major allergy centers have never used any form of endermal testing, and use *only* intradermal tests. Some use a screening battery of endermal tests first, and then do selected intradermal tests, chiefly on suspected allergens which failed to produce positive wheals on the endermal tests.

A CLOSER LOOK AT SCRATCH TESTS

It was in 1865 that scratch testing was first used experimentally for allergy diagnosis by an English physician, Dr. Charles Harrison Blackley. Dr. Blackley suffered severely from hay fever during the grass-pollinating season.

At that time the cause of hay fever was unknown, but Dr. Blackley was ill and curious about the cause of his illness. Incidentally, many of the major discoveries in the field of allergy have been made by physicians desperately seeking help for allergic symptoms suffered by themselves or one of their loved ones.

He had heard of other hay fever sufferers who had developed local wheals after being scratched by a cat which had been walking in the grass. So he made a quarter-inch scratch on the skin of his own forearm and rubbed dry grass pollen grains into the scratch.

Within minutes a large itching wheal formed. Scratch tests with substances which did not cause his hay fever did not produce such wheals.

Blackley made many careful observations and performed many meticulous experiments over a period of fourteen years. He definitely established the value of wheal formation in the diagnosis of pollen allergy.

As is typical of new discoveries in medicine, his publications aroused much disbelief, controversy, and criticism in the medical establishment. His procedure was not generally adopted until about a half-century after his death, when it was rediscovered.

However, it was Blackley's work that initiated the still-dawning realization of *the unique value of the skin as an organ of great sensitivity, specificity, reliability, and accessibility for allergy diagnosis and treatment.* Recognition of the full value of the skin for these purposes was not achieved until the past two decades, with the development of neutralization.

FOOD WHEALS ARE DIFFERENT FROM POLLEN WHEALS

It is not generally appreciated that foods do not usually produce the same kinds of wheals as inhalants. Positive food wheals are commonly not nearly as large, red, and dramatic looking as positive pollen wheals, whether produced by endermal or intradermal testing.

In instances where scratch testing produces equivocal or slightly positive wheals, only large dramatic wheals such as 3+ or 4+ are accepted as significantly positive. Such wheals are produced chiefly by pollens.

Smaller, more blanched positive food wheals, even when present, are thus often relegated to the 1+ or equivocal category and largely ignored. The more dramatic appearance of pollen wheals is one factor that has led the field of allergy to be highly pollen-oriented and virtually blind to hidden food allergy.

UNRELIABLE CONFIRMATORY FEEDING TESTS

You may have two or three food wheals which are larger than the others, and be declared possibly allergic to these two or three foods. However, attempted confirmation of this by challenge feedings is often negative.

One reason for this is that we have only recently learned that a food *and all its derivatives* must be *meticulously* avoided for *at least four days* and then fed in large quantity at one, two, or more consecutive meals to produce even moderately reliable positive challenge feeding responses. Such precision is not yet common practice.

The symptoms which follow challenge feeding tests can go unnoticed if you are busily engaged in other activities at the time symptoms emerge. Or the symptoms may not emerge at all if you are not sufficiently instructed and cooperative in meticulously avoiding the food as a hidden ingredient in other foods during the four-day, prechallenge avoidance period.

The difficulty is compounded if you are simultaneously experiencing symptoms from other foods in your diet, or minimizing the significance of your symptoms if they are relatively moderate in degree. Also, a single large feeding may not be sufficient to bring forth the symptoms.

Further, you may have a high symptom threshold or an asymptomatic sensitivity to a food which produces a positive wheal. Thus, you may not have symptoms from it on ingestion except when eating it repeatedly or also eating one or more other allergenic foods, inhaling allergenic substances, or being exposed to nonspecific triggers or stresses. So the "confirmatory" feeding tests generally used are themselves often technically inadequate.

It is easily seen why skin tests were long considered unreliable for foods and that food allergy was considered rare and of minor importance.

It is no wonder that skin testing for foods was for a long time little employed or completely abandoned by some allergists.

It is also no wonder that double-blind studies of certain types of skin testing or provocation testing in which challenge feeding was used as a control failed to correlate completely. The challenge feeding control test itself was far from 100 percent reliable.

OTHER BLOCKS AGAINST FOOD SKIN TESTING

The mystery of food allergy diagnosis was further deepened by the fact that some allergists have rarely or never performed intradermal tests to foods. If certain *inhalant* scratch tests were negative, these inhalant allergens were usually considered for possible intradermal testing. Not so with foods.

This was because of the false notions that food allergy was only of the obvious IgE-mediated type, that it was rare and minor, and that it was largely confined to early childhood. It was also thought that if a patient was allergic to a food he would almost always know it and could describe it in the medical history, and that skin tests for foods were of virtually no value by comparison with the history. Further, there was the faulty teaching that food extract immunotherapy could not be made to work reliably anyway.

The facts are that food allergies, particularly the hidden type, are *very common,* and *much more so in adults than children.* They are often unknown to the patient and undetected by the physician, yet may have prolonged, serious, and even life-altering consequences. The intradermal neutralizing system as appropriately employed is far more effective in diagnosing and relieving both obvious and hidden type food allergy syndromes.

ALL TESTS MUST BE USED APPROPRIATELY AND JUDICIOUSLY

Neutralizing testing involves injecting only one concentration of one allergen at a time, and the concentrations are carefully chosen to fit the patient's degree of sensitivity as closely as possible. In the early history of the profession, allergists tested by *simultaneously* injecting scores of food extracts intradermally, usually all of equal strength.

Under these circumstances, moderate sensitivities to several food allergens could sometimes sum up and produce severe test reactions, turning allergists away from future use of the procedure. Also, one patient can be so exquisitely sensitive to a given food that any type of skin test for this food in this patient can be truly dangerous.

All allergists know or have read about highly fish-sensitive patients who would develop severe asthma upon entering the front door of a home in which fish was being cooked in the kitchen. We also know of egg-sensitive patients who have developed life-threatening laryngeal edema when an egg was simply cracked open in the next room.

Further, we know of peanut-sensitive patients who have had acute asthma attacks when a peanut butter jar was opened nearby, and some who have died after inadvertently eating a cookie or other food containing peanut oil or a tiny fragment of a single peanut. We also have heard tragic stories of a "friend" who "did not believe in allergy," considered it "all in the mind," and therefore secretly slipped a bit of a food into his allergic friend's meal, resulting in death.

FOODS WHICH CAUSE LIFE-THREATENING REACTIONS WHEN EATEN SHOULD NOT BE TESTED

We would certainly not consider doing skin tests or feeding tests of *any* type with a food in a patient with such a severe sensitivity to that food. Fortunately, virtually all patients with such severe sensitivities already know that they have had severe reactions, and can even pinpoint the specific food that has caused them. This is one piece of information that is almost always obtainable by a carefully taken medical history. Obviously, no one should ever be skin tested by any method for a food without first obtaining a comprehensive medical and allergy history.

The extremely rare patient who has had such a life-threatening reaction but does not know its cause should be approached with great caution. Either he should not be tested for *any* foods, or he should be tested only for foods known to be tolerated in his regular diet without life-threatening reactions, such as the foods he is living on day after day. Even patients with lesser degrees of sensitivity should be tested only with the immediate availability and judicious use of the medications, equipment, and many other safeguards for protecting and relieving patients with the potential for severe allergic reactions.

A POSSIBLE BENEFICIAL USE OF THE RAST

This is one situation where the RAST may be useful. When a severe IgE-mediated food reaction is known or suspected, a blood specimen can be drawn and the serum can be RAST-tested without exposing the patient to the allergen at all. The problem with this is that no one has yet perfected a RAST or other reliable laboratory test for many foods.

A negative RAST for a given food is no guarantee that the patient is not allergic to that food. A positive RAST has value, though it may only confirm what the patient usually already knows. However, it is useful at times for convincing him that he must meticulously avoid that food and not be skin tested for it in any way.

Also, when the causative food is not known to the patient, a RAST screen for several suspected foods may reveal the culprit. Again, a negative RAST is no guarantee.

There are technical deficiencies in RAST testing for foods. Some reactions, particularly hidden food reactions, are not mediated by IgE and therefore cannot be detected by the RAST. Much research is under way to make the RAST more suitable for non-IgE mediated food sensitivities, and additional laboratory tests are under investigation which may improve this situation.

MAJOR DISCOVERIES CONCERNING WHEAL CHARACTERISTICS

In the early 1960s, I began to note a hitherto undescribed difference between food and pollen wheals. At that time, I began taking close-up photographic slides of all the wheals produced during intradermal neutralizing testing. I repeatedly examined the wheals on the patients' arms, as well as on my thousands of photographic slides, hoping to find objective distinguishing characteristics of neutralizing wheals.

One thing I noted was that about 95 percent of the dramatically positive wheals that allergists look for were produced by pollens. I call these "red giant" positive wheals. Patients who had equal or greater symptoms from foods and from most nonpollen inhalants such as dusts and molds usually produced smaller, whiter positive wheals. These I designate as "white dwarf" positive wheals.

When wheals became very red, grew 5, 10, or 15mm in ten minutes, and possibly also had very irregular margins with large broad extensions pushing into the surrounding skin (pseudopodia), they were usually produced by pollens. Such wheals were also occasionally produced in other instances such as in severe immediate-type food or nonpollen inhalant reactions, but rarely in the hidden type food allergies that usually cause headache, stomachache, and other chronic symptoms.

Positive wheals in hidden food allergies were almost always blanched paper-white rather than red, felt harder on palpation than saline control wheals, were more raised above the surface of the skin, had regular, cliff-like, sharply demarcated borders like a circular or near-circular disc cemented to the surface of the skin, and often grew only 2mm. Yet often the test symptoms and the degree of illness caused by ingested food allergens producing these small, blanched, hard, raised, discoid wheals could be as great or greater than those produced by pollens which induced red giant wheals.

This series of repeated observations continuing over all these years has led me to an astonishing conclusion. For over three-quarters of a century we allergists, not realizing the differences between positive food and inhalant wheals, have been evaluating all wheals alike.

The large dramatic-looking pollen-type wheals have been recognized as obviously positive, while the small, blanched, hard, raised, discoid food wheals have been considered negative or equivocal and thus largely ignored. No wonder food allergy has been considered rare!

Chapter 20

METHODS OF DETECTING HIDDEN FOOD SENSITIVITY:

III. ELIMINATION AND REINTRODUCTION OF FOODS

"WHAT IS FOOD TO ONE MAY BE FIERCE POISON TO OTHERS." (LUCRETIUS—1ST CENTURY, B.C.)

The simplest and oldest method for diagnosing food allergy is to eliminate totally a food from the diet for a while, then reintroduce it and see if it causes symptoms. In some patients this can provide very important diagnostic information. Foods which cause symptoms when reintroduced can then be eliminated from the diet to provide relief.

This diagnostic system works best if you have immediate IgE-mediated food allergy, particularly if you are allergic to only one or a few foods. You can benefit from an elimination diet if you have a strong will and a high level of commitment to good health. The final burden is on you to do the diagnostic and treatment procedures properly.

However, many people have hidden, delayed, or non-IgE-mediated food allergies, and other people have both types. Hidden food allergies tend to be numerous. Almost every food in the diet would have to be avoided and reintroduced, and many foods would probably have to be eliminated from the diet. This would be an extremely difficult procedure to follow.

All this assumes that simple elimination and reintroduction would be as diagnostically effective for hidden as well as immediate food allergies. In actuality, it is not. Much more careful dietary tests are usually required for hidden food allergies.

These dietary measures, to be discussed in the next chapter, are *the precision food challenge, the general rotary diet,* and *the one-food-per-meal diagnostic rotary diet.* They are more difficult to carry out, but are capable of providing more accurate diagnosis and more effective treatment if you have hidden food allergies.

NEUTRALIZATION AND DIET THERAPY

Neutralization testing and treatment can succeed when all dietary measures fail. Furthermore, you may find that it can be far less burdensome and much more effective to take a food injection twice a week covering multiple allergenic foods than to live a life of careful grocery shopping, label reading, cooking in special ways, avoiding eating in restaurants and other social settings, then still making repeated dietary mistakes and suffering the consequences. A major dietary avoidance program requires living a restricted and sometimes harrowing life.

Neutralization therapy can take much or all of this burden off many patients. Even when neutralization therapy is not totally effective for all foods to which you may be sensitive, usually it greatly reduces the number of foods which must be eliminated from the diet. A combination of neutralization and dietary therapy may be required in some complex patients to obtain maximum relief.

ELIMINATION AND REINTRODUCTION

Elimination and reintroduction is the oldest, most natural, and most obvious method of diagnosing food intolerance in general. It can be summarized as follows: If a food bothers you, or you suspect that it may, quit eating it for a while (eliminate it) and see if you get better. If you definitely improve, leave it out of your diet.

If you are still not sure, resume eating it again (reintroduce it) and see if you get worse. Do this repeatedly until you are sure. Once you are sure, keep it out of your diet entirely or eat it only in tolerated amounts and frequencies.

Elimination diets have been used in general form since the beginning of time. For example, here is the first chapter of the Book of Daniel from *The Living Bible:*[38]

> Three years after King Jehoiakim began to rule in Judah, Babylon's King Nebuchadnezzar attacked Jerusalem with his armies, and the Lord gave him victory over Jehoiakim. When he returned to Babylon, he took along some of the sacred cups from the Temple of God, and placed them in the treasury of his god in the land of Shinar.
>
> Then he ordered Ashpenaz, who was in charge of his palace personnel, to select some of the Jewish youths brought back as captives—young men of the royal family and nobility of Judah—and to teach them the

Chaldean language and literature. "Pick strong, healthy, good-looking lads," he said; "those who have read widely in many fields, are well informed, alert and sensible, and have enough poise to look good around the palace."

The king assigned them the best of food and wine from his own kitchen during their three-year training period, planning to make them his counselors when they graduated.

Daniel, Hananiah, Misha-el, and Azariah were four of the young men chosen, all from the tribe of Judah. However, their superintendent gave them Babylonian names, as follows:

Daniel was called Belteshazzar;

Hananiah was called Shadrach;

Misha-el was called Meshach;

Azariah was called Abednego.

But Daniel made up his mind not to eat the food and wine given to them by the king. He asked the superintendent for permission to eat other things instead. Now as it happened, God had given the superintendent a special appreciation for Daniel, and sympathy for his predicament. But he was alarmed by Daniel's suggestion.

"I'm afraid you will become pale and thin compared with the other youths your age," he said, "and then the king will behead me for neglecting my responsibilities."

Daniel talked it over with the steward who was appointed by the superintendent to look after Daniel, Hananiah, Misha-el, and Azariah, and suggested a ten-day diet of only vegetables and water, then, at the end of this trial period the steward could see how they looked in comparison with the other fellows who ate the king's rich food, and decide whether or not to let them continue their diet.

The steward finally agreed to the test. Well, at the end of the ten days, Daniel and his three friends looked healthier and better nourished than the youths who had been eating the food supplied by the king! So after that the steward fed them only vegetables and water, without the rich foods and wines!

God gave these four youths great ability to learn and they soon mastered all the literature and science of the time, and God gave to Daniel special ability in understanding the meanings of dreams and visions.

When the three-year training period was completed, the superintendent brought all the young men to the king for oral exams, as he had been ordered to do. King Nebuchadnezzar had long talks with each of them, and none of them impressed him as much as Daniel, Hananiah,

> Misha-el, and Azariah. So they were put on his regular staff of advisors. And in all matters requiring information and balanced judgment, the king found these young men's advice ten times better than that of all the skilled magicians and wise astrologers in his realm.
>
> Daniel held this appointment as the king's counselor until the first year of the reign of King Cyrus.

With some refinements, an elimination diet is still in vogue as a medical procedure. Even without medical advice, a great many people are already avoiding or limiting the intake of one or more foods or beverages they have found to bother them, whether their food-caused symptoms are due to allergic mechanisms or not.

Such people who continue to experience some symptoms despite meticulous avoidance of known culprit foods should consider that additional foods may also be bothering them, and try the simple elimination/reintroduction procedure for other foods. Others who suffer one or more of the idiopathic, psychosomatic, hopeless, or intractable food-type syndromes I have described, but have never realized that foods could be causative, should also consider trying the elimination/reintroduction procedure. It could at least serve as a first step in an attempt to learn about the cause of their problems.

A POSITIVE OPTIMISTIC ATTITUDE

The first requisite for any dietary program is a mind-set, a positive attitude, a willingness to change old eating habits, and a decision to take appropriate action. You must begin with an optimistic realization that your efforts may well be rewarded in the form of better health, less discomfort, increased productivity, improved social interaction, and greater enjoyment of life.

START BY TOTALLY ELIMINATING ALL *KNOWN* ALLERGENIC FOODS

Which foods to start studying first? You may already have some hard facts concerning culprit foods. You can begin by *totally* eliminating the foods that you already *know* are bothersome to you, but which you have not yet gathered the self-discipline to eliminate entirely.

The phrase, "Oh, what the heck," may be your clue as well as your downfall. When you are confronted by a food that you usually avoid, or know that you should, and think, "Oh, what the heck," you are probably about to slip and suffer the consequences.

That pernicious phrase mentally exaggerates the anticipated pleasure of eating the food or minimizes the probable consequences. It turns against you the normal pain/pleasure principle and the defense offered by your own intelligence. So start by getting rid of the "Oh, what the heck" attitude and *always do what you know is right.* The potential long-term gain far outweighs the short-term pleasure of giving in to your whim of the moment.

Often several or many foods are creating problems, but this cannot be detected as long as you are continuing to eat foods that you know are symptom-inducing. Once you have totally eliminated known culprit foods, you are in a better position to detect the cause of any additional recurrences of symptoms. A new culprit food can thus be recognized and totally eliminated, then another, and so on.

NEXT STUDY *SUSPECTED* FOODS

Second, you can consider foods which you are not sure about but which you *suspect* bother you at times. Try to find out for sure by elimination/reintroduction; and if those foods do cause symptoms, eliminate them entirely.

You can also suspect foods which seem tolerated now but which bothered you, possibly in another way, *years ago,* even back in early childhood. A food that caused vomiting, stomachache, diarrhea, eczema, hives, or hyperactivity as a child may now be causing your headache, vertigo, adult acne, mouth ulcers, drowsiness, fatigue, depression, or joint pain.

THEN STUDY YOUR *MOST FREQUENTLY EATEN* FOODS

Third, look into the foods you eat or drink now with great *frequency,* with unusual relish, or in binges. Then, if some symptoms still persist, your *staple,* dietary items should also be studied.

It is surprising how much relief this simple procedure can provide in patients with fairly simple food problems if they employ it appropriately. Here are some examples:

Chocolate: Simply eliminating chocolate (and colas, since the cacao bean and cola nut are botanically related) has worked wonders for some patients, particularly chocoholics and colaholics. I well remember one lady in her thirties who brought her daughter to me many years ago for asthma.

I was struck by the severe adult acne of the mother, so when the child's appointment was completed, I asked the mother about her diet. It turned out that she was a flaming chocoholic, eating six to eight chocolate candy bars spaced over each day.

She would also awaken every night, hot, flushed, sweaty, weak, trembly, and nervous. She would hurry into the kitchen and quickly cook a pot of fudge. Then she would proceed to eat the entire potful, and become relaxed, contented, and drowsy, after which she could peacefully return to sleep.

I pointed out this addictive relationship to her and had her go off chocolate gradually, minimizing the withdrawal symptoms. She thus soon became completely rid of her acne.

However, as is commonly the case, she could not muster the willpower to stay away from chocolate. She repeatedly yielded to temptation, resumed nibbling, then gorging again on chocolate, with repeated florid returns of the acne.

I then tested her for chocolate and provided her with neutralizing injections for temporary use. This greatly reduced the craving and still allowed her to eat moderate amounts of chocolate without acne. Whenever she stopped her injections, the acne would quickly return.

Although the chocolate/acne connection had become apparent to her intellectually, she was very slow in accepting it emotionally. Finally, knowing she had the injections to fall back on, she gradually developed the will power to eliminate chocolate completely, which allowed her to remain free of acne with no further injections.

Of course it makes more sense to avoid a nonessential food like chocolate than to take injections for it. However, the temporary use of injections to reduce addiction and provide time to muster courage to eliminate the food and develop new eating habits is quite practical. On the other hand, in instances where the food has caused life-threatening reactions, it should not be eaten or even tested except possibly in overriding circumstances.

Milk: Eliminating milk products alone can sometimes remove a great cloud from a person's life. I was once exercising in a gymnasium when a distinguished-looking elderly gentleman exercising nearby approached me and asked, "Do you know anything about nervous diseases?" He then proceeded to tell me that he had had ten or more watery stools each day for his entire life.

Further, he said, his father, who had lived to a ripe old age, had had the same lifetime problem. Both had sought expert medical care and had attended nationally known medical clinics hoping for help. Both had been told repeatedly that the problem was nerves and business pressures, but even after retirement both still had the problem.

After a few questions about his diet, it very quickly became evident that this man was addicted to cow's milk products.

He did not drink much milk as such, but he ate cheese, ice cream, and other milk derivatives repeatedly and with great relish all day. His favorite snack, which he always kept available in his refrigerator, was celery stalks stuffed with pimento cheese. I pointed this out to him and suggested he simply avoid milk products entirely for a while and see what happened.

Two weeks later, he approached me again at the same gymnasium. He was grinning broadly. "I'm well!" he exclaimed. Simply eliminating milk products had provided total relief.

He then showed me a slip of paper on which he had written many numbers including the figure "500,000." "What is that?" I asked. He said, "That's the number of unnecessary bowel movements my father and I have had in our lifetimes simply because no one had told us to avoid milk!"

Our paths crossed again many times over the next few years, and each time he assured me with gratitude that he had watery stools only when he accidentally or deliberately tried milk products again, and that he was now avoiding milk scrupulously and remaining well. I never had an opportunity to determine if his problem was allergy or another type of milk intolerance, but from the practical standpoint it didn't matter; he was happy.

Gastrointestinal symptoms are not the only ones which can clear dramatically by simply avoiding milk products. Some patients with high blood pressure, chronic muscle and joint pains, headache, hyperactivity, skin rashes, nasal congestion, asthma, and many other organ responses have noted great benefit from milk elimination.

Of course, milk is by no means the only food of which this is true. Also, any one patient may have to eliminate more than one such food to achieve this benefit.

Cereal Grains: Elimination of cereal grains (corn, wheat, rye, oats, rice, barley, and millet) can provide similar relief in other patients, even in those whose histories provide no clue that these foods may be causing trouble. Because corn and wheat cause so many people to be depressed, hyperactive, or insomniac, or to experience bizarre sensations, behave strangely, or have severe headaches, I call these the "main brain grains."

Egg: No one food has a patent on any organ or symptom. The same symptom caused by wheat in one person may be caused by egg in another. In fact, egg is a highly allergenic food and has been a frequent cause of diminished mental activity and outright depression as well as many other symptoms in my practice. Many of my patients with severe atopic eczema have marked sensitivity to egg as well as other foods.

Factory Foods: Simply eliminating "factory foods" and living on a full range of identifiable simple, wholesome, nourishing, relatively less chemicalized foods can be very helpful to some. This does not usually require living on organic foods.

Many people can tolerate a small burden of chemical additives, and these people can choose their foods wisely from any supermarket. However most people who are extremely sensitive to chemicals are also sensitive to many simple unchemicalized foods, and their attainment of relief depends upon avoidance of chemicalized foods and some nonchemicalized natural foods as well.

ALLERGY DIETS

DIET #1: The Natural Food Basic Elimination Diet

DIET #2: The Infrequently Eaten Food Diet

DIET #3: The Rotary Diet

DIET #4: The One-Food-Per-Meal Rotary Diet

DIET #1
THE NATURAL FOOD BASIC ELIMINATION DIET

Many foods may need to be studied in some individuals. If your problem is more complex or difficult than most, and you have the proper attitude and motivation, you can begin by eliminating simultaneously *chocolate and colas, milk, egg, all cereal grains, factory foods,* and all foods *known* or *suspected* to have caused symptoms in the past.

This can be your basic diet, and you can proceed from there. If symptoms clear completely in a week or two on the basic diet, some of these eliminated foods can then be reintroduced one at a time to determine which are the real problem foods.

If symptoms do not clear completely within a week or two on the basic elimination diet, some of the foods in the *basic* diet may be causing the symptoms. You may need to eliminate some of the foods in your basic diet for a while, then reintroduce them one at a time to discover the culprits.

A logical list of possible additional culprit foods to try eliminating next would include sugar, citrus fruits, tomato, peanut, soybean, beef, pork, coffee, and tea. However, no food or beverage (or vitamin pill or medication) should be permanently excluded from study if the symptoms persist.

Be sure that your diet does not become so restricted as to cause nutritional deficiencies or undue weight loss. Again, physician guidance is recommended.

This basic elimination diet deletes most of the foods which were not major factors in man's daily diet before the agricultural revolution about 10,000 years ago. Until then, man did not know how to grow and store grains or other crops, domesticate animals, obtain and store animal milks in large quantities, or manufacture synthetic foods and chemicals. Over eons of time, browsing man survived on—and adapted to—relatively simple, natural foods such as vegetables, fruits, berries, and nuts, as well as fish, fowl, and meats.

So this approximates man's "natural" diet. It can be thought of as the Garden of Eden Diet, that is, the diet of browsing, fishing, and hunting man that exemplified the preagricultural era. Although such a diet is not easy to follow in this day of restaurant eating, travel, manufactured foods, and impulse-shopping, it is nourishing and sustaining, and can be very helpful for patients who cannot tolerate the full variety of nutrients and additives on today's supermarket shelves.

Many nutrition-conscious people use similar diets by choice. However, there are many strange and not necessarily optimal diets in use today, and the supervision of a knowledgeable physician rather than a faddist is recommended.

Not all ingredients in processed foods are listed on the labels. Therefore, *most foods which pass through a factory between the farmer and the grocer must be avoided* by some people.

Common exceptions are *simple* agricultural products such as fresh, frozen, or canned stringbeans, carrots, etc. These almost certainly contain minute traces of chemicals, pesticides, herbicides, and other chemicals.

However, this minute degree of chemical contamination has been tolerated by most individuals, so far as we can determine to this point. There are definitely some patients who cannot tolerate even these small quantities of chemicals, and these patients must obtain organic foods, as discussed in the next two chapters.

DIET #2
THE INFREQUENTLY EATEN FOOD DIET

Another type of elimination diet consists of living on only a very few foods until symptoms disappear; then reintroducing one new food at a time in simple, relatively unchemicalized form to observe its effects. By simple form, I mean plain broiled pork chops, for example, rather than factory-altered pork products such as bacon, ham, or pork sausage.

In quoting Dr. Alvarez' foreword to Dr. Speer's book (Chapter 16), I mentioned his elimination diet which included only lamb, oats, rice, butter, sugar, and canned pears. Diets of this type were developed by an astute allergist, Dr. Albert H. Rowe of San Francisco, one of the early pioneers in food allergy management.

Since then, manufacturing processes and dietary habits have changed and we have also learned a great deal more about hidden and allergenic foods. Some of these foods are too frequently eaten and therefore more likely to be allergenic in the modern diet. Further, this diet may be too restricted to follow for the length of time necessary for some people to respond.

Foods which were never or rarely eaten by a given individual may be tolerated better than those which were past dietary staples. Some excellent foods not often found in the average Western diet are available.

These foods can usually be obtained from diet or gourmet sections in the local supermarkets, from health food stores, from home gardens and farms, from sport fishermen and hunters, and from specialized food shippers. A larger group of foods chosen carefully from a list of less frequently eaten, less frequently allergenic foods for the individual with hidden food allergies would be more suitable and more easily adhered to.

For example, I might allow a patient to choose a moderate number of selected foods for his baseline diet from the following list of infrequently eaten foods: lamb, turkey, duckling, local fish such as blue-fish or ling, crayfish, Alaskan King crab, lobster (Maine, Florida, South African, etc.), artichoke hearts, asparagus, avocado, beets, Brussels sprouts, carrots, cauliflower, eggplant, endive, kale, leek, okra, shallot, watercress, rutabaga, Chinese cabbage, sweet potato, American yam, fresh peeled pears, fresh peeled apricots, figs, dates, black olives canned in ferrous gluconate, safflower oil, and plain sea salt (sparingly). In addition, if obtainable, the following foods could be added: venison; squirrel; rabbit; quail; goose; goat; blackberry; kumquats; mango; papaya; persimmon; quince; certain raw nuts (for example, almond, Brazil, chestnut, hazelnut, walnut, pecan); flours and meals made from a variety of substances such as sunflower seed meal, pumpkin seed meal, lima bean flour, cassava meal, and poi; and other foods to which an individual patient has never or rarely been exposed.

If chemical sensitivity is suspected, these foods should be obtained in the least chemically contaminated forms possible. If you have been eating any one of these foods frequently it should be omitted or replaced by an infrequently eaten food.

If any food on this list has been eaten frequently or is suspected to have caused symptoms in the past, it should not be included in the diet. This list is large enough that if many of these foods must be deleted or are not obtainable in a given locale, there are still enough obtainable foods to live on for a short test period.

An "infrequently-eaten-food diet" of this type and breadth is adequately nourishing and easily sustainable for a few weeks. During these weeks, any of these foods which are noted to cause symptoms should be deleted. As soon as this diet is established as safe, new foods should be introduced on a trial basis.

The foods to be introduced first can be high protein foods such as various species of fresh or frozen infrequently eaten scale fish if previously eaten without known symptoms. Next could come raw and lightly cooked less frequently eaten vegetables, then fruits.

I have found that if allergy to fish or nuts is present, it is usually immediate and known to the patient. However, if the addition of any of these foods induces symptoms, it must be deleted.

Symptoms are usually much easier to correlate with the causative food when *only one food at a time* is added back to the diet in this manner. In general, legumes (peas and beans) are introduced late rather than early.

Peanut is a legume rather than a true nut, and is sometimes severely allergenic, so it may be omitted entirely. Mustard and cottonseed oil may also be omitted for the same reason. Of course, none of these foods should be reintroduced if they have ever been suspected of causing major symptoms.

PRECAUTIONS

Since any food can be allergenic, there is no such thing as a universally effective nonallergenic diet. You cannot theorize about "good" foods and "bad" ones; you have to go out into the real world and get the facts.

These facts can be garnered by past history, dietary manipulations, and neutralization testing and treatment with food extracts. If dietary manipulations are tried, they should be planned by and for each individual according to his own needs and problems.

Markedly restricted diets must be used only briefly. Everyone who uses elimination diets must be conscious of the need to try adding quickly to the diet a wide variety of foods that provide important nutrients such as essential amino acids, vitamins, minerals, fiber, polyunsaturated oils, essential fatty acids, and adequate calories. The diets described here are safe diets, and in fact are far more natural and healthful than the commonly utilized "eat whatever you like" diet.

These elimination diets delete most of the worst foods and retain or quickly reintroduce most of the best. They should emphasize a wide variety of vegetables, salads, fruits, fish, and poultry. They delete or minimize junk foods; refined sugars; salt; spices; cereal grains; empty calories; chemical food additives; and foods containing much saturated fat and cholesterol such as egg, butter, cream, beef, and pork.

With minor modifications, these diets could be prescribed for general good health as well as for a variety of illnesses such as obesity, diabetes, hypoglycemia, hypertension, and many cardiovascular problems. Since these diets eliminate all bakery products and junk foods—and many sweet, starchy, salty, and spicy foods—weight loss is common. Some of this loss is simply fluid loss, and some may be real fat-tissue loss.

FLUID LOSS

Cooks and homemakers know that starches such as cereals absorb water. When they add water or milk in increments to wheat flour, corn starch, or even mashed potatoes, the liquid tends to be absorbed and disappear into the thick semisolid starch mass; and then more liquid can be melded into the mass repeatedly.

The same principle applies to fluid retention in the intestines, circulation, and tissues. Sweet, starchy, salty, and spicy foods are water-retaining by nature. Eating them makes you thirsty; some of the water or other beverage you drink is held in the gastrointestinal tract, blood, and tissues and is often registered on your discomfort scale as well as your weight scale and blood pressure reading. In addition, the increased capillary permeability and subclinical edema so typical of chronic food allergy further increases the burden of retained body fluid.

Thus there are two reasons why, when you omit these foods from your diet, you may eliminate a great deal of fluid through your kidneys for a few days and thus reduce the reading on your weight scale. The decrease in empty calories and reduction of food cravings which often accompany this diet may reduce true obesity as well.

WEIGHT CONTROL

Many underweight people try to maintain their weight by eating favorite, high-calorie, or high fat-containing foods frequently. This is not a healthful diet. Reaching for these foods can become an ingrained repetitive habit.

When they go on a more sensible and varied diet, they may lose weight rapidly at first and become alarmed. My experience is that they only lose weight temporarily, quickly reaching a new plateau of steady weight maintenance with improved health, nutrition, and well-being. Of course they should be closely monitored by a physician during this period.

On the other hand, underweight patients can choose to reintroduce some high calorie foods early in the sequence. White potato, sweet potato, and other high carbohydrate-containing vegetables and fruits can be used for this purpose.

The first cereal grain to be reintroduced on a trial basis can be rice, since it is sometimes tolerated by people who cannot tolerate other cereal grains. If tolerated, rice can be eaten with a tolerated fruit or honey. Rice flour can be used as a batter for fried foods, and can now also be purchased in the form of crackers, cookies, rolls, and loaf bread. Millet cereal and millet bread are also available, and are often well tolerated.

PHYSICIAN SUPERVISION

Diets should be prescribed and fine-tuned by physicians for individual patients with various illnesses. Furthermore, diets alone should not always be relied upon as a complete treatment for such illnesses, and physician supervision of the entire treatment as well as the diet is imperative.

Withdrawal symptoms may occur, usually for about one to three days, from the eliminated foods. Therefore you may get temporarily worse before you get better. This is a good sign that you are food-sensitive and therefore will probably benefit by sticking to the program.

If any of your past symptoms have been the least bit severe, you should enter into this diet with a physician's knowledge, concurrence, and close supervision. You may also need some protective medications to keep on hand. If *your* physician forbids the reintroduction of certain foods or of the entire program, his decision must be final.

CONTINUE OBSERVING, RECORDING, AND ANALYZING YOUR RESPONSES

After about five to seven days or possibly two weeks on a restricted diet, withdrawal symptoms should be well behind you and you should be experiencing much improvement. If not, perhaps foods are not your problem, or not your only problem. Or maybe you are not following your diet meticulously, or you are slipping up on hidden ingredients. Possibly one or more of the foods in your restricted diet are causing your symptoms and should be eliminated for four or five days and reintroduced on a trial basis.

After your tolerated food list is longer, note whether or not you are completely free of symptoms. If not, perhaps you should consider living largely or entirely on the newly reintroduced foods (which you have already proved to be safe) for a brief period while you eliminate/reintroduce each of the foods in your basic diet one at a time.

If you do note marked sustained improvement, that is the time for reintroducing a new food to broaden your diet. If no symptoms arise within forty-eight hours, another new food can be reintroduced.

If symptoms do occur from any reintroduced food, no new food should be reintroduced until these symptoms have been completely clear for twenty-four hours. If a limited diet is chosen as a starting diet, the first foods reintroduced should be the ones *least* likely to cause symptoms, although they may not be the tastiest ones, so that a broader diet of tolerated foods can be attained as rapidly as possible.

Table 20-1 is a list of relatively less frequently eaten or less frequently hidden or allergenic foods. Table 20-2 is a list of more frequently eaten or more frequently hidden or allergenic foods.

Neither list is sacred; you and your physician must carefully choose which foods to include in your beginning elimination diet, which to reintroduce, and the optimal order in which to reintroduce them.

EXQUISITELY SENSITIVE PATIENTS CAN *NEVER* RELAX THEIR GUARDS

Another precaution concerns foods known or even suspected to have caused very severe or life-threatening reactions. These should be handled by elimination alone and *not* reintroduced, since reintroduction could be dangerous.

Amazingly, many people who are intelligent, mature, and fully aware of the danger of eating such a food will eventually or even repeatedly relax their guards and eat it inadvertently. Some may even try it again deliberately in the hope that this time they will not suffer the usual severe consequences. Sadly, even those who maintain maximum precautions are sometimes tripped up by the presence of a culprit food or additive as a hidden ingredient in another food.[80]

So if you are one of these rare, exquisitely sensitive people, your first mental set must be that *you must be absolutely unforgiving to yourself concerning total and permanent elimination of potentially dangerous foods.* Second, you might consider reading and studying to keep up with ever-changing agricultural processes; food manufacturing technology; and food storage, distribution, and merchandising practices.

You may have to avoid restaurant eating entirely. You may have to carry your own food with you, possibly at times in a portable cooler, so that you will never have to gamble on the possibility of your life-

TABLE 20-1
LESS FREQUENTLY EATEN AND LESS FREQUENTLY HIDDEN FOODS

lamb	artichoke hearts	kale
turkey	asparagus	leek
duckling	Brussels sprouts	shallot
blue-fish	avocado	watercress
ling	beets	rutabaga
crayfish	carrots	Chinese cabbage
Alaskan king crab	cauliflower	sweet potato
lobster	eggplant	American yam
	endive	
	okra	
venison	sunflower seed meal	black olives in ferrous gluconate
squirrel	pumpkin seed meal	safflower oil
rabbit	lima bean flour	plain sea salt
quail	cassava meal	fresh peeled pears
goose	poi	fresh peeled apricots
goat		figs
		dates
blackberry	raw nuts:	
kumquat	almond	
mango	Brazil	
papaya	chestnut	
persimmon	hazelnut	
quince	walnut	
	pecan	

TABLE 20-2
MORE FREQUENTLY EATEN AND MORE FREQUENTLY HIDDEN FOODS

milk	beef	lettuce	coffee
egg	pork	celery	tea
corn	chicken	green pea	cinnamon
wheat	potato	stringbean	mustard
malt	tomato	orange	garlic
oat	onion	lemon	peanut
rice	baker's yeast	apple	soy
cane sugar	brewer's yeast	grape	black pepper
beet sugar	honey	banana	chocolate

threatening culprit food or additive turning up as a hidden ingredient in foods prepared by others. If all else fails, it is better to suffer temporary hunger than reach for a food which might cause a severe reaction.

If you have had severe allergic reactions but have no clue as to the cause, or if you have an illness in a major organ which might be adversely affected by an unexpected severe food reaction, physician approval and close physician guidance are mandatory before you even consider the elimination/reintroduction procedure. In any event, your guiding principle must be this: *"If you are not absolutely sure, do not eat it."*

CHAPTER 21

METHODS OF DETECTING HIDDEN FOOD SENSITIVITY:
IV. PRECISION FOOD CHALLENGES AND ROTARY DIETS

> To many this has been the commencement of a serious disease, when they have merely taken twice in a day the same food which they have been in the custom of taking once. . . .
> If a patient fast for the first two or three days, and take food of a heavy nature on the fourth or fifth, he will be much injured, but that the mistake will be still more fatal if the fast be continued for the first four or five days, and if he then indulge freely in food at the end of these.
> (HIPPOCRATES – 460–377 B.C.)[36]

FIXED AND CYCLIC FOOD ALLERGY

For years there has been the mistaken notion that if you are really allergic to a food, you will have a reaction to it every time you eat it. If you do not, particularly when it has been introduced into your diet without your knowledge (so the belief goes), then it is all in your head.

A reaction with every exposure occurs in only a small fraction, perhaps 10 percent, of food allergies. When this situation exists, the food allergy is said to be "fixed," that is, permanent. Even if the food is totally eliminated for years, a fixed food allergen will still cause a reaction when eaten again. This type of food allergy was until recently considered the *only* type.

We now know that the vast majority of food allergies are dynamic, that is, changeable. The tendency to react can come and go rapidly over brief periods of time.

For example, a patient can often tolerate a food when it is eaten at only one meal every four days, but not when it is eaten more frequently. This is termed "cyclic" food allergy. For a given food, the tendency to react cycles up and down, often at intervals of about four days.

The four-day avoidance period provides time for the first portion of the food to be completely or nearly completely emptied from the digestive tract and bloodstream. Then the absorption of the second bolus does not push an already existing high blood level from the first bolus up into the symptom-causing range. In rare instances, the cycle may be seven days or longer, particularly for cereal grains and chemical additives.

Most hidden food allergies are of the cyclic type. Now that we are aware of hidden and cyclic food allergies, our concepts are better attuned to helping more of our patients.

The elimination diets discussed in Chapter 20 are useful for many people. However, if cyclic food allergies are present, a more precise dietary procedure may be utilized for accurate and effective diagnosis and treatment. This procedure, adapted to the dynamic nature of cyclic food allergy, consists of *precision food challenges* and a four-day *rotary diet.*[81]

PRECISION FOOD CHALLENGE

A precision food challenge begins with meticulously and totally eliminating for four days *all traces and derivatives* of a specific food to be tested. If the food has never caused severe or life-threatening symptoms, a large quantity of the food is then eaten at a single meal in a *simple,* preferably rapidly absorbed form, about two hours after breakfast on the morning of the fifth day.

One reason for waiting two hours after breakfast before eating the test food is to minimize confusion from immediate reactions to breakfast foods occurring within two hours or so after breakfast. A second reason is to minimize confusion with delayed reactions occurring immediately after breakfast from foods eaten the day before and being reabsorbed after breakfast. If the challenged food is truly allergenic and *no* symptoms arise after this *single* feeding, this indicates that you can probably eat it without symptoms at *one* meal every *four* days, even though you may be cyclically sensitive to it.

However, the *absence* of a reaction after this single feeding does not prove that the food is either allergenic or nonallergenic. The blood level may simply not have reached a symptom-causing level from a single feeding. To obtain that information, a second feeding must be taken about two hours after the first. When cyclic food allergy is present, the symptoms commonly emerge after this *second* feeding.

This illustrates the dynamic effect of two closely spaced feedings. The first feeding presumably elevates the blood allergen, mediator level, or mast cell reaction-tendency to a degree, but not quite sufficiently to reach the symptom threshold.

However, the first feeding seems to prime or prepare the body. The second feeding taken two hours after the first one results in sufficient additional allergen, mediator release, or mast cell reaction-tendency to exceed the symptom threshold, induce symptoms, and make the diagnosis.

FREQUENCY OF INGESTION DETERMINES EMERGENCE OF SYMPTOMS

In this instance, the patient has not reacted to an "unusual" food, but to a "usual" food eaten at two closely spaced feedings. Thus, variation in frequency of ingestion explains how a food can cause symptoms at some times but not at others.

In some instances, surpassing the symptom threshold requires more than two feedings. If by the next day no immediate or delayed symptoms have occurred, the food can be continued three times a day for at least three consecutive days while checking for onset of symptoms.

In rare instances, symptoms have not surfaced until the food has been eaten repetitively for two or three weeks. However, as soon as mild symptoms are noted, the trial should be discontinued; further feedings could worsen the symptoms unnecessarily.

Failure to react to one or two feedings of an allergenic food is more common if the prechallenge abstinence period has been too long. If the food has been avoided for two weeks or longer before being challenged, a degree of tolerance can begin to build which requires multiple frequent feedings to reach the symptom threshold. It is sometimes necessary to eat the food one to three times just *before* the four-day prechallenge avoidance period to nullify this tolerance effect.

Emptying the gastrointestinal tract with magnesium citrate solution, Epsom salts (magnesium sulfate), unflavored milk of magnesia, or another tolerated rapidly acting laxative before beginning the avoidance period enables one to eliminate previously eaten foods from the digestive tract. This can help detect if the challenged foods are the causes of symptoms.

If no laxative can be tolerated, cleansing enemas can help. However, neither laxatives nor enemas should be used excessively or chronically.

HOW TO CHALLENGE A FOOD

While undergoing precision food challenges, you should live on a stable diet of your regularly eaten, simplest, most identifiable, most nutritious, and best-tolerated foods. This often improves results by reducing confusing intercurrent reactions due to hidden food ingredients and food additives.

Ambulatory patients eating self-chosen meals, particularly at work, at school, or in restaurants, often find it difficult or impossible to carry out these required dietary restrictions. It is also difficult to properly note and record moderate symptoms occurring at work, at school, at play, or in the midst of other activities.

Further, the reaction, even if it is of the so-called acute, obvious, "immediate," presumably IgE-mediated type, may occur several hours or a day later than expected. So here is how you should probably do it most conveniently and effectively:

Take the laxative Sunday night, avoid the food Monday through Friday, do the ingestion challenge on Saturday, and remain quietly at home Saturday and Sunday to note immediate or delayed symptoms.

BINGE EFFECTS

It is not at all unusual for a person to binge on a given nonallergenic food at many consecutive feedings and then become severely and chronically allergic to it for the first time in his life. I have seen this occur in patients when fresh, ripe, homegrown tomatoes and other vegetables and fruits became available in the summer; and when large quantities of chocolate candy, fresh oranges, figs, nuts, and other foods were received as gifts.

Binges of this type can not only create sensitivity to the food being eaten repetitively but may seriously impair the immune system in certain patients. This may initiate a prolonged, even life-long tendency to become extremely sensitive to a great many other foods and to other substances as well.

Prolonged generalized sensitivity can also be initiated by other factors. These include virus infections, chemical exposures, and hormonal changes including puberty and postpregnancy.

There may well come a time when this cyclic phenomenon is sufficiently well recognized that a degree of diet simplification and rotation will be recommended for large populations, or at least for people with personal or family histories of allergy syndromes. It might be worthwhile meantime to study changes in population behavior in mental institutions, penitentiaries, hospitals, nursing homes, and even school cafeterias. Dieticians can simply design wholesome tasteful meals for a four-day rotation in a manner that the population involved is well satisfied without even being aware of the rotation of the foods they are served.

There may also come a time, hopefully, when a laboratory test or other parameter can predict which specific people are at risk. Then at least these can be advised to avoid a repetitive eating pattern as well as to eliminate complex and chemicalized foods.

CHALLENGE PRECAUTIONS

Challenge feedings are well suited for patients with moderate symptoms, such as itching, headache, stomachache, muscle-joint pains, reasonable degrees of hyperactivity, and other such nonlife-threatening symptoms. They may *not* be suitable, especially for home use, in patients with a tendency to anaphylaxis, laryngeal edema, severe attacks of asthma, tongue or throat swellings, epilepsy, heart disease, and other such potentially serious conditions.

If you have *ever* had such symptoms or other severe reactions of a life-threatening degree, *challenge feedings could be dangerous.* Do not undertake challenge feedings without first consulting a physician experienced in food allergy management.

Great judgment must be exercised as to whether or not to challenge a specific food, to challenge any foods at all, to do the challenges in a hospital setting, and so on. You must be aware that food reactions can be extremely and unpredictably severe, and that avoiding such reactions is far more preferable than treating them.

If the *physician* judges that challenge feedings should be used in an extremely sensitive patient, he may decide to modify the procedure for safety. He may prescribe a very tiny feeding of the suspected food on the morning of the first challenge day.

Ideally such a patient should spend hours or the entire day in the office or some other relatively safe area where he can be closely observed and treated if necessary. The symptoms can be severe, and may not occur until many hours after the feeding, possibly in the middle of the night. In some instances, overnight stay in the hospital may be desirable.

A comprehensive emergency kit can be supplied in the event that a reaction should occur at home. You can be instructed carefully in the use of the kit, which would probably include some form of injectable epinephrine (Adrenalin®) as well as other oral or injectable antiallergy medications.

If possible, a spouse, relative, or friend should be instructed in the use of the kit also, and should spend the evening with you. In the event of a severe reaction you can use your emergency medications immediately, inform your physician, and go directly to the emergency room of a hospital in case further treatment is needed.

After the first challenge feeding, if no symptoms occur in the next day or two, your physician may instruct you to try a slightly larger portion of the food four days later, and so on. Even so, there are some patients so sensitive to a given food that even this careful test system *should not be utilized* for that food.

These patients must rely solely on strict and total *avoidance* of that food, with the backup of the emergency kit for *unintended or accidental* exposures. Hopefully, effective preventive medications for life-long use will become available to minimize the risk of such exposures.

PROMPT RELIEF OF FOOD REACTIONS

Whenever an ordinary food-caused symptom occurs, the symptom will often subside more quickly if you take a heaping teaspoonful of bicarbonate of soda in a glass of ice water, followed by another glass or two of water. Continuing intake of water helps clear the allergen out of the bloodstream through the kidneys. The elimination of the food from the body can be accelerated by deliberate induction of vomiting, the use of enemas, the administration of a laxative, or combinations of these.

Vomiting is by far the most rapid method for acute symptoms following shortly after ingestion of the allergenic food. Bicarbonate in *warm* water may help induce vomiting. Syrup of Ipecac will usually induce vomiting within 30 minutes.

Incidentally, patients with chronic grogginess or depression are often pleasantly surprised at how rapidly their minds clear when a laxative takes effect, signaling that their problem may be more allergenic than psychiatric. The same thing is true to some extent with cleansing enemas.

However, none of these measures should be relied upon alone by patients with potentially severe reactions. A tendency to acute severe reactions of any type requires advance arrangement for physician involvement.

DIET #3
THE ROTARY DIET

As mentioned, if you have had severe allergic reactions, or even if you have had some nonallergic complicating or debilitating illness such as cardiovascular disease or convulsions, you should exercise caution concerning whether or not to use feeding challenges. In such situations, *challenge feedings can be omitted* and a rotary diet entered into directly *without challenges* to reduce allergic symptoms for treatment rather than temporarily exacerbate them with challenges for diagnosis.

In this instance, you should simply omit "factory foods" and mixtures and live on a rotary diet of the less frequently allergenic foods in recognizable simple form (Appendix I). You should not eat any given food more often than at one *meal* every four days. To reduce withdrawal symptoms and get used to the rotary system, *one-day,* then *two-day* rotations can be used for the first few rotations.

After a few symptom-free four-day rotations you should then add, one at a time, additional simple foods which you wish to reintroduce into your diet, eating each at only one meal every four days. You should save for last the ones you have eaten most frequently or suspect have ever caused mild symptoms, and entirely omit those suspected of ever having caused severe symptoms.

When using a rotary diet without preliminary food challenges, the first meal of a new food should be very small in patients with histories of severe food reactions or vital organ involvements. If the first meal is tolerated, the food can be eaten four days later in larger quantity.

In such sensitive patients, it may require several four-day rotations to fully prove the ability to tolerate a single food. The idea is to carefully and gradually build a rotary diet of symptom-negative foods on which to live, avoiding challenge symptoms as much as possible.

The four-day rotary diet serves three purposes:

(1) It *eliminates symptoms* from the foods which can be tolerated when eaten once every four days but not when eaten more frequently (your "cyclic" foods).

(2) It helps in the *identification* of fixed food allergens, consisting of the foods which induce symptoms even when eaten only once in four days, and which must therefore be eliminated entirely.
(3) It enables you to *continue* tolerating most of the currently tolerated foods presently in your diet, since, over time, people with food allergies tend to become sensitive more readily to foods eaten more frequently.

For example, if you simply omit milk, chocolate, and cola drinks, you might start drinking more orange juice, grape juice, tea, or coffee instead. Then you may develop new allergies to these previously tolerated beverages and foods through sheer frequency of ingestion. You then must avoid these foods to which you have developed new allergies, so you may tend to eat some of the remaining foods more frequently and develop still more allergies.

In this way, you may rapidly become sensitive to virtually all of the foods in your normal diet. Since the development of new food allergies is much less common when foods are repeated only at intervals of four or more days, you can usually preserve most of your remaining food tolerances by following a diet in which you eat any one food at only one meal every four days.

For example, if beef is eaten at dinner on Monday, it should not be eaten again (as hamburger, roast, steak, gravy, soup, or in any other form) until dinner on Friday. If chicken is eaten at dinner on Tuesday, it should not be eaten again in any form (such as in chicken soup or salad) until dinner on Saturday. If pork is eaten at dinner on Wednesday, it too should not be eaten again in any form (for example, ham, bacon, sausage, nonvegetable shortening, gelatin desserts, and other pork-containing products) until dinner on Sunday. Similarly, turkey can be eaten on Thursday, and not repeated until Monday, and so on.

In the rotary diet, you must take into account the presence of one food as a hidden ingredient of other foods, the multiple forms and derivatives of foods, and the presence of chemical food additives. This is why prepared mixtures and factory foods must be eliminated in order to achieve relief through diet rotation.

AIDS TO ROTARY DIETS

The home freezer is a great aid to those on rotary diets since large amounts of a food can be prepared at one time, for example, on a Saturday, and the leftovers stored frozen in multiple meal-size por-

SOME AIDS TO ALLERGY DIETS

1. Home Freezer
2. Food Grinder
3. Special Cooking Utensils
4. Diet Diary
5. Food Ledger
6. Label Reading
7. Source Lists of Special Foods
8. Avoidance of Alcohol, Caffeine, Chemicals, Spices, and Mixtures with Unknown Ingredients

tions. One such portion can be thawed and eaten every four days.

Thus the freezer shelves can serve like supermarket shelves from which the precooked foods can be selected for each meal. The shelves can even be numbered: Shelf #1 is for Diet Day #1, and so on. The packages can be color coded or labelled so that you can make suitable choices. Or an entire meal can be stored in one container (like a home-made T.V. dinner) and thawed in the oven or microwave.

Rotary diets cannot be followed casually. They must be committed to paper. Meals must be planned, written out, and shopped for in advance. Three or four meals a day for four days requires twelve or sixteen menus to be constructed. The same meals can be used again the following four days, with planned variations.

One planned variation consists of omitting a food which caused symptoms or aroused suspicion on the preceding four days. Another planned variation consists of adding a new, hopefully tolerated, food from time to time. This provides for the final "fine-tuning" of the diet.

Rotation can be done successfully, but requires constant label reading, careful shopping and cooking, no or very cautious eating in restaurants, and regular note-keeping. Surprisingly, some patients prefer a seven-day rotation so that they know exactly which foods they will eat each Monday, etc. They feel that this simplifies their diet and their note-keeping, and they generally do quite well.

Fortunately, a rotary diet is necessary only for the patient who has multiple severe sensitivities. *The need for it can usually be greatly reduced or entirely eliminated by food extract injection therapy.*

FOOD FAMILIES

Some knowledge of food families (Appendix II) is often helpful in the management of food allergy in some broadly sensitive people. If you are sensitive to one member of a food family, you may be sensitive to another member of the same family, although this is by no means always true.

For example, cross-reactivity may exist within the grass family (Graminneae), which includes cereals, sugar cane, sorghum, bamboo sprouts, bamboo shoots, and Chinese water chestnuts. Patients sensitive to an edible member of the grass family, such as wheat, may react to wheat as a food or to wheat flour in inhaled particulate form, as in "baker's asthma."

They also may react to inhaled cooking odors of this and related foods, and to related grass pollens. Patients with cereal sensitivity may have grass hay fever, and they may note increased symptoms from grain ingestion during grass season.

It is for this reason that it is sometimes necessary to rotate an entire family so that only one member of the food family is taken every four days. The rotation of entire families is not usually necessary, and it is often possible to eat one member of a food family every two days, or even daily, so long as no *individual* food is eaten more often than once every four days.

Every food family containing foods considered to be acceptable, nutritious, and reasonably obtainable has been listed in the rotary diet charts (Appendix I). Each food family has been enclosed in a *box* in the charts. The *underlined* foods are those to be omitted in the natural-food basic elimination diet (which eliminates chocolate, colas, milk, egg, cereal grains, factory foods, and foods known or suspected to have caused symptoms in the past).

Additional foods which can complicate the rotary diet in the beginning, such as spices and caffeine-containing foods, are also *underlined* as a reminder to omit them until the diet has been well established. Each box in the four-day rotary diet contains the common edible members of one family; no family is repeated in the entire four-day diet list. Milk and chocolate have been excluded from all four days of the rotary diet, but may be reintroduced later on a trial basis when the four-day rotation and freedom from symptoms have been achieved.

Food family classifications (Appendix II) have been listed alphabetically and assigned numbers. These numbers correspond to the numbers of the family boxes on the rotary diet charts (Appendix I) and to the numbers of the individual simple foods (Appendix III). This will allow you to easily identify the family name of any given food. However, it is not necessary to know the names of the food families to follow the rotary diet charts.

Food families may play no role in your illness. You may simply be allergic to a great many foods, and it is inevitable that some of these foods just accidentally happen to belong in the same family. So, although I think the importance of food families has sometimes been overemphasized, I have included this information simply for your awareness of the possibility.

MAINTAINING GOOD NUTRITION

As mentioned, high protein-containing foods are available every day. Fish is an excellent source of protein and one or more species may be eaten daily, as long as fish from any one fish *family* is not eaten more frequently than once every four days. Later, family rotation can usually be dropped, and a given family can be used daily as long as any one *species* from that family is still used only at four-day intervals.

Some people simply cannot manage a four-day rotation. In these instances, a two-day rotation may be achievable and can often reduce symptoms considerably. The diet can sometimes also be made easier without penalty by totally ignoring food families and simply rotating foods individually.

The goal is to seek the most convenient way to keep the total body burden down to the lowest possible level consistent with good nutrition, minimal symptoms, and maximum safety. A great deal of thoughtful trial and self-observation may be required to suit your food intake to your personal needs.

VITAMINS AND MINERALS

Most commercial vitamin and mineral preparations are better avoided at first because of the substances from which they are made, the chemical residues of processing, and the excipients and fillers in the finished products. Side effects from commercial vitamins and minerals are common.

Ascorbic acid and ascorbates are usually made from corn which is a common cause of food reactions. New sources of vitamin C have become available, but it is still a matter of trial and error for each person.

Residual chemicals used in manufacturing may require omitting all commercial forms of vitamin C.

Raw brewer's yeast is a relatively natural source of B-complex, but may not be tolerated by the yeast-sensitive patient. Yeast-sensitive and corn-sensitive patients can usually tolerate some preparations of non-yeast derived B-complex if the latter do not also contain vitamin C.

Some mineral tablets are also made without corn starch so may be tolerated by corn-sensitive patients. A patient who wishes to use such nutritional supplements must shop carefully and consider a trial-and-error approach, just as when adding a new food to the diet. Any product that exacerbates symptoms should be deleted. Many manufacturers now label which of their vitamin or mineral products are wheat free, corn free, yeast free, sugar free, and so on.

Most simple, wholesome foods contain a relatively high content of vitamins and minerals. An adequate vitamin-mineral intake usually can be obtained by most people by eating only the foods in the natural diet. This is aided by daily stressing a wide variety of fruits and salads in the raw state, by cooking vegetables with a minimum of water for a minimum amount of time, and by utilizing the cooking water containing water-soluble vitamins and minerals for soups and sauces.

Slow-cooking, low-temperature, minimum water-requiring utensils and steaming racks are convenient tools for achieving these ends. Inexpensive food grinders allow small amounts of ordinary cooked foods to be pureed. Thus, many of the safe, simple, natural foods prepared for the family can be fed, possibly on a rotary schedule, to the allergic or potentially allergic infant.

The need for calcium supplementation in patients on milk avoidance is a subject of controversy. If the diet is deemed deficient in calcium, extra calcium can be taken. It may be helpful to avoid colored calcium capsules, calcium tablets or wafers containing corn starch or corn sugar, and liquid calcium preparations containing sugar or corn syrup. Exquisitely beef-sensitive patients may have to avoid medications in beef-derived gelatin capsules.

Charts showing four days of suggested menus for the rotary diet, in which entire food families are rotated, are outlined in Appendix I. Each patient, however, must sit down with a pencil and paper and draw upon these four days from over four hundred listed foods to select and construct his own meals. An aware nurse, allergy technician, dietician, or nutritionist can be helpful in planning menus and special recipes.

DIET #4
THE ONE-FOOD-PER-MEAL ROTARY DIET

A second type rotary diet for a patient with unusually broad sensitivities is the one-food-per-meal rotary diet. Three to five meals a day are allowed, but only one food is allowed at each meal.

Plain sea salt is the only seasoning allowed, and can be used in moderation unless contraindicated by the presence of some salt-negating illness such as high blood pressure. Any one food cannot be eaten again until at least four days later. If an oil is needed in the preparation of a food, four or more less frequently eaten oils should be purchased, and only one oil used per day, and only at one meal of that day.

For example, breakfast the first day can consist of several bananas *or* apples (raw or baked, peeled) with no sugar or other additives. Lunch the first day can consist of plain baked white potato, sweet potato, *or* plain rice (with sea salt). Dinner can be plain broiled beef steak *or* plain broiled chicken. A fourth meal if desired can consist of any one plain noncombined food, such as raw tomatoes *or* celery. A fifth meal or snack could consist of raw pecans, almonds, walnuts, Brazil nuts, *or* other nuts (not cooked in oil), *or* one species of berry.

The amount of each food taken per meal is usually not restricted. For example, one may eat as many apples as desired at the apple meal, and the same goes for each of the other foods. However, this is not necessarily true of every food. A food that has caused symptoms when eaten in a single large feeding, but not when eaten in a single small feeding, must be limited to the tolerated quantity. One food each day should be a meat (beef; pork; lamb; chicken; turkey; goose; duck; water-packed tuna; salmon canned in glass jars; fresh or frozen fish; shell-fish; or game such as venison, squirrel, rabbit, quail, or partridge). One fruit, one vegetable, one starch, one nut, and one berry can also be taken each day.

Thus, although no one meal is balanced, each day's total intake is generally balanced well enough for the brief period required. Each meal is a test meal for one food. Each food that causes no symptoms is added to the list of tolerated foods.

During such a diet, you should try to remain in a quiet environment and keep records. In this way you can note and record brief periods of ear-ringing, pulse-racing, cloudy thinking or other subtle symptoms.

In some patients, the cardiovascular system is an allergic shock organ. The mediators released by eating an allergenic food may cause an increase or decrease in the pulse rate of 15 or more beats per minute.

If no change except in pulse rate occurs shortly after eating any one food, and a delayed symptom of another type occurs that night, the delayed symptom may have been caused by the pulse-changing food. Knowing this may help you suspect and later try again this specific food for confirmation.

As the list of tolerated foods grows, two proven tolerated foods can be eaten at each meal, then three, four, etc. The four-day rotation should be carefully adhered to, since eating a given tolerated food at two or more closely spaced meals can cause return of symptoms and confusion in the progression of the trial diet.

These diets require a great deal of self-discipline, repeated trials, and a closely-kept diet diary. However, they can solve many obscure, difficult medical problems.

THE DIET DIARY

When utilizing a rotary diet of any type, it is essential to keep an accurate record or diary of all foods eaten and the time they are eaten, preferably in *blue or black* ink. On the same diary a record of symptoms *and their time of occurrence* (especially which meals they followed) should be written in *red* ink below or beside the meal (Appendix IV).

Errors in choice of foods and in frequency of ingestion of allowed foods will show up almost automatically. Thus, the correlation of symptoms and their causative foods will be more easily made.

This is especially important in the early weeks of the diet, since it may take you a while to get completely focused on your diet. It is natural to make many inadvertent mistakes and dietary slips at first.

In addition, if you have problems from inhalants, chemicals, and nonspecific triggers, you should record in your diary all significant activities. These should include exposures to inhalants, including dusts; molds; feathers; fur-bearing animals; cooking odors; and chemical odors like after-shave lotions, perfumes, etc.

You should be aware of the problem of "outgassing" or evaporation of chemical molecules from things such as new clothing, new cars, new carpets, new home furnishings, fiberboard walls, foam insulation, paint, structural materials, janitorial-type products, cosmetics, sprays, and the clicking on and off of the home heating system. You should also record nonspecific stresses such as chilling, overheating, weather changes, undue fatigue, or inadequate sleep.

Menstruating women should record on the diet diary the dates of onset of menstrual cycles, and also of ovulation (which can be calculated retroactively as approximately two weeks before onset of menses). In addition to increasing the total body burden, these chemical, hormonal, and other nonfood stresses can also trigger addictive eating, resulting in symptoms from the culprit foods.

As described, symptoms from an allergenic food may not occur immediately after eating it; but may occur later that day, during the night, or even on the following day. Symptoms from a single exposure are prone to occur on two or three consecutive nights, often with milder or no symptoms during the intervening daytime hours. These delayed reactions have to be taken into consideration in order to pinpoint causative foods. Detailed notes in the diet diary are a most valuable reference source for these correlations.

THE FOOD TOLERANCE LEDGER

It is also important to set up and maintain a food tolerance ledger consisting of a single sheet of paper with four columns (Appendix V). The first column should list all the foods which are proven by the diagnostic diet to be tolerated. The second column should list all foods which *questionably* produce mild symptoms. These eventually must be tried again and moved either to the first or third column.

The third column should contain all foods which *definitely* cause mild symptoms. These ordinarily should be avoided, but some can be eaten occasionally if the list of tolerated foods remains very limited.

The fourth column should list all foods which have *apparently* caused severe symptoms. These foods should be totally eliminated for at least three months; after which some foods from this list (but not those suspected of causing life-threatening reactions) may cautiously be tried again, one at a time, in very small quantities. If tolerated, such a food can be reintroduced into the diet but only in limited quantity and no more frequently than at one meal every four days.

Tolerance to some foods changes, and it may be necessary to move a food from one column to another from time to time. If tolerance does not build within three months, the food should be eliminated and possibly tried again in a year. In an adult, if it is still not tolerated in a year despite careful avoidance, it is not likely ever to be tolerated.

FASTING AND CHALLENGING IN THE HOSPITAL

Some physicians have successfully managed patients with extremely complex food and chemical sensitivities by first evacuating their gastrointestinal tracts and hospitalizing them for close observation in a less chemically contaminated environment. They then clear the symptoms by having them fast in the hospital for four to five days on only a carefully chosen spring water bottled in glass containers. Control of both inhaled and ingested chemicals is an important part of the hospital fast program.

After patients' symptoms clear, they give them individual natural, less chemically contaminated or organic foods, one food per meal, three to five meals per day, under close observation to detect food sensitivities. After sensitivities to natural foods have been diagnosed, they then switch patients onto the same foods but employ ordinary commercially available chemicalized forms of the foods to detect chemical sensitivities. This determines if they can eat ordinary chemicalized foods, or must eat less chemicalized or organic foods.

The next step is to discharge them from the hospital and observe their responses to the home inhalant environment. Hopefully, the home environment has been appropriately modified before discharge from the hospital.

Modification consists of the elimination or at least the minimizing of household products and furnishings which out-gas chemical fumes or produce floating particles such as dusts, mold spores, or lint. If symptoms still occur, greater modification of the entire home or of at least one or more rooms in the home will be needed.

This hospital procedure is an application of the one-food-per-meal diet described earlier in this chapter. If these patients turn out to be sensitive to a great many foods which are difficult to avoid, they can sometimes be allowed a broader diet through food extract injection therapy.

ORGANIC FOODS

Even simple foods purchased in supermarkets may contain minute amounts of unintentional contaminants such as pesticides, herbicides, antimicrobial agents, and other chemicals. Some of these may cause reactions in the extremely sensitive patient. If this turns out to be the case, it may be necessary to purchase organic foods.

Lists are available of shippers of foods reputed to be simple, organic, or otherwise desirable for the patient who is sensitive to common foods, hidden ingredients, or chemical contaminants.[82,83] A comprehensive encyclopedia is available for study of the technology of food production.[84] A monthly journal of food technology is also available.[85] Not all organic foods are equally uncontaminated or less contaminated with chemicals, so the organic food buyer must still be aware and alert to unsuitable food sources or changes in reliability of such sources.

I am not mentioning organic foods because such foods are necessarily "healthier," "better," or "nutritionally superior." They may not be any of these. Their value is that they contain no, or less, chemical contaminants, and so you may simply tolerate them better if you are very chemically sensitive. You can eat them without so much likelihood of getting sick from chemical ingredients.

LABELLING PROBLEMS

It is difficult to keep track of the changing contents of processed foods because the labels on such products are often incomplete and confusing. In the case of "standardized" foods, the labels may offer no ingredient information whatsoever.

A standardized food is one for which the FDA has prescribed a broad general list of allowed ingredients. Examples are ice cream; solid white shortenings; and alcoholic beverages such as beer, wine, and hard liquors.

The specific ingredients in such foods need not be listed on the labels, except ingredients not included in the FDA standardized ingredient list. The consumer does not have possession of these lists, and certainly should not be expected to carry such lists to the supermarket each day.

Standardized lists may help manufacturers but they place a heavy burden on the allergic patient. It would be helpful if labels on all products revealed the entire list of ingredients, and we as consumers could then know what we are paying for and putting into our bodies. Our health, and even some of our lives, could depend on it.

FOODS WITH PHARMACOLOGIC EFFECTS

Alcohol-containing beverages should initially be avoided by patients on this diet, because they contain many ingredients, most of which are proprietary secrets. Alcohols may also cause pharmacologic effects that complicate symptom evaluation. Some alcohols are less complex than others, and these may be introduced on a trial basis later. Foods to be omitted are underlined in the Rotary Diet Charts (Appendix I).

Caffeine-containing foods, such as coffee, tea, and colas, should also be omitted. Aside from the possibility of allergic sensitization to coffee and other caffeine-containing foods, nonallergic sensitivity to caffeine itself can cause many problems, such as hyperactivity, difficult behavior, irritability, irregular heart beats, indigestion, diarrhea, and insomnia. Some "difficult" problems become much more tractable by simply eliminating caffeine.

SOME HAZARDS IN RESTAURANTS AND AT PARTIES

1. Cooking Odors
2. Natural Gas Odors
3. Steak Tenderizer
4. Bisulfites and Metabisulfites
5. Monosodium Glutamate
6. Hidden Food Ingredients
7. Oils of Unknown Origin
8. Chemical Preservatives and Contaminants

THE PATIENT'S ROLE

The successful management of your diet is largely dependent on your attitude and cooperation. You must follow dietary instructions meticulously. Restaurant meals may have to be avoided, either temporarily or permanently; since restaurant flavorings, chemical additives, oils, or other materials cannot always be identified.

Some people are made sick by the odor of natural gas or cooking odors each time they go to a restaurant, and this must be distinguished from reactions due to the foods eaten. If restaurant eating cannot be avoided, selections must be simple, such as a plain broiled steak or fish (no butter, oil, seasonings, or tenderizer), a dry baked potato with natural gravy from the broiled steak, a plain sliced tomato *or* head lettuce salad, and melon, berries, or other fresh fruit for dessert. Be aware that monosodium glutamate may be a hidden symptom-causing ingredient of restaurant and other foods.

Complex salad dressings must be avoided; olive oil with lemon wedges or wine vinegar (grape, yeast, and coloring material) can be used if tolerated. Self-carried fresh or dried fruits and nuts are nourishing and convenient "fillers," although care should be taken to avoid dried fruits treated with additives and fumigants, if these are a problem.

Salad bars can be a hazard. Foods possibly contaminated by bisulfites or metabisulfites may need to be avoided. Oils in salad dressings at the salad bar may consist of peanut, soy, cottonseed, or other oils to which you may be exquisitely sensitive.

Previous customers may have dripped some of these dressings on the lettuce or other foods at the salad bar without your knowledge. Artificial "bacon bits" and many other such substances make salad bars extra hazardous for some people.

Many patients ask what to do about food at parties. Parties themselves should not be avoided if possible, but it is best to satisfy hunger at home before and after the party, and then eat only safe known foods at the party, or none at all. You should avoid diet deviation. However, if some carefully chosen foods are eaten, they should be noted in your diet diary. Thus, if symptoms occur, the causative foods may be pinpointed.

If you are exquisitely sensitive to preservatives, you must be extremely careful about your choice of foods; and you simply cannot eat at all in restaurants or at parties. For example, sodium and potassium bisulfite and metabisulfite are known to have caused life-threatening reactions, yet are commonly used in some beers and most vinegars and wines. They are also sprayed on or added to a variety of restaurant foods such as salads, fried potatoes, seafoods, fresh fruits and vegetables, avocado dips, shellfish, dried fruits and vegetables, fruit juices, purees, syrups, concentrates, and condiments.

These preservatives may cause immediate or long-delayed "mysterious" reactions of a severe degree. There should be a strict requirement for restaurants as well as food producers to either completely *avoid* the use of these chemicals or clearly inform their customers if they are following such practices.

Chapter 22

HIDDEN FOOD INGREDIENTS AND INCOMPLETE LABELS: INTOLERABLE BURDENS ON CONSUMERS

In 1970, I sent my office personnel into five different supermarkets—with the consent of the managers—to copy the labelled ingredients off the container labels of every product on the shelves. In 1976, we repeated the entire process. We continue to monitor individual label changes.

Each time my staff assembled the information, we categorized all products by their type and contents. This was an invaluable source for gaining a broad perspective on the labelling problem, for teaching our patients, and for sorting out the specific ingredients which might be causing given reactions.

Since products and manufacturing processes do change, consistent label reading must become a way of life for some in order to at least be aware of varying *labelled* ingredients. However, one of the foremost obstacles encountered by patients on allergy diets is the problem of hidden *unlabelled* food ingredients.[84,86,87]

Many foods available in our supermarkets are processed, packaged, or canned with hidden food ingredients or additives. Food labelling is usually incomplete and often misleading. Furthermore, there are no labels available to reveal products added at the supermarket or in restaurants.

Sugars, starches, oils, split protein products, alcohols, and other derivatives of natural foods usually carry the allergenicity of the specific food from which each is derived. Such foods and their derivatives often contain chemical additives deliberately introduced at the factory to achieve certain desired ends, like uniform texture, color, flavor, and long shelf life.

Some also tend to retain residues of insecticides, herbicides, and other chemicals used on farms, orchards, ranches, dairies, poultry houses, and fisheries; in raw product storage, food transportation, cleaning of vats and tubes, control of bacteria, fungi, insects, and rodents in factories;

and packaging and merchandising of finished products. These chemicals may be natural or synthetic, the synthetic ones being most commonly of petroleum, coal tar, and cellulose origin.

HIDDEN NATURAL INGREDIENTS

Among the natural foods commonly incorporated into other foods as labelled or unlabelled ingredients are egg, milk, soy, cottonseed, pork, beef, yeast, corn, wheat, and peanut. However, many other natural ingredients may be present without specific labelling.

Even when products are labelled, the patient may be confused by the unfamiliar labelling terms sometimes used by food technologists. For example, vitellin, ovovitellin, livetin, omomucoid, ovomucin, and albumin are all egg derivatives.

EGG

Egg derivatives are commonly found as labelled or unlabelled ingredients of baking powder, cakes, pancakes, prepared cake and pancake mixes, cookies, doughnuts, pastries, waffles, pretzels, French toast, pies, muffins, meringues, souffles, fritters, noodles, some ice creams, mayonnaise, Hollandaise sauce, tartar sauce, and some salad dressings (for example, Caesar salad). They are also used in icings, marshmallows, many candies and candy bars, and some sausages and luncheon meats. Egg albumin is often used in root beer for producing foam, and in coffee and some wines to remove floating particles.

MILK

Casein, caseinate, lactose, and whey may not be recognized as milk. Most "nondairy" creamers surprisingly contain milk products (sodium or calcium caseinate and lactose), and all of them contain ingredients from other unexpected sources such as corn, soy, animal and vegetable fat, and petrochemicals.

Powdered artificial sweeteners usually contain lactose (milk) or dextrose (corn) as well as saccharin (derived from coal tar). Disodium cromoglycate inhalant powder for asthma contains lactose. Milk is absent from kosher bread (challah) and from some French, Italian, Syrian, and other special breads.

Milk derivatives are found in butter, most margarines (including some—not all—labelled as 100 percent corn oil margarines), cheese, cottage cheese, ice cream, sherbet, junket, yogurt, creamed soups, puddings, custards, most nondairy creamers, cakes, pancakes, waffles, and candies (including chocolate). Milk powder is used as a filler in many products.

Coffee Rich® and Mocha Mix® do not contain milk derivatives. Soybean formulas are free of milk, but some milk-sensitive infants are also sensitive to the soy, corn, and other ingredients in these formulas. Margarines and cheeses are further complicated by the various dyes, flavors, preservatives, and other additives introduced at the factory to produce a uniform product with an appealing taste and appearance and a long shelf life.

Blue label Mazola 100% Corn Oil Margarine® contains milk, but green label Mazola 100% Corn Oil Margarine® does not. Nucoa Margarine® contains no milk. Shedd's Spread® contains no milk but does contain citric acid. Shedd's Willow Run Margarine® contains neither milk nor citric acid. Hain's Unsalted Safflower Margarine® (green label) contains no milk but does contain citric acid. Hain's Safflower Margarine® (yellow label) contains cottonseed oil but no milk, corn, or citric acid, and no preservatives. All contain soy.

SOY

Soy is another common hidden ingredient in foods. Lecithin, food "extenders," and factory-made low-cholesterol food substitutes are derived largely from soy and also contain a multitude of spices and chemicals.

Soybean flour is used in some breads, cakes, rolls, pastries, doughnuts, and crackers. Soy is used in cereals, as a nut (roasted soy beans), and in sauces (soy sauce, Lea and Perrins Sauce®, Heinz Worcestershire Sauce®, Teriyaki Sauce®, La Choy Sauce®, etc.).

Tuna, sardines, and other foods are often packed in soy oil. Popcorn, potato chips, processed fried fish, and other substances are frequently fried in soy oil. Soy oil is used in salad dressings and mayonnaises which are often simply labelled as containing vegetable oil.

Soy is also added to sausages, lunch meats, hard candies, chocolates, caramels, and margarines. As mentioned, soy is also the base of many infant formulas.

COTTONSEED OIL

Cottonseed oil is used in virtually all the same products listed above as containing soybean oil. Cottonseed flour is also used in some bakery products and to make gin. Cottonseed sensitivity has been responsible for some of the most severe reactions reported in medical literature.

VEGETABLE SHORTENINGS

Vegetable oil labelling covers soy, peanut, coconut, cottonseed, corn, olive, palm, safflower, sunflower, almond, sesame, and any other oil not of animal origin. The type of vegetable oil used in many products can be changed without notice and without changing the label.

Liquid shortenings labelled as to the specific source of the oil must contain oil only from that source. Solid white vegetable shortenings are mixtures of oils; and the oils used vary from time to time, depending chiefly on the current market prices of individual oils. These changes are not revealed on the labels.

Liquid Crisco Oil® is labelled as pure soy oil with BHA and BHT (butylated hydroxy-anisole and butylated hydroxy-toluene). Louanna® is labelled as containing cottonseed oil, with no preservatives. Oils without preservatives can be obtained from some supermarkets, health food stores, and specialized food shippers.

OILS REALLY ARE ALLERGENIC

There have been some recent research reports which state that oils are not allergenic. This flies in the face of common day-to-day experiences of many of my patients who experience reactions, sometimes extremely severe, from inadvertent exposure to oils to which they were sensitive.

Possibly if oils could be inexpensively refined so completely that *no traces whatsoever* remain of the proteins or protein break-down products of the peanut, corn, soy, or other substances from which they are derived, this could conceivably be true. But such refinement is not used in commercially available foods, and the human immune mechanism can be sensitive enough to react severely to even a few parts of proteinaceous substances per thousand, per million, or even per billion parts of the oil.

Oils are most certainly allergenic to some people. However, the reactions may sometimes be delayed by the slow digestion and absorption of oils as compared to sugars and other foodstuffs.

PORK, BEEF, LAMB

Shortening not labelled as of vegetable origin is usually derived from pork (lard), beef, or lamb fat. Gelatin capsules are of animal origin also. Almost all gelatin desserts, such as Jell-O®, are now made from both pork and beef except Knox® gelatin, which is made exclusively from beef.

However, some chemically sensitive patients are unable to tolerate beef-derived gelatin. This is apparently due to residual chemicals from processing, since many of these patients can tolerate fresh nonchemicalized beef.

YEAST

Yeast is found mostly in bakery products; alcoholic beverages; products which contain vinegar (such as catsup, mayonnaise, and barbecue sauce); products containing yeast-derived vitamins of the B-complex series (including some packaged "enriched" cereals); and black tea, the leaves of which are yeast-fermented. Torula, listed in some processed and smoked foods, is also a yeast.

WHEAT

Wheat includes everything made from the wheat grain, including wheat flour, wheat germ, wheat bran, etc. Of course this includes all bakery products such as bread (even rye breads and pumpernickel usually contain much wheat), crackers, cookies, pies, doughnuts, matzos, and pretzels.

It also includes spaghetti; macaroni; noodles; dumplings; alphabet soups; wheat batters on fried foods; and wheat cereals such as Wheaties®, Cream of Wheat®, Grape Nuts®, and farina. Additionally, wheat is found in dressings and gravies thickened with wheat flour, frankfurters and sausages in which wheat flour is used as a filler, and most products labelled as containing gluten.

Special wheat-free breads and crackers (such as rice crackers, 100 percent rye bread, and Ry-Krisp®) may be used by some patients, but many wheat-sensitive patients are also sensitive to rye. Recipes for wheat-free, corn-free, and milk-free breads for allergic and celiac patients are published in special cookbooks available in libraries, bookstores, and health food stores.

CORN

Corn products are found in a great number of foods both as known and as hidden ingredients. Examples are products which contain corn meal, corn starch, corn oil, corn oil margarine, corn sugar, corn syrup, corn sweetener, dextrose, glucose, dexin, dextrin, dextrimaltose, and corn alcohol (beer, bourbon, Scotch, blended whiskeys, vodka, gin, fortified wines, and many liqueurs).

Commercial fructose is now also made from corn (not from fruit). Malt is generally yeast-fermented from corn and wheat as well as barley.

Almost all factory-processed sweets and spicy foods contain corn-derived products such as corn syrup, corn sugar, corn sweetener, citric acid, or monosodium glutamate. These include candies, cakes, cookies, pastries, ice cream, canned fruits, canned juices, frozen juices, powdered fruit drinks, ham, bacon, luncheon meats, salami, frankfurters, jams, jellies, syrups, peanut butters, catsups, chili, barbecue sauces, salad dressings, soft drinks, ices, powdered sugar, cake icings, gelatin desserts, chewing gum, tacos, tortillas, enchiladas, Fritos®, and Chee-Wees®.

It also includes most infant formulas. Examples of corn-free, milk-free formulas are Cho-Free® and I–Soyalac®. Many medications contain corn derivatives, for example, cough syrups, cough drops, lozenges, pills, tablets, suppositories, and baby powders.

Corn meal is often used as a dry lubricant on the floors of bakery ovens and becomes cooked into the under surfaces of rolls and bread loaves. Corn meal and corn starch are used in some paper milk cartons; in baking powders; in the glue of some stamps, envelopes, adhesive tapes, and other stickers; and as fillers and thickeners.

Vinegar on a label, unqualified as to source, usually means white grain vinegar. White grain vinegar carries the allergenicity of wheat, corn, and other grains, and sugars, as well as yeast.

The primary vinegar in Great Britain is malt vinegar, made chiefly from barley, sometimes with adjuncts of other grains such as corn and rice. Wine (grape) vinegar is most commonly used on the Continent. Grape wine vinegar and apple cider vinegar are free of corn and wheat.

Olives canned in vinegar contain wheat and corn, but black olives canned in ferrous gluconate and water do not.

Many foods which cannot be eaten by grain-sensitive patients because of their vinegar content could be tolerated if manufacturers made them available with wine vinegar or apple vinegar. Virtually all vinegars and wines contain sodium bisulfite or sodium metabisulfite, although these chemicals are not listed on the labels.

Citric acid employed commercially is usually made from corn starch or sugar beet molasses fermented by a microorganism, Aspergillus niger. It may also be derived from lemon and pineapple wastes.

Interestingly, one of my patients is sensitive to Aspergillus niger, not to corn or beet. He can tolerate foods containing citric acid only when using neutralizing injections for Aspergillus niger.

The more rapid absorption of corn alcohols and sugars explains why some patients have no detectable symptoms from whole corn but do develop symptoms when challenged with corn alcohols or corn sugars. The glucose loading dose used for the glucose tolerance test often produces a corn sensitivity reaction, but its significance is usually overlooked.

The same is true to a lesser extent of intravenous glucose solutions, which are more highly refined. The glucose used for the glucose tolerance test may also contain a cola flavoring.

There are many substitutes for wheat and corn, such as rice flour, brown rice flour, potato flour, tapioca, arrowroot starch, lima bean flour, soy flour, and other flours that can be found in some supermarkets and health food stores. Food can be fried in a substitute batter or placed in Pyrex dishes or aluminum foil and baked in their own juices, thus eliminating the need for a batter and a frying oil or butter.

Either no salt need be added or plain sea salt (available in health food stores) can be used sparingly. Most table salts contain corn sugar (dextrose) as well as sodium silico-aluminate and iodide, and may cause symptoms in some corn-sensitive, chemical-sensitive, or iodide-sensitive patients.

The presence of "food starch" or "modified food starch" on a label can indicate a starch of wheat, corn, sorghum, arrowroot, tapioca, or potato origin. Arrowroot and tapioca are much less frequently allergenic than wheat or corn.

Manufacturers could do some of their customers a service by using these nongrain-derived starches more often in their products. They could also help by using only one source of starch in each product, and by designating on the label the exact starch used.

ALCOHOLS

Alcoholic beverages are derived from foods and carry the allergenicity of their food origin. Most beer is made from corn grits; and all beer contains barley, malt, hops, yeast, and other ingredients which are often industrial secrets. Many are made from both rice and corn products.

Michelob® beer is made from rice and apparently contains no corn. Malt may be fermented from barley, corn, wheat, or other grains.

Whiskeys, including "straight corn whiskeys," contain an impossible number of ingredients. One popular brand is advertised as "containing 94 ingredients for your taste pleasure." Gin is equally complicated.

Aquavit® is made from potatoes. Many people believe that vodka is made from potatoes, but this is not true. Vodkas in general are almost as complex as blended whiskeys. Gin and even imported vodkas are usually clearly labelled as derived chiefly from neutral grain spirits rather than potato.

Rums are made primarily from cane sugar. Most are corn-free. Bacardi® rum is said to contain grape but is free of corn. By law, Jamaican rums must be free of all noncane alcohol.

Grapes and other fruits used in making wine and brandy do not naturally ferment beyond about 14 percent alcohol concentration. Most table wines contain about 9 to 12 percent alcohol. A patient who can tolerate yeast and grapes, or whatever other fruit the product is made from, can usually tolerate table wine and brandy. However, some products with greater than 14 percent alcohol listed on the label contain additional alcohol from other sources, often from corn.

Since alcoholic extracts of foods are absorbed very rapidly and cause more immediate, more severe, or more noticeable reactions, they can sometimes be used to pinpoint sensitivities not otherwise apparent. For example, a patient who gets symptoms from most beers, whiskeys, and fortified wines but not from Michelob, Bacardi rum, or table wine is almost certainly corn-sensitive. One who gets symptoms from Michelob but not from nonrice-containing beers may be rice-sensitive.

Symptoms from Aquavit alone would cast suspicion on potatoes. Symptoms from Jamaican rum suggest cane sugar sensitivity. Symptoms from Bacardi Rum and from grape-derived table wine but not from Jamaican rum suggest grape sensitivity. A patient who exhibits symptoms from virtually all fermented beverages may be sensitive to yeast; or he may have multiple sensitivities, possibly including corn, wheat, rye, barley, potato, rice, and grape.

THE CHOCOLATE FAMILY

"Pure" chocolate is a highly complex, chemicalized, and processed product. It can contain very allergenic substances, such as finely ground peanuts, cereals, coffee, milk, and other ingredients which *need not be mentioned on the label.*

Synthetic chocolate is also now widely used. When true chocolate sensitivity exists, cola drinks and karaya gum (often listed on labels as "gum" or "vegetable gum") should also be considered since the cacao bean, cola nut, and karaya gum (derived from Stericula trees of East India) are all in the same botanical family.

CHEMICALS

We have already discussed that patients with multiple food and chemical sensitivities usually do better to avoid all foods which have passed through a factory on the way to the supermarket. However, this does not guarantee freedom from inadvertent exposures, particularly to chemicals.

Fresh fruits and vegetables, which would ordinarily appear to be very good food choices, may present problems to the chemically sensitive patient because of unexpected processing procedures. Nearly all fruits and vegetables available from commercial grocers have been treated somewhere along the line with insecticides, many of which have been found to cause reactions in hypersensitive patients.

Peaches, apples, and cherries are the most seriously affected, often being sprayed or treated with insecticides 10 to 15 times per growing season. Although the fruits and vegetables may be washed or even peeled, the chemicals have often penetrated the pulp.

In addition, fruits are sometimes sprayed at the market counter to prevent fruit fly infestation. Sulfites and metabisulfites are sprayed on lettuce and other salad vegetables in salad bars of restaurants to preserve their appearance of freshness, and have been reported to have caused extremely severe sensitivity reactions.

Although awareness of this problem is fairly recent, the practice has been around for a long time and may have been responsible for many puzzling reactions over the years. A comprehensive study should be made of such practices in restaurants, butcher shops, fruit and vegetable stands, and other sites where nonlabelled additives can be introduced into foods.

Cosmetic alterations of foods also may cause difficulties. The appealing shine on many fruits and vegetables is often due to coating with vegetable or mineral oils or petrochemically derived waxes. Since these chemicals are not water-soluble, washing is not an effective method of removal.

Among the types of produce which may be treated in this manner are rutabagas, cucumbers, green peppers, apples, parsnips, and squash. Peeling can reduce chemical exposures but does not entirely eliminate them; and some foods, for example, green peppers, do not lend themselves to peeling.

All commercially dried fruits are treated with sulfur dioxide unless otherwise stated on the package. All dates crossing state lines are fumigated with methyl bromide in accordance with federal regulations.

Bananas, which are picked green, are usually exposed to a petroleum-derived gas, ethylene, which destroys the green chlorophyll and hastens apparent ripening. Such bananas may not be tolerated by the petrochemically-sensitive patient. Some patients have said that they can distinguish these bananas from nongassed ones by the fact that more heavily gassed bananas develop large brown spots as they ripen and have a "green" taste, whereas nongassed or less-gassed bananas ripen with small, stippled brown spots and have a sweeter taste.

Apples, pears, oranges, and tomatoes are also often exposed to ethylene gas and other ripening agents. In addition, oranges are frequently dyed with artificial colors.

Eggs may be dipped in penicillin solutions to retard spoilage. The penicillin penetrates the shell and contaminates the contents. Patients with severe penicillin sensitivities should be aware of this.

Chicken can also be a problem. Antibiotics, coccidiostats, hormones, and other chemicals (including arsenic for growth stimulation) are often added to their feed. Killed, plucked, eviscerated chickens are sometimes placed in an ice slush bath containing antibiotics to retard bacterial growth. The patient who is exquisitely sensitive to antibiotics and other chemicals may be bothered by the traces of these and other materials remaining in the marketed chicken.

CANNED AND PACKAGED FOODS

Some foods in cans cannot be tolerated by some patients who can tolerate the same foods in glass jars. A major cause of this is the plastic or phenolic resin liner of the inner surface of the can. Since corn sweetener is sweeter and less expensive than sugar, it has largely replaced cane and beet sugar in commercial canned and packaged products.

Some methods of storing and preparing foods may also cause symptoms in hypersensitive patients. The plastic solvents in soft plastic wrappers used to cover foods have produced reactions in certain patients.

Some patients who have an apparent allergy to coffee report that they tolerate coffee roasted with electric heat but not coffee roasted with a gas flame. Others cannot tolerate decaffeinated coffee, presumably due to residues of the chemicals used to remove the caffeine.

FROZEN FOODS

Frozen fish is often dipped in antibiotics before freezing to retard spoilage. Preservatives such as bisulfites are used by commercial shrimpers and fishermen.

Frozen potatoes are often treated with chemicals such as sodium acid pyrophosphate and sodium EDTA to prevent discoloration. They may also be coated with methylcellulose to harden when subjected to frying, so as to produce a crisp outer shell with a tender, moist interior. Bisulfites are used to keep frozen french fries from turning brown.

Coatings or batters on frozen fried chicken, fried shrimp, and similar products often contain not only wheat flour and corn meal, but sometimes egg, seasonings, monosodium glutamate, chemical modifiers, and preservatives. Sugar is highly chemicalized and bleached, in addition to being filtered through lime which is said to be derived from bone char (beef, pork, lamb), and reputedly also from oyster shells.

ARTIFICIAL SWEETENERS

Sugar substitutes often contain chemicals and corn-derived ingredients. One popular powdered low-calorie sugar substitute (Sweet 'n Low®) is labelled as containing nutritive dextrose (corn sugar), 4% soluble saccharin (derived from coal tar), cream of tartar (derived from grapes), and calcium silicate, an anticaking chemical.

Another popular powdered low-calorie sugar substitute (Equal®) is labelled as containing dextrose with dried corn syrup, the sweetener aspartame, silicon dioxide, microcrystalline cellulose, tribasic calcium phosphate, and cellulose gum. The labelling print is so fine and so difficult to read on some of these packages that there are undoubtedly many people whose visual acuity is not adequate to discern the ingredient list.

UNINTENTIONAL CHEMICAL CONTAMINANTS

It is inevitable that some chemicals used in food factories to control bacteria, mold, insects, and rodents should accidentally drift onto or otherwise enter the foods. This is also true of detergents and organic solvents used to clean food vats and pipes, and lubricating materials used for food manufacturing equipment.

Cleansers and antiseptics used in cleaning milking equipment and tubing at dairies enter the milk. While the amounts may not be above currently allowed levels of contamination with regard to toxicity in the general population, they can cause sensitivity reactions in some patients.

WATER

Water is also a problem for increasing numbers of people. In these days of bacteriologically and chemically contaminated streams and water sources, municipal water undergoes a great many chemical processes before it reaches the consumer. Some patients are sensitive to the contaminating chemicals or to the chemicals used in water-processing.

Distilled water occasionally can be helpful, but distilled water carries over some of the contaminants and is not tolerated by some patients. When distilled water is bottled in plastic containers, it is often symptom-inducing because the plastic solvents leach out into the water and cause the symptoms.

Commercially available water bottled in glass is often tolerated, but even here the chemicals used for washing the bottles before filling and heat sterilizing can sometimes leave sufficient residues to bother some patients. The caps may have a plastic inner lining and the water may have been filtered through resins. Trials may be necessary of a variety of waters bottled in glass in order to find one that is well tolerated.

Some patients who cannot drink freshly drawn tap water can sometimes tolerate it if they boil it for thirty minutes. Or they can draw it into a glass pitcher and leave it uncovered, or covered with a large strainer, overnight or for several days to allow some of the volatile chemicals to evaporate.

Some patients find that they can only tolerate water derived from a spring or well. Spring water for such patients is best stored in glass bottles with natural cork stoppers. Empty unstoppered glass water containers can be sterilized without chemicals by baking in an oven.

MEDICATIONS

Medications often contain hidden food and chemical ingredients. A particular capsule or tablet may contain starch as a filler, derived from corn, potato, sorghum, arrowroot, tapioca, or other sources. Medications may also contain a binder such as calcium or magnesium stearate made from the stearic acid of pork, beef, or lamb fat.

Color is usually derived from coal tar and complex synthetic compounds. Flavoring is usually made from aromatic hydrocarbons derived from petroleum. Artificial colors, flavors, preservatives, and other chemicals have been incriminated as causative agents in hyperactivity, behavioral problems and learning disorders, as well as asthma, urticaria, and other allergic syndromes.

In addition, clinical experience has repeatedly implicated many other additives in both foods and medications. Such additives include thickeners, gums, suspending agents, emulsifiers, surface active agents, chelating agents, sequestrants, buffers, acidulants, texture modifiers, antioxidants, freshness preservers, antibacterials, antibiotics, mold retarders, humectants, organic solvents, enzymes, vitamins, minerals, alcohols (for example, glycerol, sorbitol, and mannitol), and nonnutritive sweeteners and flavor potentiators (for example, sugar, salt, monosodium glutamate, citric acid, eugenol, nucleotides, and maltol).

A final coating or glaze on hard tablets may contain either corn syrup or plastic films of petrochemical origin. Liquid medications may also contain synthetic alcohol derived from petroleum. If the medication is thick it often contains natural gums (karaya, acacia, tragacanth, arabic, guar, or carob bean gum), methylcellulose (derived from wood or plant pulp), carrageenan (derived from dried Irish moss, a seaweed), or suspending and emulsifying agents derived from petroleum.

CONSUMER/MANUFACTURER/GOVERNMENT INTERFACES

Self-nourishment presents a hazardous obstacle course for many exquisitely or broadly sensitive patients. Some must virtually pick their way through a menacing jungle of allergens in supermarkets and restaurants.

Manufacturers should use minimum concentrations of less toxic and less sensitizing additives, and choose natural rather than synthetic ingredients whenever possible. They should also minimize or omit chemicals which add nothing to the nutritional value of the product. Food processors who do not label their products completely place an unacceptable health burden on a rapidly growing vulnerable segment of the public.

Labels should include comprehensive listings of all ingredients and their sources. Growing, transporting, processing, merchandising, and restaurant practices should be reexamined with greater attention to the needs of the sensitive consumer.

The primary concern of the government should be to maintain an adequate national food supply without unduly jeopardizing an increasingly sensitive population. Since restaurants display no labels, a greater awareness of restaurant practices by patients, and closer regulation of hidden restaurant additives such as bisulfites must be forthcoming.

Chapter 23

INHALED PARTICLES: CAUSES OF ALLERGIES OF THE NOSE, SINUSES, THROAT, EARS, BRONCHIAL TUBES, AND LUNGS

The main allergic syndromes which are caused primarily by inhalant allergens are seasonal hay fever, perennial allergic rhinitis, and allergic asthma. Inhalant allergic syndromes may lead to obstructive and infectious complications such as sinusitis, sinus headache, Eustachian tube block with resultant serous otitis, repeated ear infections, postnasal drip, bronchitis, recurrent upper respiratory infections, and recurrent pneumonia.

Recurrent laryngeal edema and laryngitis with hoarseness or croupy cough can also be caused by inhalants, often combined with exposure to cold or dry air, or secondary infection. However, acute severe layngeal edema is usually due to food, chemical, or drug reactions. The inhaled particles that most often produce allergic illnesses are pollens, dusts, molds, and epidermals (animal skin scales and feathers).

NEUTRALIZATION OF INHALANT SYNDROMES

Neutralization with extracts of inhalant allergens usually produces the same remarkable beneficial results as with extracts of foods. When symptoms are induced with a given test-concentration of an inhalant extract, they are relieved by another test-concentration, just as with food extracts.

As with foods, marked response to treatment injections often begins within one to three weeks. Once this relief is begun, a recurrence of symptoms caused by undue inhalant exposure or delaying of an inhalant treatment injection can usually be relieved within thirty minutes by a subcutaneously administered inhalant injection.

Most patients in my practice with seasonal pollen symptoms are also allergic to some perennial inhalant allergens, such as dusts, molds, or epidermals. Each contributes its portion to the total allergic burden.

It is truly gratifying to watch the rapid and continued relief that usually ensues in patients when broad and continued antigenic coverage is utilized. This minimizes the total allergic burden and maximizes the ongoing beneficial response.

NEUTRALIZING TREATMENT SCHEDULES

Neutralizing treatment injections can be kept in your possession. Thus you can self-administer them on a regular schedule and also whenever an extra or booster injection is needed. A booster injection can be taken whenever inhalant symptoms arise from an undue inhalant exposure, and relief often occurs in thirty minutes.

A commonly used regimen for new patients consists of administering injections three times a week for the first two weeks, and then twice a week. On the other hand, the injections can be given daily the first few days to hasten response.

If the patient first enters the office with seasonal symptoms in the middle of an inhalant season, or if very rapid results are desired for any other reason, he can be directed to use two or three injections *each day* the first day or two of treatment. In this way much relief can often be noted within one or two days.

This is an unusually rapid and practical method of therapy. Each injection contains a beneficial and well-tolerated treatment dose for each of the allergens in the injection, as already proved by prior intradermal testing.

Even when daily injections are not used, most patients experience marked improvement within two to three weeks of therapy. Many are better after one week, and some are better after the first one, two, or three treatment injections. Some start improving while still undergoing testing.

THE VALUE OF "SINGLES"

Usually, a treatment solution containing ten treatment doses is made at the end of testing and provided the patient for home administration. However, while testing, a "single" injection is generally prepared and administered in the office at the end of each test day.

The initial workup and the tests for inhalants normally require about three days. At the end of the first test day, we administer in the office a single subcutaneous treatment injection containing the neutralizing doses of all inhalant antigens tested thus far.

At the end of the second day, the single treatment injection includes all the antigens tested on the first *and* second days. On the third day, inhalant testing is usually completed; then the vial of ten all-inclusive injections is prepared and the patient is administered one of these in the office. Meanwhile, he is being instructed and supervised in the procedure of self-administration of injections. An important point is that many patients begin improving day by day while still being tested!

In our office, there is a morning and afternoon test session each day, with a break for lunch. In the case of very sick or complex patients, or patients who come from great distances, we sometimes administer a single cumulative treatment injection at the end of both the morning and afternoon test sessions to further speed onset of relief.

We use the same system during food testing for patients with severe broad food sensitivities who are in desperate need of relief and nourishment. They are thus often able to tolerate many formerly symptom-causing foods while still being tested.

THE VALUE OF "BOOSTERS"

Once a satisfactory level of protection has been established, most patients feel markedly better as long as they continue taking their injections on schedule. However, symptoms may begin to return when an injection is skipped. When the patients then belatedly take the treatment injection, they usually note relief or marked improvement within thirty minutes.

If the injection is taken at bedtime, relief is often noted on arising in the morning. If symptoms recur between regularly scheduled injections from an unusually large exposure to dust, mold, grass, ragweed, or any of the other allergens in the treatment solution, one or more self-administered booster injections often provide marked relief. The same is true of food extract booster injections in food-sensitive patients. In asthma and other complex syndromes, supportive and relieving medications are provided in advance for additional benefit if needed.

ADVANTAGES OF INHALANT NEUTRALIZATION THERAPY

In inhalant neutralization therapy, relief often comes rapidly, it occurs in a high percentage of patients, and the degree of relief is usually great. Patients deeply appreciate the economy, convenience, control of suffering, and prevention of absenteeism from work accompanying self-administration at home.

Many of my own patients who were only partial responders on my conventional inhalant therapy have exclaimed that they obtained more relief of nasal or chest congestion after two or three weeks of neutralization therapy than after two or three years of my previously administered conventional therapy. The effectiveness of neutralization therapy has enabled us to almost totally avoid the use of long-term daily or alternate-day steroid therapy.

Most patients who have been sent to us on long-term steroid schedules could be weaned off regular steroid therapy within a few months of beginning neutralization therapy. However, these patients are particularly vulnerable to allergic and other stresses. In such instances there is no substitute for an occasional five to seven-day course of steroids along with other indicated measures to tide them over acute situations if such should occur.

FINDING THE BEST TREATMENT DOSE

Conventional skin testing does not determine the diagnosis or the *treatment* dose of any of the allergens tested. A conventionally derived positive or negative wheal provides *some* diagnostic evidence that a given antigen is either allergenic to this patient or not, depending on the history and other factors, but does not provide the answer as to what is the best *treatment* dose.

When I was practicing only conventional allergy, I used the same methods as my conventional colleagues to find the best treatment dose I could for each patient. This dose was arrived at by long-term subcutaneous buildup therapy.

Obviously, some allergens require stronger doses than others. Neutralization testing can usually determine this with precision for each allergen in each patient at a given time. The very first treatment injection contains the optimum treatment dose for each allergen in the solution. No buildup of dosage strength is required. If the body changes its dosage needs at any time, these needs can be determined again by retesting, and the beneficial response immediately restored.

THE PRECISION OF INHALANT NEUTRALIZATION THERAPY

Thus neutralization is neither a high dose nor a low dose method. It is a *precise, individualized, allergen-specific, patient-specific,* and *time-specific* method, with each dose being just right for each allergen in each patient's solution for the state of his immune mechanism at a given time. It utilizes the maximum tolerated objective *intradermally determined* dose of each allergen, and each subcutaneous treatment dose is not only tolerated but is usually rapidly symptom-relieving. It provides higher doses for allergens which require higher doses, and lower doses for allergens which require lower doses. So for inhalants as for foods, neutralization offers a different approach to a sometimes puzzling problem.

PROBLEMS

Inhalant neutralization, however, cannot work miracles. No form of medical treatment yet devised for any disease has produced 100 percent results or been 100 percent free of side effects.

Complicated Patients: Some patients may be so sensitive to one inhalant or food allergen that they cannot be successfully or safely tested and treated for it. Some inhalant patients may also be complicated by allergies to a tremendous number of foods, chemicals, and drugs.

Some may be sensitive to as-yet undeterminable self-substances. Some may have immunodeficiencies; poor cellular immune responses; infections; impacted bronchial mucus; susceptibility to chill; physical exhaustion; adrenal atrophy from prolonged cortisone therapy; poor heart, lung, liver, or kidney function; or other adverse immunologic or nonimmunologic factors in their internal or external environment.

Some may be suffering overwhelming allergenic exposures in the home, such as an indoor dog, cat, or bird; a feather pillow which may also be old and moldy; a mattress full of dust mites; an old dusty carpet; a bookcase full of old books; a new carpet or other house furnishing that gives off chemical vapors; insecticides; or a formaldehyde-based type of insulation in the walls.

Some may be trapped in an intolerably contaminated occupational environment. Allergic teachers and allergic school children are often helpless to recognize or remedy the unendurable allergenic hazards present in almost all schools.

Noncompliance: Noncompliance is another common problem. This term means the inability of the patient to comply with the physician's instructions concerning such things as the timely taking of medications, remembering to maintain the schedule of injections, keeping office appointments, and instituting required life-style changes.

It is amazing how many chronically ill severe asthmatics who receive badly needed relief through neutralization therapy with or without additional medications will go off on trips without packing their injections and medications. Others feel so well after a while that they think—or hope—they are cured and become erratic or even stop their injections and medications altogether—and have a sudden, severe relapse.

THE GOLDILOCKS ANALOGY

Sometimes an analogy or mental image is helpful in understanding and remembering an idea. I have already mentioned the Goldilocks analogy or "just-right" dose. Remember the picture in your mind of Goldilocks at the breakfast table of the three bears? One porridge is too *hot,* another is too *cold,* and yet another is *"just right."*

The "just-right" phenomenon is a basic and universal principle of life. We understand it because it fits our lifelong experiences. Each of us automatically seeks what is "just right" for us as individuals, whether it be food, clothes, abode, education, occupation, recreation, art, entertainment, life style, climate, or whatever. We want things to be not too hot, not too cold; not too hard, not too soft; not too loud, not too quiet; not too fast, not too slow; not too strong, not too weak; and so on, as our *individual* needs require. Each of us is unique, and we vary in our needs and desires for each of these individual facets of life. Thus neutralization makes sense. It feels right and works right.

So the neutralizing method is a method which determines the "just right" dose for each allergen in each individual. Each dose has to be strong enough, but not too strong. When a mosquito lands on your arm, you do not swat him with either a sledgehammer or a feather!

CHAPTER 24

NEUTRALIZATION OF CANDIDA YEAST SENSITIVITY AND CANDIDA YEAST INFECTION

We are just now becoming increasingly aware of a sometimes mild, sometimes serious disease caused by a microbe called Candida albicans. This is a yeast, a member of the mold family.[88]

Candida has always been with us, and was even described by Hippocrates. However, it was generally considered a benign, relatively friendly microbe that usually caused only minor illnesses if any.

A well-known example of these illnesses is oral thrush, especially common in the first few weeks of infancy. Another is yeast vaginitis, which formerly occurred only sporadically in some women between puberty and menopause.

However, certain recent medical breakthroughs and changes in diet and life style tend to inhibit body defenses or stimulate Candida growth. For these reasons it has become a more frequent factor in medical illness.

A UBIQUITOUS DISEASE WITH MANY FACES

The disease that Candida is causing now in ever-greater numbers is called candidiasis. This is not really one disease but many. Which combination of symptoms shows up in an individual depends upon whether or not he is suffering an active Candida *infection* of the bloodstream or of one or more organs, or is reacting *allergically* in one or more shock organs.

Allergic reactions are probably caused by Candida antigens produced in the digestive tract or vagina and absorbed into the bloodstream. The extra burden of circulating Candida products is precipitating recurrent and chronic dysfunctions of many organs.

TRANSMISSION OF CANDIDA

Where is Candida found in nature? Can we avoid it? Candida organisms float around in the air along with many other microbes in the sea of germs in which we live.

Like other such microbes, it drifts downward because of gravity. It settles on various surfaces, landing on our skin, our hands, our food, our eating utensils, anything.

It also readily passes from one person to another by simple casual contact. Since one of its favorite breeding places is in the vagina, many women are potential carriers.

Most transmission then is from person to person: mother to infant, wife to husband, husband back to wife, child to child. It is ubiquitous and there is no way to avoid it. But with an undisturbed resistance/burden ratio, we can usually live in peace with it, as with many other organisms.

CANDIDA IN INFANTS AND CHILDREN

Infants begin their passage through the birth canal without Candida on their skins or in their systems. Their first contact with it may be in the birth canal or soon thereafter. Despite any and all precautions we might take, virtually all infants contract it to some degree. Candida can be identified by laboratory tests in the mouths of 90 percent of infants by four weeks of age.

It may even show up as visible cottony-white thrush colonies in the mouth within days or weeks after birth. By six months, almost all infants have positive Candida skin tests. This means that living Candida are already present in the body and the body has already mounted an immune defense against it. It is this immune defense that turns the skin test positive.

The little white Candida colonies of oral thrush look like milk curds, about pinhead in size, on the gums, tongue, and other inner linings of the mouth. They can be distinguished from milk curds by the fact that wiping off thrush colonies with sterile swabs leaves little red or slightly bleeding surfaces where the colonies were attached to the mucosa.

In older children and adults, it is one of the common causes of cracks at the sides of the lips (cheilitis); redness and swelling of the tongue; and roughened tongue surfaces described as fissured tongue, furrowed tongue, or geographic tongue (resembling a topographic map). Some people note a slick or slimy feeling in the mouth.

Thrush can be contracted from the organisms settling from the air on the baby's lips, food, or utensils; or it can be transferred by feeding bottles, or the mother's hands or breasts. It is sometimes transferred by a wash cloth used to clean the inside of the infant's mouth.

Wash cloths are used by the mother also and are not sterilized by ordinary laundering, so they should not be used for cleaning the baby's mouth. The sad thing about this is that the baby's mouth is naturally self-cleaning anyway.

Candida on the skin is also one of the most common causes of recurrent diaper rash and recurrent infant rashes in general. Candida in the colon can overgrow during antibiotic therapy which suppresses ecologically competing organisms in that area, and can cause "antibiotic diarrhea."

CANDIDA IN WOMEN

Once in the body, Candida takes up permanent residence. It lives chiefly in the intestinal tract, particularly in the colon or large bowel.

From the anus, Candida can be transferred to the vagina or to the urethra which is the bladder opening just in front of the vagina. In the vagina, it can cause itching, sometimes burning, and sometimes a discharge. In the urethra, it can cause burning on urination, frequency of urination, and other discomforts often mistaken for bacterial cystitis.

None of these problems sound so dangerous. However, they can make a woman miserable, need repeated medical attention and pharmacy visits, and result in expenditure of much money and of time which might be spent on the job or in other productive ways. But this is only the beginning of the story.

THE ETERNAL STRUGGLE BETWEEN DEFENSE AND OFFENSE

We are faced again with the old resistance/burden ratio which is so basic in the body's attempts to keep us in good health. Candida organisms usually remain only on surfaces, causing merely superficial infections, if any.

Our defense mechanisms keep them from invading more deeply and causing dangerous, even lethal infections. They are kept in check by the skin and mucosal linings, backed up by defensive cells such as lymphocytes, macrophages, and neutrophils, and a variety of chemicals including antibodies and complement.

So why is candidiasis becoming a serious epidemic disease? Because the resistance/burden ratio has been disturbed in many people by our new life styles and the use of new medications. These medications are often necessary to help us over many serious diseases, but they can also sometimes open the door to allow Candida organisms to do their dirty work.

ALTERED ECOLOGIC BALANCE

Here is an example of how it works. Our digestive tract, other mucosal surfaces, and skin provide homes for many kinds of competing microbes. Each microbe holds the others in check to a degree, in the same manner that ecologic balance is achieved among creatures in the wilderness and in the oceans of the world.

These microbes live in competitive balance, in relative numerical appropriateness, in and on and with their hosts, which are us. Our defenses adapt to this natural dynamic balance, not eradicating the microbes entirely, but constantly fighting them off and keeping them from invading our tissues.

Then we catch a viral cold, get bacterial secondary infection of the sinuses, ears, bronchi, or lungs. Or we get bacterial cystitis or vaginitis or whatever. So we take an antibiotic.

The antibiotic kills off the invading bacteria which are the immediate threat. It also kills many of the relatively harmless antibiotic-susceptible bacteria that live in our digestive tract and on our skin and mucosal surfaces.

This reduces the microbial competition and allows Candida, which is not killed by antibacterial antibiotics, to grow more profusely. Then the Candida organisms form a much larger proportion of our microbial population.

This upsets the microbial balance and adds a greater burden to the Candida controlling part of the defensive system. The defensive system must now work harder to keep the multiplying Candida and its absorbed products under control.

THE CONSEQUENCES OF IMBALANCE

At this point, three alternative conditions may occur. The antibiotic can be stopped or an anti-Candida antibiotic added, and the preantibiotic *balance* can be restored gradually. Or the flood of *chemicals* produced by the large population of growing and dividing Candida organisms can enter the bloodstream in greater than usual quantities and overwhelm the defensive cells and antibodies, producing symptoms. Or finally, the Candida *organisms* themselves can enter the bloodstream and travel to distant organs such as the kidneys, lungs, or brain and cause serious, even life-threatening, infections in these organs.

Before you become too alarmed, let us realize that the third alternative is extremely rare. It occurs in only exceptional circumstances, such as in major immunologic impairments.

It is the second alternative, the excessive absorption into the circulation of antigenic *chemicals* produced by Candida in the digestive tract that adversely affects many people. If the body's defense mechanisms can be strengthened and the overgrowth of the Candida can be checked, most or all of this harm can usually be ameliorated.

THE LINEUP OF OPPOSING FORCES: THE BAD GUYS FIRST

We can approach this problem tactically by lining up the two opposing forces and analyzing their relative roles. Candida overgrowth is stimulated by *antibacterial antibiotics,* and by nonspecific powerful *immunosuppressive drugs.* The latter are used deliberately to knock down the entire defense system in treating certain autoimmune diseases and cancers, and in preventing rejection in transplantation surgery.

Candida overgrowth may also be stimulated by *cortisones* (steroids), especially after long-term usage. Cortisones also have some immunosuppressive effects, and are used in a much greater variety of conditions than the other immunosuppressives mentioned.

In addition, *birth control pills* increase the availability to Candida of a carbohydrate, glycogen (a precursor of sugar), in surface cells of the vagina.[89] This provides extra nourishment for increasing the growth rate of Candida organisms.

Carbohydrates in our diet also stimulate Candida growth by providing it extra nourishment. The most growth-stimulating carbohydrates are refined sugars and sweets such as cane sugar, beet sugar, dates and date sugar, corn sugars and sweeteners, all kinds of molasses, maple sugar or syrup, and honey. In some patients a minute amount of sugar in the diet can produce organ dysfunctions. Potatoes, natural cereal grains, and other complex carbohydrates are also Candida-stimulating, although usually to a lesser degree.

When yeast antigen is in our bloodstream in such high levels, eating *mold-containing or yeasty foods* can cause increased symptoms, apparently by further increasing these blood levels. Yeasty foods are chiefly bakery products (baker's yeast); vinegars and alcoholic beverages (brewer's yeast); and B-complex vitamins when made from brewer's yeast, which is their most common source.

Mushrooms are also members of the mold family. In addition, mold and yeasts get into many naturally sweet foods we eat, particularly fruits and processed fruit juices which have become contaminated by yeasts and molds during processing. It is for the control of these and other microorganisms that preservatives such as bisulfites are so often added to these products.

Fresh peeled fruits and fresh fruit juices generally contain far less mold or yeast. However, even the air we breathe contains yeasts and other airborne molds which can add to our total mold/yeast burden.

Diabetics have a tendency to high blood sugar and relatively poor resistance to infection. They are thus more prone to persistent and recurrent Candida infections.

Premenstrually, the progesterone naturally present tends to increase the available glycogen, the sugar precursor in the cellular lining of the vagina.[89] This results in a tendency to increased vaginal yeast growth and symptoms at that time of the month.

The same is true of *pregnancy,* when progesterone levels are naturally high to keep the uterus quiet and protect the pregnancy. Others note flare-ups a few weeks after termination of a pregnancy, when blood and tissue levels of several elements of the immune and endocrine systems seem to subside below baseline after having been super-elevated all during pregnancy, with a resultant change in resistance/burden ratio.

Finally, some people have a definite *genetic deficiency* in their ability to mount a defense against Candida organisms. This makes them more susceptible than others to the products of Candida growth, and in rare instances to serious deep tissue invasion by Candida organisms themselves.

AND NOW THE GOOD GUYS: IMMUNORESTORATIVE NEUTRALIZATION THERAPY

Here's where *Candida neutralization therapy* comes in. We often can quickly increase our defensive capability against Candida and its secretions by skin testing to find the precise neutralizing dose of Candida extract. This will usually relieve Candida vaginitis patients from most or all of their vaginal itching within thirty minutes during testing.

In resistant cases, the itching returns, usually within twenty-four hours in the early stage of treatment. Another neutralizing injection can be self-administered every day for a while if needed to keep the itching under control and improve the resistance/Candida ratio.

If we treat with neutralization alone in patients whose chronic candidiasis has repeatedly resisted all other forms of therapy, the patient will usually require one injection daily for about twenty days to reduce Candida colonization and maintain marked or complete relief of itching. Then each injection begins to provide longer relief. They can subsequently be spaced farther apart, say every other day for a few weeks, then twice a week for a few weeks, then once a week.

Each decrease in the injection schedule is predicated on obtaining continuing relief on the new schedule. Otherwise, reverting to a more frequent injection schedule again for a while may be needed. In any event, if itching does recur, it will usually improve markedly or clear completely in thirty minutes after a neutralizing injection.

When the itching fails to recur, the injections can be stopped. Even resistant cases can generally discontinue Candida injections after a two or three-month course of treatment, although in rare instances, treatment must continue longer.

Many patients with the Candida problem have inhalant sensitivity symptoms also and are receiving regular neutralizing injections for inhalants. As soon as the Candida neutralizing test is completed, the Candida neutralizing dose is added to the regular inhalant treatment set.

Then separate Candida injections can be skipped on days that the regular inhalant injection is given, and finally omitted altogether. By continuing only the regular inhalant injections, ongoing long-term protection is thus provided for Candida as well as for the other antigens in the inhalant treatment set.

If you are not suffering a resistant chronic Candida infection at the time of Candida testing, but give a history of having had repeated

Candida vaginitis in the recent past, the daily injections are not needed. The Candida neutralizing dose in the regular allergy injection is usually all that is required for protection from future attacks.

However, if an antibacterial antibiotic is prescribed at some future time, or if excessive sweets are eaten, a beginning flare-up may be noted. Then a few daily self-administered booster injections of the regular inhalant treatment are often enough to control the Candida flare-up.

At the other end of the spectrum are women with such severe vaginal candidiasis and irritative vaginal discharge that the entire vaginal orifice and the skin around it are reddened, swollen, and exquisitely painful. I have seen women with inflammatory skin lesions extending half way down the thighs and around the anus. Some have had to walk into the office with their legs spread apart in a broad, waddling gait because of the pain suffered when the sides of the vaginal orifice or the thighs rubbed together. Some have had painful ulcers of the vaginal orifice, and fissures around the anus where these areas had been irritated by the discharge.

These patients have had to have as many as four neutralizing doses of Candida extract per day for weeks. They also have had to apply soothing cortisone creams for several days, followed by antibiotic creams for the secondary infection. They were able to use anti-Candida vaginal inserts once the vaginal inflammation subsided enough that they could tolerate the insertion of medications into the vagina. They were also put on diets free of sweets and yeasts, and given a prescription for mycostatin tablets.

Response in such cases has been slow but steady. Complete resolution of the problem has been achieved in each case so far. A most gratifying response has been the change in facial expressions and outlook, from pained, grim, and desperate to smiling with delight.

The neutralizing dose is the mainstay of the treatment; and even after the lesions are no longer present, the neutralizing doses must be continued four times a day for weeks to prevent relapse. Reducing the dose too soon to three times a day has sometimes been sufficient to allow return of the itching, which promptly clears when the dose is increased again to four times a day.

During the course of the treatment, the neutralizing dose has sometimes changed one or more times with return of itching despite the neutralizing doses. Whenever this has occurred, retesting and using the new neutralizing dose has provided rapid relief of itching and resumption of healing.

All of this sounds like a lot to go through, but these patients have already received all that the gynecologist has to offer, and in fact have often been referred to me by the gynecologist. They have been suffering without respite for months and are happy to have a treatment that finally restores them to freedom from discomfort and disability.

ANTI-CANDIDA ANTIBIOTICS

What else do we have on our side? There are *anti-Candida antibiotics* which can be taken by mouth to reduce the Candida population in the lower gastrointestinal tract, which is its main den or home base. The most commonly used one is *mycostatin,* marketed also as Nilstat® or Nystatin®.

Mycostatin in the usual dosage needed passes along the gastrointestinal tract virtually unabsorbed into the circulation. It does its beneficial work in the digestive tract and then leaves the body. So if an anti-Candida antibiotic is needed, this is usually the first to be prescribed. Even so, it is not tolerated by some people. It is not needed very often in patients receiving Candida neutralizing treatment.

Mycostatin's benefit may not show up for days or weeks, although some patients report improvement within hours after a given dose. It may have to be continued for a long time, depending partly on what else is happening in the patient's life, such as sugar intake, the repeated use of antibacterial antibiotics, cortisones, birth control pills, immunosuppressives, diabetes, and endocrine changes.

There is a second anti-Candida antibiotic, *ketoconazole* (Nizoral®). I have not yet needed to prescribe it, but others report having used it judiciously and successfully in severe resistant cases. Some report combining long-term mycostatin therapy with one or more short courses of ketoconazole.

Amphotericin-B is a third anti-Candida antibiotic for oral use which has been employed for many years in other countries. It is available in the United States for intravenous use to help kill Candida organisms that have invaded the bloodstream or penetrated deeply into vital tissues. It is not available in its simple oral form in the United States, although it has been marketed here for some time in capsules in combination with tetracycline as Mysteclin-F®.

Tetracycline tends to increase Candida growth, as do all antibacterial antibiotics. However, Amphotericin-B is combined with tetracycline in

Mysteclin-F to nullify or at least decrease the tendency of tetracycline to increase the Candida population.

DIET

Another factor on our side is the *diet.* Simple sugars, and to a less extent complex carbohydrates, feed the yeast. If you cut refined sweets completely out of your diet, at least for a while, the response to neutralization or mycostatin or any other therapy usually will be much more rapid.

In resistant cases, mold and yeast-containing foods and possibly the more complex carbohydrates, including potatoes and cereal grains, may need to be removed for a while also. Some patients who are highly disciplined and organized about the diet may obtain marked relief from diet alone.

This diet contains only raw and cooked vegetables, fish, poultry, and meats. After this diet is established and relief obtained, each patient may add additional complex carbohydrates and fruits one at a time in a trial-and-error fashion. As the diet enlarges, red meats can be eaten less frequently for other health reasons if desired.

PROGESTERONE NEUTRALIZATION

Another weapon in our arsenal is *progesterone neutralization.* If the added hormonal burden causes premenstrual or menstrual flares of candidiasis, progesterone neutralization can often provide marked relief of both hormonally and yeast caused premenstrual symptoms. When needed, a combination of progesterone and Candida neutralizing doses can be even more effective.

NEUTRALIZATION OF FOODS, INHALANTS, AND CHEMICALS

The body is all of one piece. In fact, patients with allergies and multiple sensitivities to inhalants, foods, and chemicals seem to be the very ones who are most prone to Candida and premenstrual, menstrual, and other gynecologic problems. A combination of genetic tendency and altered resistance/burden ratio often disturbs multiple body functions simultaneously.

Most of the patients I see with premenstrual tension and Candida problems have really come to me primarily for their allergic rhinitis, sinusitis, asthma, skin allergies, food-caused syndromes such as migraine or colon problems, and other such illnesses in various combinations. Many children are brought with recurrent ear infections secondary to nasal allergy. Menstrual, yeast, and urinary discomforts are often present as secondary "nonallergic" complaints.

Gynecologists who use neutralization therapy tell me they have noted the opposite side of the same phenomenon. The patients who come to them primarily for yeast vaginitis, premenstrual and menstrual problems, infertility, and other hormonal dysfunctions and urinary complaints often turn out to have allergic rhinitis, sinusitis, asthma, food syndromes, and chemical susceptibilities as well.

They even tell me that toxemia of pregnancy is more prone to occur in these same type people and that toxemia can be exacerbated during periods of high pollen counts and by many of the same triggers we have noted in asthma, migraine, and other resistance/burden syndromes. Some pediatricians who use neutralization therapy feel that mothers with allergic syndromes seem more prone to produce offspring with many of these same problems, even including respiratory distress of the newborn (hyaline membrane disease) and respiratory allergies such as croup and asthma.

We are all becoming more and more aware that there is a large population out there attending a number of different specialty clinics, and receiving many different descriptive diagnoses, whose primary problem is really the altered resistance/burden ratio manifesting itself in a variety of syndromes. Most of these can be greatly helped by neutralization therapy and other measures described in this book. The yeast problem is just one aspect of a broader imbalance.

So we have other weapons to use when we need them. We can favorably alter the resistance/burden ratio in yeast patients and other indicated patients by neutralizing them to *inhalants, foods,* and *chemicals* when needed, as well as to the *Candida* and *progesterone* already mentioned.

THE PHYSICIAN'S ADDITIONAL ROLES

Allergists and environmentalists can also help you learn how to minimize your exposures to dusts, molds, animal skin scales, pollens, and chemicals to reduce the total body burden. We can teach you to read and understand food labels so as to reduce sugar and hidden food-allergen burdens.

We can also encourage you to live on simple, natural, wholesome nutritious foods obtained chiefly from the ordinary supermarket, foods which supply essential amino acids, essential fatty acids, possibly some complex starches, vitamins, minerals, and fiber. We can help you learn how to identify junk foods: factory-made foods with artificial colors, artificial flavors, preservatives, and thousands of other chemical ingredients that no cooks add to the foods they prepare in their own kitchens.

When antibiotics are needed, we can consider prescribing *narrow-spectrum antibiotics,* although we must remain aware that broad-spectrum antibiotics are sometimes required for the infection being treated, and that narrow-spectrum antibiotics can also cause overgrowth of Candida in many patients. We can prescribe *mycostatin* along with the antibacterial antibiotic when indicated in patients with the Candida tendency to minimize or nullify its Candida-stimulating effect.

We can also prescribe *anti-Candida vaginal creams or inserts* for temporary use under these circumstances when indicated. We can further prescribe *oral mycostatin suspensions* for infants. This suspension is also useful in some adults, to be vigorously swished around in the mouth, gargled, and then swallowed to reduce Candida in the mouth, pharnyx, and esophagus as well as the lower digestive tract.

LAXATIVES AND ENEMAS

We have already discussed the use of *relatively nonallergenic laxatives* (such as unflavored milk of magnesia, Magnesium Citrate Oral Solution, Fleet's Phospho-Soda®, and Epsom salts) or *cleansing enemas* to rid the body more quickly of allergenic foods. By cleansing enemas I mean repeated enemas until the final enema produces only relatively clear fluid, such as when being prepared for an x-ray of the colon. Since the greatest concentration of Candida is in the colon and lower small intestines, the same procedures can quickly reduce the Candida burden.

I am not advocating that one throw dietary precautions and other treatments to the winds and try to maintain relief with regularly taken laxatives and enemas. In the first place, it would not work. Second, it could be harmful. But in specific indicated infrequent times of increased need, it can be a very useful adjunctive treatment to provide greater and more rapid relief.

Dr. Denis Burkitt, the famous British researcher who described Burkitt's Lymphoma and popularized the value of dietary *fiber,* has also pointed out that bowel transit time can be speeded up by eating more fiber and starch and less fat and sugar. This should result in larger and more frequent bowel movements, and provide less time for food allergens, Candida, and carcinogens to exert their adverse effects on the colon.

In countries with high-fiber, low-fat, low-sweet diets, cancer of the colon is very infrequent. When people move from those countries to Western countries and partake of Western diets, their tendency to colon cancer greatly increases.

RESTORING BALANCE BY INDIVIDUALIZING TREATMENT

Many additional positive steps can be taken. However, very few patients need the entire range of treatment. Some need only one or two modalities. Each case is individualized.

The important things to remember are that we are all different, that we are bothered by different things to different degrees, that usually no one of these causative factors does it all, and that the final common pathway to illness is the disturbed overall resistance/burden ratio. Conversely, the road back to health is restoration of a better overall balance.

THE IMMUNORESTORATIVE SPECIFICITY OF NEUTRALIZATION THERAPY

The neutralization part of the treatment is specifically protective only for the adverse causative factors. It does not in any way suppress the entire immune mechanism like immunosuppressive drugs, but relieves it of many burdens. In fact, it leaves the defense mechanism *better* able to cope with intercurrent infections, allergy exposures, and other stresses. Thus neutralization is not immunosuppressive but *immunorestorative.*

THE DEVASTATING CEREBRAL EFFECTS OF CANDIDA SENSITIVITY

Up to this point, I have focused chiefly on oral and vaginal thrush. However, the Candida problem can be far greater than this.

A pioneer in this field, Dr. C. Orian Truss of Birmingham, Alabama has been collecting data for over twenty years on the effects of absorbed Candida antigens on the brain and other organs, and has published his observations in an excellent book, *The Missing Diagnosis.*[90] Another excellent book on this subject has been published by Dr. William Crook, *The Yeast Connection.*[91]

Both Dr. Truss and Dr. Crook point out that the brain seems particularly susceptible to Candida antigens. They cite cases of patients who show marked deleterious effects on their personalities, mood, and mental abilities when plagued with candidiasis; and who return toward normal when the Candida problem is controlled.

Some of the most characteristic symptoms described by Dr. Truss and Dr. Crook in Candida sensitivity are depression, irritability, anxiety, and uncontrollable crying, especially premenstrually. Intellectually, these patients may note difficulty concentrating, reasoning, and remembering.

In my experience, when these symptoms are limited to the premenstrual time, they are usually neutralizable by progesterone alone. When the symptoms are not related to the hormonal cycle, they are generally neutralizable by food, inhalant, and chemical extracts.

However, Candida-prone women do frequently suffer vaginal itching, urinary burning, and urinary frequency. The addition of candidiasis seems also to add to the total body burden in some.

This increase in body burden tends to cause other potential problems to surface or worsen. These include depression; migraine; irritable bowel syndrome; allergic asthma and hay fever; and all the food, inhalant, and chemical problems we have discussed in this book.

In occasional instances, management of candidiasis alone can decrease the total body burden sufficiently to result in marked relief. However, the *comprehensive* management system that considers each stress factor and its role in the individual patient is usually needed.

CAUGHT IN THE PSYCHOSOMATIC TRAP

When patients with so many problems are examined and tested by the finest of diagnosticians, the physical exam and the laboratory results are almost always negative or irrelevant to the problem. They not only fail to lead to a diagnosis, but also give no indication whatever of the real causes of the symptoms.

So these women are often labelled "functional" or "neurotic." The physician may reassure them, "You're just as healthy as I am." If tranquilizers fail, as they often do since they do not get at the cause of the problem and often cause side effects or allergic reactions in these patients, the women may be referred to a psychiatrist.

However, years of fine psychiatric treatment may be to little or no avail if the true organic etiologic factors remain unrecognized. This entire field is one in which psychiatrists as well as other physicians should become deeply interested and well informed.

CANDIDA IN MALES

This resistance/burden syndrome is more frequent in females, but occurs in males also. Candida antigens in the bloodstream add to the boy or man's total body burden.

However, in males it is expressed more commonly as bowel symptoms, easy fatigability, and cerebral symptoms. Memory, ability to concentrate, libido, and career potential may be affected.

Allergies and autoimmune diseases may be aggravated by the increased total burden. Other than the menstrual hormonal problems, men's symptoms are very similar to the symptoms of women.

PROBLEMS

Not all vaginal itching is due to Candida. Non-Candida organisms and many different strains of Candida itself can cause the same symptom. The husband may have Candida or other infections, and treatment of both husband and wife simultaneously may be necessary. A gynecologist or urologist may be needed for organisms or conditions for which no neutralizing extract is available.

The extra burden of dietary yeasts and airborne skin molds may in some instances require that neutralizing doses of these be included. A tip-off that dietary yeasts are involved may be supplied by a history of flare-ups from alcoholic beverages, bakery products or B-complex vitamins, or immediate relief of vaginal itching due to masking when these substances are ingested. The same may occur after entering a moldy basement, raking moldy leaves, or working in a moldy hothouse.

THE POSSIBLE NEED FOR RETESTING

The neutralizing dose of Candida required by the body tends to change more often than with foods and inhalants. When a patient has been doing well on Candida neutralizing injections and then the injections no longer work, it is not the fault of the treatment system but rather the change in the body's requirements.

However, there is no need to abandon the method or switch to less effective treatment systems. Retesting determines immediately the body's new neutralizing dose needs and provides quick relief again. Several such retestings may be necessary over a period of time.

"DIE-OFF" REACTIONS

Some patients note worsening of symptoms when they begin to take mycostatin or any other anti-Candida antibiotic. The worsening can be due to direct sensitivity to the drug but is often thought to be due to the killing of Candida by the mycostatin, with increased absorption of the products of killed Candida into the circulation.

This is usually a transient phenomenon, and the symptoms are generally those previously caused by Candida, not allergic reactions like hives. They gradually disappear quickly even when Candida treatment is continued, although the dose may need to be markedly reduced for a while.

This type reaction to a microbe-killing drug is called a "die-off" reaction. It is apparently a temporary reaction to the increased flood into the circulation of chemicals from the newly killed organisms.

However, some start the diet several days before starting the mycostatin in order to reduce the Candida population in advance. Some also use a laxative or cleansing enema a day or two before starting the mycostatin. The idea is to minimize this type reaction by reducing the Candida, carbohydrate, and food allergen content of the colon.

Obviously, we need much more research on neutralization therapy and the relative role of each substance that increases the total body burden. This should lead to greater understanding and more rational employment of various methods of therapy.

CHAPTER 25

NEUTRALIZATION OF MENSTRUAL AND PREMENSTRUAL SYNDROMES

If neutralization is so effective in food, inhalant, Candida, and so many other conditions, what could some of its other potential applications be? I spent a great deal of time in medical libraries seeking answers to these questions. Then some of my patients inadvertently supplied me with astounding breakthroughs.

NEUTRALIZATION OF INSULIN SENSITIVITY

The first patient, a five-year-old boy, had both asthma and diabetes. Then he became allergic to his insulin. Each time he took his daily therapeutic insulin injection he developed a severe headache and swelling of his face, eyelids, and parotid glands (the glands on each side of the jaw, the same glands that become swollen in mumps). His insulin was vital to his well-being, yet he was beginning to resist the injections because they made him so ill.

Faced with this serious problem, I made serial concentrations of his own vial of insulin and tested him in the neutralizing manner. I was able to provoke his headache and facial swelling with one concentration and relieve them with another.

I then had his mother give him a daily neutralizing dose of insulin about fifteen minutes before his regular insulin treatment injection, thus keeping him free of his symptoms. As far as I know, this was the first time in history that a sensitivity to insulin or any other hormone had been neutralized.

At first, any day that he failed to receive his neutralizing injection of insulin, he would again experience his headache and facial swelling after his therapeutic insulin injection. His mother became very careful to administer his neutralizing dose before every therapeutic dose of insulin, thus providing complete protection from insulin sensitivity reactions.

After a few months, she inadvertently failed to do so on one occasion, and he evidenced no ill effect. I then advised her to start spacing his injections out to whatever was the minimum frequency of need. After about five months he required his neutralizing injections only once a week, despite the fact that he was receiving therapeutic injections of insulin daily.

Surprisingly, by the end of a year the neutralizing injections were no longer needed! He could take his therapeutic insulin injections without preceding neutralizing injections. This was an unexpected indication that a very high degree of *long-lasting* protection, improved homeostasis, or favorably altered resistance/burden ratio had occurred.

NEUTRALIZATION OF PROGESTERONE-RELATED SYMPTOMS

At about this same time I was testing a young lady with food extracts for severe headaches. One morning when she arrived at the office for testing she complained that she was having very severe menstrual cramps.

Although she had hoped to be able to test that day, she now felt that she would have to go back home, take a pain pill and lie down with a heating pad on her abdomen. She said, "I wish you had something in your bag of tricks for my menstrual cramps."

What could be causing her menstrual cramps? It was certainly related to hormones; and I had already discovered that I could neutralize symptoms due to a hormone, insulin.

Two weeks before each menstrual period, at the time of ovulation, an egg is released from the ovary and the blood level of progesterone starts rising rapidly. If the egg is not fertilized, the progesterone level rises for only one week after ovulation and then starts falling. At the onset of menstruation the progesterone level is falling most rapidly and is approaching its original low baseline level.

Could progesterone withdrawal be responsible for premenstrual symptoms during the last few days before menstruation? Could the resistance/burden equation to progesterone be knocked out of kilter by the rapid decline of the progesterone level?

Progesterone is probably the most innocuous hormone in female gynecology. It is often beneficial, rarely harmful. It is self-made by the ovaries each month, present in all healthy adult females from puberty to menopause, and produced by the placenta in about fifteen times the usual amount for the full nine months of pregnancy.

I did not know if my concepts were correct, or if progesterone neutralization would be effective. However, I discussed it thoroughly with my patient and her gynecologist. Together, we decided we could do no harm with the tiny amount required for testing, and might well do much good.

I made serial dilutions of the standard progesterone suspension and performed the neutralizing test. When the neutralizing dilution was administered, her cramps began lessening in three minutes and by thirty minutes they were completely gone!

One amazing thing about neutralization is that such tiny doses provide such large benefits. The dose of progesterone that provided relief was about one six-thousandth the dose that is ordinarily used in gynecologic practice.

She remained symptom free for eighteen hours and then returned to the office the next day with cramps again. I repeated the neutralizing dose. This again relieved her completely within thirty minutes and the pain did not recur during that monthly cycle.

During the next four cycles she required only 2 to 4 neutralizing injections per cycle to maintain complete freedom from cramps. After the fourth cycle, she remained ready to use the injections whenever the cramps should return, but they never returned! Again a strange and unexpected *long-lasting* homeostasis, favorably altered resistance/burden ratio, or recurrence prevention had occurred.

Although this long-lasting relief has been a surprising phenomenon, it is impossible to doubt. It has been confirmed in many patients by me and other physicians including gynecologists who use progesterone neutralization. The vast majority of patients—not all—develop virtually total, long-lasting, or apparently permanent prevention of recurrent premenstrual and menstrual symptoms after three to six months of neutralization therapy, usually using only a few tiny but precisely quantitated injections of progesterone with each monthly cycle.

THE USES OF PROGESTERONE NEUTRALIZATION

Progesterone neutralization seems to be effective for most of the discomforts that occur each month in relationship to the menstrual cycle. It usually provides great relief from all or most of the premenstrual syndrome with its many discomforts. These include premenstrual breast tenderness, irritability, headache, fluid retention; and monthly flareups of other syndromes such as migraine, asthma, nasal congestion, urticaria, cyclic menstrual acne, and many bizarre mental and behavioral reactions.[4]

It also often provides great relief from menstrual cramps and the various other symptoms that occur during the menstrual period itself. It generally increases scant flows toward normal, and reduces heavy flows toward normal as well.

In addition, it usually relieves the pain of endometriosis, and shrinks the swollen endometrial nodules. This can obviate the need for surgery to remove the nodules which would otherwise enlarge with each period and press painfully against adjacent organs.

It usually alleviates the nausea and vomiting of pregnancy, as well as intolerance to birth control pills. For a great number of suffering women, it is a welcome source of relief.

It is sometimes, but not always, effective for ovulation pain. Ovulation pain might respond better to neutralizing doses of the pituitary hormones that control ovulation.

As mentioned earlier, adult acne can be cyclic, and is then relieved by progesterone neutralizing injections administered during the cycle as described. Adult acne can also be chronic, that is, not related to menstrual cycles; in which case it is usually caused by foods and is relieved by regular administration of food extract neutralizing injections, or avoidance of the causative foods.

Adolescent acne responds to neither. If we had an extract of the causative self-substance in adolescent acne, this situation might well be remedied and adolescent acne be greatly reduced or eliminated.

ESTROGEN NEUTRALIZATION

Progesterone does not always relieve all of the symptoms surrounding the menstrual cycle. At times, despite great relief with progesterone neutralization, there are slight secondary residual symptoms, such as a feeling of frigidity or mild depression. These residual symptoms can sometimes be cleared with estrogen neutralizing doses. The estrogen I have used most commonly has been Premarin®. But Premarin has been of little or no value for the primary symptoms of the premenstrual or menstrual period.

However, Premarin neutralization has turned out to be very effective in most cases of chronic cystic mastitis, that is, fibrocystic breast disease. Here the breast pain is not related to menstrual cycles.

When the neutralizing dose of Premarin is administered during testing in chronic cystic mastitis, the breast pain and tenderness which has been present daily for months or years usually becomes markedly better or completely clear in thirty minutes! Whenever the pain returns, another dose administered at home provides relief again in thirty minutes. The breast masses shrink in size hour by hour or day by day, until soon they are usually completely gone.

While progesterone neutralization is effective for premenstrual breast tenderness, it is not helpful in the breast tenderness of chronic cystic mastitis. Conversely, Premarin neutralization is of no value for premenstrual breast tenderness. In chronic cystic mastitis, Premarin neutralizing doses seem to give the same rapid and *long-lasting* relief as does progesterone for premenstrual mastitis, and usually only a few tiny doses have been needed to provide years of relief.

ESTRONE NEUTRALIZATION

Neither progesterone nor Premarin neutralization has been effective in relieving menopausal symptoms. I was puzzled by this until I was reminded by Dr. Richard Mabray, a board certified gynecologist of Victoria, Texas, that the predominant circulating female sex hormone of menopausal women was estrone.

Sure enough, neutralizing doses of estrone were found to relieve many of the discomforts of menopause not relieved by oral estrogen therapy. Estrone is marketed under the trade names of Theelin® and Urestrin®.

Incidentally, Dr. Mabray has developed a great deal of experience in neutralization therapy. He and his four gynecologist associates have confirmed my results in more than a thousand patients over the past ten years.

They have published a paper in the journal *Obstetrics and Gynecology*[92] to make other gynecologists aware of the benefits of progesterone neutralization. The same beneficial results are being obtained by many gynecologists, psychiatrists, internists, allergists, and other physicians who use these procedures.

SUBCUTANEOUS PROGESTERONE TESTING

Large conventional-sized doses of progesterone have been reported to sometimes cause local reactions in the tissues, such as redness, tenderness, and swelling at the site of injection. Progesterone concentrate has been observed to occasionally cause a similar local reaction when used intradermally in testing.

When injected in the arm subcutaneously in the tiny doses required for neutralizing testing and treatment, I have never seen a significant local reaction. Therefore I perform this test with subcutaneous test injections in the deltoid area of the upper arm.

A second reason I use subcutaneous test injections for progesterone is that progesterone does not produce reliably positive or negative wheals when used intradermally. There is thus no advantage in the intradermal route of testing for progesterone.

Since the test is performed subcutaneously, there is no wheal guide to the neutralizing dose, so symptoms are the only guide available. Therefore the patient must come to the office while she is experiencing her *natural* symptoms.

The subcutaneous dose that best relieves the natural symptoms in the office within thirty minutes is the neutralizing dose. This is the treatment dose that will be used by the patient for self-administration at home whenever the symptoms recur.

RELIEVING SEVERE MENSTRUAL CRAMPS

Menstrual cramps can be excruciating. It is very difficult for some women to sit in the office for testing at the height of their pain.

These women almost always have some milder premenstrual symptom before the onset of cramping, and this milder symptom can be used as a guide for finding the neutralizing dose. The dose that relieves the premenstrual irritability, headache, or breast tenderness is the same dose that will prevent and relieve the severe cramps which come later.

Therefore these women are tested premenstrually when possible. The treatment injections are thus begun before the severe cramps would be expected to occur—and the cramps are often prevented or minimized.

If no such premenstrual symptoms are available as test guides, a tolerated pain pill for menstrual cramps can be given if necessary to take the edge off the pain during testing. The neutralizing concentration is the concentration that finally makes the relief of cramps complete or most nearly so.

These women are extremely grateful patients because their pain was usually so incapacitating and unbearable before using treatment injections. There are literally millions of such women with little hope in sight, and with no awareness of the relief they would likely obtain with progesterone neutralization therapy.

TESTING FOR ADULT PREMENSTRUAL ACNE

Another variation in testing has to do with adult premenstrual acne. This presents no test problems if the acne is accompanied by premenstrual symptoms, as the dose that relieves the premenstrual symptoms also helps the acne.

But acne alone does not produce a symptom that can be neutralized in thirty minutes. Rather the acne lesions or "bumps" occur on a day-by-day basis just before and during the menstrual period. Therefore, if acne is the only manifestation which occurs, only one test strength can be given per month, and it is given once daily premenstrually for a few days to determine if this is the neutralizing dose.

For example, the first test dose is given daily in the office beginning the first day that cyclic acne lesions would be expected to occur, or when in fact some do first occur. The same dose is repeated each day until the menstrual flow is established. If no further acne lesions occur, this is the neutralizing dose.

If the first test concentration does not prevent the occurrence of daily lesions in that particular cycle, then at the following cycle, when acne lesions are expected to occur or in fact do begin to occur, a different test dose is administered daily for three or four days in the office to see if this will prevent the occurrence of acne. If not, then the following month yet another concentration is used, and so on. Most patients require only one or two such monthly test sessions.

This test requires that the patient count and record the *new* bumps each morning. She reports this "bump count" to the physician so he can assess the value of each preceding day's test injection.

After the neutralizing dose has been determined, the patient can then self-administer one injection daily for 4 or 5 days per cycle. This series of daily injections should begin on the day that acne lesions would be expected to begin or when they in fact do begin. This usually prevents the acne from occurring. After four or five cycles, the acne often does not recur, and the injections can be discontinued.

A similar one-test-dose-per-day procedure in the office is sometimes needed with estrone testing for menopausal symptoms. This is because menopausal symptoms may occur at night or at other times than during office hours. The physician may need to choose the neutralizing dose based on reported freedom from menopausal symptoms the night before due to the dose given the previous day. Since menopausal symptoms occur daily rather than monthly, the neutralizing dose can usually be determined in just a few days.

"MORNING SICKNESS"

If the egg is fertilized, the progesterone level does not decline after one week. Rather, it continues to rise. The placenta then forms in the womb and becomes a giant progesterone factory, producing fifteen times the blood level of progesterone as was produced by the ovary.

This extra progesterone makes many pregnant women feel great. Others seem to be made sick by it. They may develop "morning sickness," the nausea and vomiting of pregnancy.

This may last for many months, and some women are virtually housebound by this problem. The nausea can be relieved in thirty minutes by progesterone neutralizing testing in the office, and each recurrence of nausea usually can be eliminated in minutes by a self-administered subcutaneous neutralizing injection.

Women can thus go about their usual activities, and working women can ordinarily keep working. They may begin to feel nausea returning one or more times a day while on the job, but can obtain relief in minutes each time by self-administration at work of one of their tiny progesterone neutralizing doses.

NEUTRALIZATION OF INTOLERANCE TO CONTRACEPTIVE PILLS

Progestins are not the same as progesterone. Progesterone is a natural hormone, destroyed by digestion, and is therefore not effective when taken by mouth. Progestins are synthetic progesterone-like compounds which can be administered by mouth in contraceptive pills and in other formulations to achieve some of the benefits of progesterone.

It is these orally effective progestins that make contraceptive pills possible. Interestingly, many of the unpleasant side effects of contraceptive pills can often be relieved with progesterone neutralizing doses. Again, a *long-lasting or permanent* protection is soon usually achieved which allows the continued use of contraceptive pills without requiring long-continued neutralization treatment.

PRODUCT PROBLEMS

There are several potential problems in therapy with progesterone of which everyone should be aware. A few studies have led the FDA to suggest that progesterone should not be administered during the first four months of pregnancy. According to some researchers, it may possibly cause a delay in spontaneous abortion in case the fetus is defective, and possibly it may also seriously affect a normally developing fetus.

However, these studies were not performed using the tiny doses employed in neutralization therapy. Furthermore, many factors can cause birth defects. It is difficult for me to believe that progesterone, a beneficial and even necessary hormone for establishing and maintaining a pregnancy, can be responsible for birth defects, especially when administered in such tiny doses as in neutralization therapy. In fact, gynecologists have told me that many of their infertility cases were enabled to conceive and deliver normal infants once they had undergone progesterone neutralization therapy for premenstrual or menstrual problems.

Even so, the possibility of pregnancy should not be a problem in treating either an already established premenstrual syndrome or menstrual cramps. The presence of these symptoms indicates that the egg has *not* been fertilized, the patient has *not* become pregnant, the progesterone level is declining, and in fact the menstrual cycle is imminent or already under way. However, the premenstrual symptoms must be carefully distinguished from the breast soreness, increased frequency of urination, and morning sickness which often occur in early pregnancy.

Until this conflict has been resolved, if you are going to be tested with progesterone, you must be sure that you are not pregnant. Also, if you become pregnant while taking progesterone neutralizing doses, you must consult your physician about possibly discontinuing the neutralizing doses. I do not believe that the FDA position presents a problem in the use of progesterone neutralizing injections for morning sickness after the first four months of pregnancy.

In neutralizing doses, the benefit/risk ratio for a severely nauseated or vomiting woman in early pregnancy may be in favor of using the progesterone anyway. However, this is a decision to be decided jointly by you and your obstetrician.

Second, progesterone usage should be avoided in the face of undiagnosed vaginal bleeding or a missed period. The cause of the bleeding or the miss should be determined before progesterone use is considered. Vaginal bleeding may be caused by a more serious problem requiring a higher priority for treatment.

THE MAGNITUDE OF PROGESTERONE-CAUSED ILLNESS

Not everyone with premenstrual symptoms or menstrual cramps has severe enough problems to warrant therapy. On the other hand, these cyclic changes make many women extremely miserable.

Every woman should read the book *Once A Month* by Dr. Katharina Dalton.[93] This distinguished British physician is an acknowledged authority on "the part played by menstrual dysfunction in confused and criminal behavior, accidents, drug abuse, and morbidity" (Foreword). The first sentence in the book is, "Once-a-month, with monotonous regularity, chaos is inflicted on American homes as premenstrual tension and other menstrual problems recur time and again with demoralizing repetition" (p. X1).

Dr. Dalton estimates that over 5.5 million American women suffer severely with incapacitating monthly problems (p. XII). The number is far larger than this when we include those who are made extremely uncomfortable, though not totally incapacitated.

The premenstrual syndrome is said to be "the commonest cause of marital breakdown" (p. XII). There is "a seven-fold increase (in suicide rate) in the second half of the menstrual cycle" (p. XII). "Shoplifting is thirty times commoner in the second half of the cycle" (p. XII). "Half of all women's attempts at suicide are made during the four days immediately before or the first four days of menstruation" (p. 25).

She also cites figures showing increased mental hospital admissions, attempted homicides as well as suicides, alcoholism, baby-battering, criminal behavior, epilepsy, and asthma in the second half of the monthly cycle. She describes patient after patient with severe depression, tiredness, irritability, sleep disturbances, violent dreams, heart pounding, manic behavior, "stupidness," or apathy (pp. 3–32).

She also states, "In Britain, a survey of 156 newly committed women prisoners revealed that half had committed their crime during the paramenstruum (the four days before and the four days during the period), and in fact the premenstrual syndrome was present in two-thirds of these women who committed their crimes during the paramenstruum." She also cites studies done in Paris and New York that confirm the British findings (p. 32).

Dr. Dalton further points out that human and economic losses are caused by the premenstrual syndrome. Absenteeism from work and school occurs during the paramenstruum. Production rates fall off. The manual dexterity and dependability of production workers decline.

Time and monetary loss result from misfiling, mistyping, and lack of inspiration suffered by people in creative professions. They also result from irritability and bad tempers in receptionists, salespeople, waitresses, and others in the public eye. There can be poorer judgment and poorer decision-making ability in teachers, legislators, business women, attorneys, judges, jurors, and others in responsible positions. Imagine the many problems of children whose mothers or baby sitters have this syndrome, and of school children who have teachers with it.

SIMILAR OBSERVATIONS AND DIFFERENT TREATMENTS

It is interesting how Dr. Dalton's observations closely parallel mine, and how we both were moved to make these observations by our own personal symptoms. Her symptom, like mine, was migraine.

The difference was that my migraine was an everyday matter for three years and was due to foods. Hers was an every month problem, occurring premenstrually. Her only time of prolonged relief had been during her pregnancies (p. 50). Just as I was enabled to grasp that migraine can be due to food allergy by my own migraine/food correlation, she was enabled to connect migraine with premenstrual progesterone imbalance because of her own premenstrual migraine flareups.

During her first month in practice she saw two women with premenstrual asthma, two with premenstrual epilepsy, and one with premenstrual migraine. Suddenly, she became aware of the great frequency and major problems involved with the menstrual cycle.

This was quickly followed by observation of many other premenstrual complaints including bouts of allergic rhinitis, hoarseness, loss of sense of smell, vertigo, fainting, joint and muscle pains, acne, boils, styes, herpes, conjunctivitis, food cravings, alcoholic bouts, and mouth ulcers. She also noted the onset of attacks of symptoms after a long interval without food (food withdrawal symptoms) during the premenstruum.

These are the types of symptoms my own patients are relieved of, chiefly through neutralization with progesterone and foods. Inhalant neutralization may be useful in premenstrual allergic rhinitis, asthma, hoarseness, and other respiratory syndromes. But progesterone neutralization alone is all that is needed in many cases.

All this should be great news for women with paramenstrual problems, the world's most common disease. *If women are looking for liberation, they should look first for liberation from the physical and mental tyranny so often imposed by their improper bodily responses to their own hormones.*

THE DISTURBING NEWS ABOUT PROGESTERONE AVAILABILITY

Yet Dr. Dalton's book, like this chapter, ends on a sad note. Progesterone aqueous suspension is no longer manufactured in America.

Many products containing natural progesterone or synthetic progesterone-like compounds are used in tremendous quantities in the United Sates and throughout the world. They are available in such forms as suppositories, tablets, depot injections, and birth control pills. Even the aqueous suspension is still manufactured in other countries.

Why is such a safe, sorely needed, and remarkably effective product no longer produced in America? It disappeared from the market when the FDA, during a study of progesterone in a long-term review of all old drugs, announced that manufacturers must file an N.D.A., a New Drug Application.

An N.D.A. is very expensive. Manufacturers avoid filing one when possible. Until neutralization was discovered, the market for the aqueous suspension was small and there was little profit in it.

Hopefully the potentially tremendous new market afforded by neutralizing usage can bring progesterone aqueous suspension back to America, especially in the extremely limited dosage and manner required in neutralization therapy. Many highly potent and potentially far more dangerous drugs are marketed with limitations and precautions simply printed on the labels or package inserts. I see no reason why progesterone aqueous suspension could not be handled similarly.

THE NEED FOR PROGESTERONE AVAILABILITY

Many people have a great stake in the renewed availability of progesterone for suffering women and the impact of their recurring monthly problems on the women themselves and others around them. This would include not only female support groups but also those who employ or deal with female personnel, such as giant corporations, municipalities, regulatory agencies, storekeepers, restaurant chains, law enforcement and penal institutions, gynecologists, pediatricians, and other medical groups, school boards, teacher organizations, PTA's, children support groups, personnel managers, marital counselors, perplexed husbands, divorce lawyers, and judges.

As mentioned, there are many drugs on the market which are much more powerful and potentially much more dangerous. Physicians are allowed and expected to use their own judgments in prescribing these, as well as in performing hazardous surgical procedures, using high-powered radiation therapies, and handling life-threatening illnesses and invasive diagnostic procedures and treatments of all kinds.

Natural progesterone is one of the safest drugs imaginable. It is a constituent of every normal woman's body, and every woman who has ever been pregnant has been exposed to very high blood levels of her own progesterone for nine months. It is unique and invaluable, not in a rare disease but in the world's most common disease.

Progesterone neutralization can spare women hospitalization and surgery for removal of excruciatingly painful breasts, for removal of unbearably painful endometrial nodules, and for hysterectomies because of severe recurrent menstrual cramps. It can save lives, careers, marriages, families, wife-battering, child-battering, office and emergency room visits, hospitalizations, crime problems, court proceedings, jail sentences, mental institutionalizations, and industrial and financial losses.

Weighing possible risk against possible benefit, the decision is obvious. *Progesterone aqueous suspension must be made available again.* It is one of the least harmful and most beneficial drugs around. The doses required are almost infinitesimal, and the course of treatment is usually brief.

ADDITIONAL BENEFITS

As important as progesterone relief is, a still greater ultimate benefit might well lie in the use of progesterone neutralization to demonstrate to researchers that self-substances in general can cause illness, and that neutralization with extracts of self-substances can restore health. Investigators may well find answers to many other ills once they focus on these phenomena and begin studying the adverse effects of various hormones, immune complexes, and other self-substances and the role of neutralization in providing relief.

Chapter 26

NEUTRALIZATION OF INFLUENZA AND HERPES VIRUS INFECTIONS

In the fall of 1968, the news media issued repeated warnings from the United States Public Health Service of an imminent epidemic of "Hong Kong Flu." The epidemic was expected to occur during the winter of 1968–69.

Strong recommendations were made for all elderly patients and those with chronic or debilitating diseases to be immunized. The vaccine to be used was the newly available Hong Kong Flu vaccine (Influenza Virus Vaccine, Monovalent, Type A_2, A_2/Aichi/2/68 Hong Kong Variant, 400 CCA units per cc).

Many of my patients with asthma and other chronic allergic illnesses responded to these requests for immunization. The very cooperative mother of a bright-eyed eleven-year-old girl brought her daughter for a "flu shot" on December 5, 1968.

This was a child I knew quite well. I had tested and treated her very successfully for multiple inhalant, food, and chemical sensitivities. I gave her the immunizing injection as requested, and expected to hear nothing further.

The next day, mother and daughter were back in my office. The formerly grateful mother was now angry and critical. "You've given my child the flu," she raged. Sure enough, the child was obviously suffering influenza-type symptoms, with bleary eyes, runny nose, sore throat, foggy mind, feelings of great weakness and malaise, and typical painful aching in the muscles of her back and neck.

Apparently the child's symptoms were a reaction to the previous day's immunizing injection, a not uncommon occurrence. However, the viruses in the vaccine are not living viruses, and could not have caused an active virus infection.

I explained to the mother that I had not "given her child the flu," but that her child was most likely having an immunologic reaction to the protein of the killed viruses in the vaccine. In further explanation, I used the analogy of provocation of test symptoms. This was something with which she was very familiar because her daughter had been very clearly provoked and neutralized during testing with many allergenic extracts.

"It's like a neutralizing test," I explained, "with symptoms from the provoking dose of an allergen."

"Well," she snapped, "go ahead and *neutralize* it!"

My mind nearly exploded. Neutralize a reaction to a *virus* vaccine? But then, why not? I had already neutralized many allergic reactions to extracts of various foods, inhalants, and other substances. I had seen innumerable patients with resistant vaginal Candida yeast *infections* obtain relief of vaginal itching within thirty minutes from a neutralizing dose of Candida extract. Patients with skin infections due to Candida yeast as well as to Trichophyton and Epidermophyton molds had responded similarly. Patients with "ringworm" (fungus infections of the skin caused by species of Microspora molds) had noted marked improvement from neutralization with Microspora extracts.

I had been thinking about the implications of this for neutralizing other viral and fungal infections, pneumococcal and other bacterial infections, and parasitic infestations, but had not yet had an opportunity to explore these possibilities. The more we discussed this, the more insistent the mother became. Here was a golden opportunity to use a perfectly safe vaccine in tiny dosage on a consenting and even demanding patient, with no risk of harm and with possible great future benefits for her and many others.

I immediately made 1:5 serial concentrations of Influenza Virus Vaccine, and performed the test. *The neutralizing dose completely cleared all her symptoms in thirty minutes!*

The same symptoms returned each day for three additional days, and each day a single neutralizing dose in the office completely cleared the symptoms in thirty minutes or less, under my unbelieving eyes. The mother was grateful but not nearly so impressed as I; she had seen her daughter neutralized to so many other materials that she regarded this as a natural, expected phenomenon. She was solely interested in her daughter's release from the grip of illness, being unaware and doubtless uncaring of the key role she and her daughter were playing in what might become a historic health breakthrough for mankind.

Over the next two weeks, I confirmed this thirty-minute neutralizing response in twelve patients suffering symptoms from Influenza Virus

Vaccine immunization. Then on December 18, 1968, a fourteen-year-old boy was brought in with typical active influenza virus *infection,* with much malaise, fever, weakness, and "aching all over."

When I entered the examining room, he was lying listlessly and uncommunicatively on the examining table. This child, too, was an old patient. He had been tested and treated by the neutralizing method for asthma and allergic rhinitis and had made the typical rapid response. When I recounted my experiences to his mother, she was eager to seek rapid relief of her son's symptoms.

Again neutralization was achieved quickly. *In thirty minutes* he was free of all malaise, weakness, and aching; and was sitting up, chatting, and alert. However, his fever was unchanged.

Over the next three days, his symptoms recurred five times, and each time a neutralizing dose cleared them in thirty minutes. The fever disappeared the first night, after the third injection, a fairly typical pattern I have observed many times since.

The epidemic that winter was a fairly large one. In all, I neutralized thirty-five patients in the same manner. Complete or partial relief was obtained in 96 percent of patients.

THE CONFIRMATION OF MY DISCOVERY BY OTHERS

I then described my experiences to Dr. Carleton Lee of St. Joseph, Missouri; to Dr. Edward Binkley of Denver, Colorado; and to Dr. Sterling Hardt of Harlingen, Texas. All three were intrigued by my story, and all very quickly confirmed my results in their own practices.

In March, 1969, I presented my first seminar on neutralization therapy in Mobile, Alabama. Approximately a hundred physicians attended. I described my results in influenza and asked those physicians to join with me in an informal clinical study of Influenza Virus Vaccine neutralization.

Could they duplicate my results in influenza? Was it effective for *only* influenza, or could this represent a nonspecific stimulant of the immune mechanism for many virus infections and possibly other immunologic problems?

Over the next few months, telephone calls and letters from excited physicians began arriving. (Such communications are still coming in.) Their experiences duplicated mine!

What they reported was that Influenza Virus Vaccine neutralization was not effective in the common run of virus infections seen in everyday office practice, but was usually highly effective for influenza. Furthermore, it was similarly effective for herpes-caused fever blisters! Some mailed me before-and-after pictures of herpes patients, including one with herpes of the eye.

Next, reports started coming in of similar responses in patients with genital herpes. Then Dr. Pete Brown of Gadsden, Alabama, informed me of his successful neutralization of shingles (herpes zoster). I confirmed all these responses in my own patients with these conditions. I also produced similar responses in patients with chickenpox (varicella), "mono" (infectious mononucleosis), and a severe long-lasting disease called chronic Epstein-Barr Virus infection. All of these are caused by herpes viruses. My findings in these syndromes have been confirmed by my colleagues.

I then organized a group of eight physicians in various cities to join with me in a study of active influenza virus infections, using a common protocol. We pooled a total of 125 influenza patients and obtained moderate to complete relief in 87 percent.

Since then I have continued using this method successfully every year during influenza virus epidemics, and throughout the year for various herpes virus infections. The same beneficial results have continued to occur.

I have presented this material at international, national, regional, state, and local medical symposia. I have also sponsored many internationally attended seminars in which I have described these results.

These seminars have been attended by a growing number of physicians. In addition, many physicians from the various states and from other countries have visited my office each year to learn neutralizing procedures first-hand. I have published two papers on Influenza Virus Vaccine neutralization in internationally circulated medical journals and two additional papers in state journals.[5,12,13,94]

So I have reached over two thousand physicians personally in my seminars and office courses, and many thousands more through lectures and publications. I believe that there are at least three thousand physicians in the United States using this procedure, and know that there are physicians in foreign countries using it also.

All the physicians I have discussed this with have had the same general results as I, and I have heard of no contradictory reports. However, no treatment is effective in 100 percent of patients, and we all experience occasional nonresponding and poorly responding patients.

RETESTING

Dose Change: This is all good news for such sufferers; but, as with all medical therapy, there is a bit of bad news also. The dose must be precise, and the body can inexplicably change its dosage requirement at any time.

Dose-change can even occur within hours after the initial test, although this is rare. Therefore, the test may need to be repeated at any time.

Of course, if each treatment injection using the dose determined by the first test continues to provide marked relief in thirty minutes, retesting is not necessary. If there is any question of this, or if the patient comes from a great distance, I usually repeat the test at least once, preferably the next day.

This greatly reduces the dose-change problem. However, I remind the patient to return for a retest any time his injections fail to provide adequate relief or cause worsening of his symptoms.

SENSITIVITY TO VACCINE INGREDIENTS

Influenza Virus Vaccine is made from viruses grown in living chick embryos. If a patient is very sensitive to egg, chicken, or feathers, or to any ingredient in the vaccine, such as thimerosal (a mercury derivative), he probably should not be tested. If he has ever had a severe reaction to an immunizing injection of Influenza Virus Vaccine, great judgment must be exercised before deciding to test. However, these are all uncommon situations, and most people can be safely tested and treated.

CHAPTER 27

INFLUENZA AND HERPES TREATMENT AND RESPONSES

Now let us focus our attention on the specific situations in which Influenza Virus Vaccine neutralization can be effective. In this chapter, we will first consider aspects of treatment of influenza virus infections, and then of herpes virus infections.

I. INFLUENZA VIRUS VACCINE FOR INFLUENZA NEUTRALIZATION

As I have described, a patient with an adverse allergic reaction to an *immunizing* dose of Influenza Virus Vaccine usually can be markedly or completely relieved by the *neutralizing* dose. *One* neutralizing dose is usually sufficient to permanently terminate the entire adverse reaction. Only in occasional instances have symptoms recurred, and these symptoms have usually been eliminated by one or two additional neutralizing doses.

INFLUENZA VIRUS INFECTIONS

When the symptoms are caused by a live influenza virus *infection*, symptoms tend to persist longer, so additional neutralizing doses are needed. They should be repeated whenever symptoms begin to recur. The times of symptom recurrences are variable, but each recurrence usually can be quickly diminished or eliminated in thirty minutes by self-administration of the neutralizing injection.

Often three such injections are needed the first day, two the second day, and one the third day. After that, if further doses are required, each dose will usually relieve in thirty minutes and last about twenty-four hours.

When I describe this schedule, some say, "Influenza is just a three-day illness anyway, so what have you accomplished?" The fact is that influenza is usually a problem for far more than three days. The fever may subside in three days; but the discomforts, weakness, and secondary complications tend to linger much longer.

Absenteeism from work, school, and normal activities is often prolonged. Some patients have persistent weakness for weeks or months; some seem to get well and then relapse with full return of the original symptoms; and some develop persistent secondary infections of the sinuses, ears, bronchi, or lungs.

Pneumonia is a serious and highly fatal complication in infants; the elderly; and patients with chronic illnesses or on chemotherapy, immunosuppressives, or long-term cortisone therapy. Most of these complications and other problems seem to have been markedly diminished in patients who have been neutralized early in the illness. Such patients have been spared much prolonged suffering and expense.

In addition, neutralized patients do not have to experience even the initial three days of misery. Usually they are nearly or completely protected from symptoms during the first three days, except for the few minutes in which they begin to perceive symptoms returning. They can immediately self-administer a neutralizing dose which usually will abort these symptoms in thirty minutes.

PERSISTENCE OF INFLUENZA VIRUS INFECTION

Even if influenza symptoms tend to persist, you usually can keep yourself relieved throughout the persistence by continuing your neutralizing injections. Each such additional injection ordinarily provides twenty-four hour relief.

As long as complete relief is obtained after each injection, the dose is correct and retesting is not necessary. If relief is not complete, or nearly so, retesting can be performed to seek the optimal dose.

INFLUENZA RELAPSE

If you become completely free of all signs of influenzal illness for days or weeks and then symptoms return, this is a relapse. The neutralizing injection can be readministered and, if the dose is still correct, total and permanent relief of the relapse usually occurs after *one* such injection. If symptoms should recur later, the neutralizing injection can be repeated with each recurrence until the symptoms no longer recur. If symptoms do not respond maximally, your body's dosage needs may have changed, indicating the need for retesting.

DOSE CHANGES

If a patient with acute influenza obtains complete relief from the first few neutralizing doses and then incomplete relief or worsening of symptoms from subsequent injections of the same dose, his neutralizing dose needs have probably changed during therapy. Retesting determines the new neutralizing dose, which then usually provides complete or near-complete relief again. Of course, secondary bacterial infections or other complications must also be sought for and treated appropriately.

OFFICE AND HOSPITAL USE OF INFLUENZA NEUTRALIZATION

If your physician prefers office administration of treatment doses, he can simply repeat the neutralizing dose injection daily in the office. In more severe cases, he can have his patients come to the office for treatment injections twice daily the first day or two.

In grave situations, the patient can be hospitalized and administered the injections on a regular schedule such as every three hours day and night, or even more frequently. Each dose is usually beneficial for the viral part of the illness, and the cumulative effects of frequent multiple correct doses have often been even more beneficial. In some instances, antibacterial antibiotics, cardiopulmonary medications, and other supportive measures may also be needed.

II. INFLUENZA VIRUS VACCINE FOR HERPES NEUTRALIZATION

The test procedure and the achievement of relief when the neutralizing dose is administered usually are the same in herpes as in influenza. Patients who are experiencing pain from fever blisters, herpetic eye or ear lesions, genital herpes, or shingles often note marked or complete relief in thirty minutes when the neutralizing test injection is administered.

The same is frequently true for the malaise or prostration of chickenpox, and the severe sore throat and debility of infectious mononucleosis.

As in influenza, herpes symptoms do tend to recur, but the symptoms of each recurrence are usually relieved in thirty minutes by self-administration of a subcutaneous injection of the treatment dose at home. Response occurs in both local symptoms (such as pain at the site of a blister) and generalized symptoms (such as malaise and listlessness). The lesions of herpes simplex I and II usually show progressive healing within a few hours after each such injection and reach the dry scab stage much more rapidly than in previous recurrences, thus greatly shortening the attack.

In my experience, about 90 percent of patients with herpes simplex I respond, 70 percent of patients with herpes simplex II, and 80 percent of patients with shingles. Patients usually respond better if treatment is begun in the early days of the attack.

TYPICAL RESPONSES OF HERPES SIMPLEX

A typical example of favorable response of fever blisters was my first patient, an attractive fifteen-year-old girl. She had a history of having large crops of herpes blisters over her lower lip and chin *every month* for two years. Each attack lasted *ten to fourteen days* and was very painful and disfiguring. At her age, it was also emotionally devastating.

After neutralization in the office, her response was typical. The pain cleared thirty minutes after each neutralizing injection and the lesions dried, scabbed over, and healed in four days.

Her next attack did not occur until five months later, and the next was eighteen months after that. Both attacks were mild and brief, and required only two or three neutralizing injections. During an additional two-year follow-up, she had no further recurrences.

Not every patient with fever blisters responds this well. However, the majority follow this general pattern. Genital lesions usually also follow this pattern. However, the response of genital lesions appears slightly less dramatic, and females seem to respond somewhat more rapidly and consistently than males.

NEUTRALIZATION OF CHICKENPOX

In chickenpox, the normal progression of the disease involves the appearance of repeated crops of chickenpox blisters day after day during the active illness. In the chickenpox patients I have neutralized, this progression has usually ceased abruptly after the first one or two neutralizing injections; few or no new blisters have appeared. Of course, the old blisters take several days or a week to scab over and heal.

This rapid cessation of lesion occurrence suggests the importance of early treatment to minimize or prevent facial lesions and possibly lifetime chickenpox scars, particularly in girls.

As chickenpox blisters are not accompanied by pain so much as by itching, each recurrence of itching is used as the signal for another neutralizing injection. This usually stops the itching in thirty minutes. Relief in thirty minutes of the severe malaise and prostration suffered by some patients with chickenpox has been one of the most dramatic and gratifying responses in this field.

AN EXAMPLE OF RESPONSE IN CHICKENPOX

Adults with chickenpox are usually very sick people. One of the most marked responses I have ever seen in any illness was in a twenty-three-year-old woman with such extreme prostration and weakness from acute chickenpox that she had to be carried into the office by her husband. She could not communicate sufficiently to provide a history of her illness; but her husband reported her recent exposure to chickenpox, and she was covered with typical chickenpox blisters.

On the neutralizing test dose of Influenza Virus Vaccine, she cleared virtually completely of all malaise and discomfort, and in thirty minutes was an alert, smiling, chatting patient! After a few additional minutes, she was able to get up and walk out of the office without her husband's support.

She used her neutralizing injections twice daily when itching recurred the first two days, then once daily for itching for five more days. During this time she experienced no malaise or other symptoms and developed no new blisters. At the end of this time, the itching did not recur, and the lesions had healed. She then discontinued the injections and remained well.

NEUTRALIZATION OF SHINGLES

In shingles, the *duration* of blistering lesions is highly variable, so it has been impossible to determine whether or not the lesions clear in individual patients any more quickly with neutralization than without. A large series of cases comparing lesion-clearing time in treated and untreated patients would be required to make this determination. The untreated "average" course usually requires several weeks for lesion clearing, and the same may be true when neutralization is used.

PREVENTION OF SUFFERING AND NEED FOR HOSPITALIZATION

However, in about 80 percent of patients with shingles, neutralization provides rapid, marked, and welcome relief from pain. These patients are often in excruciating misery, requiring prolonged expensive hospitalization and frequent injections of narcotic drugs, sedatives, and tranquilizers day and night. In addition, they may need pills by mouth for relief between injections. Even so, they may still suffer much discomfort.

This 80 percent get sufficient relief from neutralizing injections that they can almost immediately reduce or forego their narcotic injections and use far fewer pain pills. Many need no treatment other than neutralization. Unfortunately, 20 percent do not respond.

To achieve relief, the patient may require four or more neutralizing injections daily, especially in the first few days of treatment. However, this often provides great benefit in cost-effectiveness and convenience. Most can be treated at home rather than in the hospital. Those who are already in the hospital can be given a pass to come to the office for testing; if response occurs, they can usually be discharged from the hospital and kept relatively pain-free by home injections of neutralizing doses.

Many patients feel so well after a few days on the neutralizing injections that they think the attack is over, and start skipping their injections or stop them altogether. This often brings on an unnecessary painful relapse. It is better to continue the injections regularly until all the shingles lesions are healed, and to then start spacing injections apart gradually before stopping altogether. No patient that I have treated early in the active stage of shingles has yet developed postherpetic neuralgia.

Shingles patients under treatment who awaken during the night with recurrent pain are tempted to take just a strong pain pill and try to go back to sleep. It is better to take the neutralizing injection to stimulate the immune mechanism rather than using the pain medication for symptomatic relief. This is preferable, regardless of the time of day or night, in order to keep the virus from gaining on body defenses. Then if necessary, a milder pain pill can be used if relief from the neutralization injection is not quite complete.

POSSIBLE PREVENTION OF UNNECESSARY DIAGNOSTIC TESTS AND EXPLORATORY SURGERY

Shingles often causes severe pain in the face, eye, ear, chest, back, abdomen, groin, or leg for days before any lesions appear and before the cause of the pain is known. Abdominal pain can be so acute that it suggests a "surgical abdomen," meaning that exploratory abdominal surgery may be considered to determine the cause of pain. If such a patient could promptly be relieved of most or all of his pain by neutralization with Influenza Virus Vaccine, the diagnosis would be made and surgery might be avoided.

Even if surgery was not a consideration, the origin of the puzzling pain could be determined by prompt neutralization. This might save many unnecessary diagnostic tests and x-rays for "heart attacks" and other possible illnesses. The patient could be spared days of suffering, as well as the need for prolonged hospitalization for the diagnostic workup or for the purpose of administering major pain-relieving injections day and night.

Of course, the judgment and experience of the physician are very important in making such decisions. Benefit/risk ratios for all procedures must always be considered.

AN EXAMPLE OF RESPONSE IN SHINGLES

A recent patient of mine from another city went through an experience that illustrates this. A major executive in a large industrial plant, he missed four weeks of work because of a shingles attack. First he had only excruciating back pain for five days, during which time he was kept in the hospital; tested exhaustively; and given injections of Demerol and Vistaril every two hours, day and night. Even this did not provide complete relief, and he had to be given codeine-containing pain pills as well.

To minimize suffering, he had to be kept heavily sedated. On the sixth day the shingles blisters appeared, making the diagnosis but not relieving the pain. He continued to need hospitalization and the same medications for three additional weeks.

His wife, with the concurrence of his physician, then checked him out of the hospital and brought him to my office. We neutralized him with Influenza Virus Vaccine, and he walked out of the office *free of pain.* He remained entirely pain-free by self-administering four neutralizing doses daily. The pain shots and pills were discontinued and the clouding of his mind immediately cleared. He could again function normally, and returned to work the very next day.

After about ten days of complete freedom from pain, he felt so well that he stopped his injections. His pain returned; so, after a telephone call to me, he again reverted to the four-a-day injection schedule. He obtained prompt and complete relief again, and then decreased his injection schedule more gradually, with no further relapses.

POSTHERPETIC NEURALGIA

In postherpetic neuralgia, only about 30 percent respond if treated in the first year after the shingles attack, and only about 10 percent if treatment is delayed for several years. So far, none of the patients whom I have treated in the active phase of shingles have developed postherpetic neuralgia. The severe, prolonged, even lifetime, suffering and expense of postherpetic neuralgia suggests the desirability of initiating treatment during the early active phase of shingles, or as soon thereafter as possible.

NEUTRALIZATION OF HERPES OF THE EYE

Herpes lesions of the eye can be a recurrent painful nuisance, or can destroy the eye. Herpes virus infection of the eye is the leading infectious cause of blindness in this country. To save the eye, the injections should be given much more frequently than when only the skin is involved. The idea is not to wait until pain returns, but to "stay well ahead of the virus."

I had a telephone call several years ago from my good friend and noted allergist, Dr. Julia Baker. She has long employed neutralizing procedures in her practice and has written and spoken on this subject repeatedly.

Her interest began when she came to me as a patient in 1977. She had severe intestinal symptoms from so many common foods that she was becoming alarmed about her steady weight loss. She was barely able to sustain herself nutritionally, and managed only by eating rare and exotic foods, such as shark and octopus, to which she had not yet become allergic.

After her second day in my office, she started tolerating corn and other foods I had tested her to the first day. Within a couple of weeks after starting her food injections, she could eat a virtually normal diet, and has continued to do so.

At any rate, her telephone call was about a patient with severe herpes of the eye who had been referred to her by two eminent ophthalmologists who had exhausted all their therapeutic efforts fruitlessly. The lesion was progressing and the eye was in danger of destruction.

She had already determined the neutralizing dose, and had started the treatment injections on the usual as-needed basis for pain. This stopped the progression of the lesion. After two days, the eye was no worse but was also no better. She was barely holding the virus in check.

When she called me, I suggested that she hospitalize the patient for close observation and give the injections every three hours day and night. She called me back two days later to tell me that the pain had responded quickly and was now entirely controlled. Furthermore, the ophthalmologists had already noted marked evidence of healing of the lesion. The eye did go on to complete healing, and the ophthalmologists agreed that the saving of the eye was entirely due to the neutralization therapy.

Such stories could be multiplied ad nauseum but are "anecdotal," that is, they are reports of individual patients rather than a double-blind controlled series. However, such patients have been numerous, and the same patterns of response have been occurring in my practice for over twenty years. The same patterns are confirmed by the personal experiences and clinical observations of many other physicians using this form of treatment. Further, the increased effectiveness of *frequently* repeated neutralizing injections when needed has been true in symptoms due to foods, inhalants, and other substances, as well as in herpes.

HERPES ZOSTER OF THE EAR AND BELL'S PALSY

Herpes zoster of the ear (Ramsay Hunt Syndrome) is a very painful herpetic infection of the outer ear. It also often causes palsy (paralysis) of one side of the face. Many ear specialists have reported dramatic results from neutralizing treatment with Influenza Virus Vaccine. Bell's Palsy is a different condition, only rarely caused by herpes, so it is only rarely helped by neutralization therapy.

MORE FREQUENT DOSAGE

As discussed, in severe herpes virus infections giving neutralizing injections frequently enough to "stay well ahead of the virus" is apt to lead to more rapid and greater response. In patients with herpes simplex lesions of the lip or genitals, however, there is generally no need to space the injections so closely.

Each recurrence of symptoms usually can serve as the signal for another injection. Herpes simplex infections often require just three or four injections the first day, two or three the second day, one or two the third, and possibly one injection daily for another few days.

RECURRENT HERPES ATTACKS

Neutralization usually is particularly effective in aborting and relieving *recurrent* attacks of herpes. Often a single injection is all that is needed. Recurrent attacks usually can be aborted by early administration of one or two treatment doses during the early prodromal or preblister stage of an attack. The pain, burning, or tingling which often precedes a blistering attack usually disappears in thirty minutes and the blisters generally do not form.

If blisters are allowed to form before beginning the injections, some extra injections will often be needed to heal the blisters. Even so, the duration of the blistering attack usually can be reduced to only a few days, rather than possibly a couple of weeks.

When a patient has had one or two attacks treated by neutralization, subsequent attacks usually tend to become much less frequent. Recurrent attacks also tend to produce fewer blisters; the pain is less severe; and the blisters often clear with unusual rapidity. Even when treatment has been omitted in some recurrences, patients have often noted that the attacks have been milder and briefer as though their body defenses were continuing to act more efficiently than before their initial treatment.

Chapter 28

THE IMPORTANCE OF INFLUENZA VIRUS INFECTIONS AND THE ABILITY TO NEUTRALIZE THEM

The influenza virus has been causing recurrent epidemics of febrile respiratory disease every one to three years for at least the past 400 years.[95,96] In addition, thirty-two known epidemics of worldwide scope, called pandemics, have occurred.

The greatest pandemic occurred in 1918–19, when 549,000 deaths were recorded in the United States and 21 million deaths were recorded worldwide.[97] This was the worst single epidemic *of any kind* in recorded history.

Influenza epidemics characteristically occur worldwide, alternating between the northern and southern hemispheres. Epidemics of influenza A occur every one to three years and affect all age groups. Epidemics of influenza B occur every three to five years. During epidemics, at least 10–30 percent of the population—and probably up to twice that many—become infected. In schools or other institutions, as many as 50–60 percent may develop influenza.

Influenza results in a tremendous amount of absenteeism. The maintenance of vital utilities and services in a community or a military group may be seriously curtailed by the rapidity of the spread of the disease to a critical number of essential persons.

During the Asian virus pandemic of 1957–58, an estimated 70,000 excess deaths occurred in the USA. During the 1968 pandemic caused by the A/Hong Kong virus, an estimated 34,000 excess deaths occurred here.

The economic cost of these influenza A epidemics and pandemics cannot be precisely calculated. However, the cost for the 1968 pandemic, which could not be considered a major pandemic, was estimated to exceed 3.9 billion dollars.

Even though the incidence of complications, especially those of a serious nature, is relatively low considering the number of cases, the absolute number of patients with complications may be relatively large. This is because of the high attack rate of epidemic influenza.[98–102]

It was estimated by the Center for Disease Control that 275,000 deaths associated with influenza occurred from 1957 to 1970 in the United States and an additional 86,800 from 1971 to 1976.[103–105] More than half of these were persons with cardiovascular-renal disease and over two-thirds of the total were sixty-five years of age and older. Case fatality rates for influenza A in the last few decades have been about 10 deaths per 100,000.

The people who are at greatest risk of severe pneumonia and fatality include the older age group and persons of all ages with chronic debilitating diseases. The following conditions predispose individuals to such risks:

(1) Acquired or congenital heart disease.
(2) Chronic pulmonary disease.
(3) Chronic kidney disease.
(4) Diabetes.
(5) Chronic severe anemia such as Sickle Cell Disease.
(6) Conditions that compromise the immune mechanism, including certain malignancies and therapy with immunosuppressive drugs, and to a lesser extent those on long-term daily high-dose cortisone.
(7) Older persons, particularly those over age sixty-five.

DIAGNOSING THE EPIDEMIC

Diagnosing sporadic cases of influenza is not easy. However, during an influenza epidemic, there is little difficulty in diagnosing characteristic influenza with a reasonable degree of accuracy. Other virus epidemics tend to occur each winter, but they are usually distinguishable from influenza.

Epidemics of rhinovirus ("nose colds") and other runny-nose type illnesses cause nasal symptoms but *not the generalized muscular aches* (myalgia) of influenza. In winter, people with nose colds suddenly appear in physicians' offices in droves, and the similarity of the various cases makes it apparent that the physician is dealing with a "common cold" virus.

There may also be an epidemic of a gastrointestinal virus infection, with vomiting and diarrhea. These too occur in great numbers, and the similarity of cases within an epidemic makes this diagnosis apparent also.

Then many patients begin appearing with a different set of symptoms, emphasizing myalgia ("aching all over"). Epidemics of influenza are usually distinguished from other viral epidemics by this characteristic myalgia.

The illness begins suddenly, and the patient can often tell the first moment he fell ill. His temperature rises sharply and he is very soon incapable of carrying on. He goes to bed and rapidly feels that he is in the grip of some prostrating illness. He may then begin to shiver and become aware of smarting in his eyes, stuffiness in his nose, and soreness in his throat. He often develops a cough accompanied by hoarseness and pain under the breastbone.

When the illness is fully developed his main feeling is one of great malaise accompanied by cough, fever, headache, backache, and pain throughout the entire body. He has no wish to eat, he may become dizzy, and occasionally he may vomit. In my experience, diarrhea is very rare except in patients with preexisting colon disease.

In most healthy young patients the temperature falls on the third or fourth day; the patient is up and about on the fifth or sixth day; and he is usually fit to return to work inside ten days. In a few cases the fever persists somewhat longer, and patients with cough and other complications may be sick for an additional week or so.

Older patients may take even longer to recover; and in them, weakness and lassitude may be quite marked for many weeks, even months. Some develop postinfluenzal depression, which may also last for weeks or months.

COMPLICATIONS

Influenza may be complicated by pneumonia caused either by the influenza virus or by bacteria which act as secondary invaders in the respiratory tract. Bacterial pneumonias are somewhat less serious because of the availability of antibacterial antibiotics. Influenza virus pneumonia is highly fatal, as there is no really effective antiviral drug available for it.

The Guillain-Barré Syndrome is a form of generalized paralysis which seems to be caused by a delayed immunologic reaction within the spinal cord against the protein of an invading virus. It has been observed occasionally following influenza.

Reye's syndrome also seems to involve a toxic or immunologic reaction, but the reaction is more acute and is greater in the brain and liver. It is accompanied by severe vomiting, coma, and often death. It has been commonly associated with influenza B and chickenpox.[103,106]

Whether or not aspirin is associated with Reye's Syndrome has been a subject for much ongoing research.

It is interesting that the two major viruses incriminated in Reye's Syndrome (influenza and chickenpox) might both be neutralized by Influenza Virus Vaccine. To my knowledge this has not been tried as a preventive for Reye's Syndrome. Effectiveness might well be dependent on very early administration, before liver and brain damage have progressed.

In such cases, it might be necessary to administer neutralizing injections every thirty minutes or so in the beginning. Some of the treatment injections could be administered intradermally, say every tenth dose or so, in order to produce a wheal. This would provide evidence of a possible dosage change requiring retesting.

RESEARCH IMPLICATIONS OF INFLUENZA VIRUS VACCINE NEUTRALIZATION

In my experience, the ability to neutralize ordinary active influenza virus infections with Influenza Virus Vaccine is a clinically established fact. Those who have tried it know. It usually provides effective, reliable, safe, and rapid relief from the symptoms and signs of influenza virus infection, and seems to shorten and moderate the entire attack.

Influenza patients with known cardiac, pulmonary, renal, and other diseases which predispose to fatality from influenza might well be prime candidates for neutralization therapy. However, neutralization is still an untried tool for influenza virus pneumonia and Reye's Syndrome.

These are areas that cry out for study. Unfortunately, it is impossible for me to do the type of controlled study that would be required to provide scientifically acceptable proof of effectiveness in ordinary influenza virus infections, much less the complicated types. The technical problems are insurmountable to a practicing physician. A million-dollar virology laboratory, a team of skilled research assistants, and access to large numbers of cases over a reasonably short period of time would be required.

However, I have made the initial findings, reported them repeatedly to my colleagues, and carried this to the farthest point of which I am now capable. The next move is up to the experts in the field who have the facilities, personnel, and funds required to put this to the acid test.

SAFER IMMUNIZATION

An additional use of Influenza Virus Vaccine neutralization is in the safer administration of *immunizing* doses of Influenza Virus Vaccine in elderly patients, patients with chronic debilitating diseases, and patients who have had flu-like reactions after previous immunizing doses. The neutralizing dose can be determined and administered thirty minutes *before* the immunizing dose. This will usually completely or partially prevent immunizing dose reactions.

I also supply such a patient with several additional neutralizing doses to take home, so that if postimmunization symptoms arise at all, they can be quickly neutralized at home. However, I would not consider using any test or treatment dose of Influenza Virus Vaccine in patients who have had *major or life-threatening* reactions to previous immunization with this vaccine or to any of its ingredients such as egg, chicken, chicken-feathers, and mercurials, except in extreme or overriding circumstances.

POSSIBLE NEUTRALIZATION WITH OTHER VIRUS VACCINES

As mentioned, I have also seen a few cases of mumps in my practice, and these have all responded markedly and rapidly to neutralization with mumps virus vaccine. Since mumps virus vaccine contains live viruses which might overwhelm an immunosuppressed or immunodeficient patient, it should not be used in such cases.

However, I would expect it to be perfectly safe in persons with normal immune mechanisms. Further, killed virus vaccines for mumps, measles (rubeola), whooping cough (pertussis), and innumerable other virus infections could easily be made available by manufacturers for therapeutic (neutralization) purposes.

NEUTRALIZATION OF BACTERIAL AND OTHER ORGANISMS

Good immunizing bacterial vaccines for specific bacterial infections are as yet untried. I have tried neutralization with mixed respiratory bacterial vaccines and usually have found this to be ineffective. They are generally weak or ineffective for immunization also.

However, specific bacterial vaccines which have been proved to be potent immunizing vaccines for infections caused by the specific bacterium for which each vaccine is prepared might be useful. At least it seems worthy of judicious trial. The same principle may also apply to invasive fungi, rickettsiae, protozoa, worms, insect larvae, and other invasive organisms.

NEUTRALIZATION FOR DIAGNOSIS

Another possible additional use of virus vaccine neutralization is in the diagnosis of the causative virus in a sick patient with a febrile flu-like illness of unknown cause. If the symptoms of the illness markedly improve or disappear within thirty minutes after administering a neutralizing dose of Influenza Virus Vaccine, this would suggest the diagnosis.

The diagnosis would likely be influenza or a herpes family virus infection such as infectious mononucleosis, chronic Epstein-Barr Virus infection, or cytomegalovirus infection. As another example, the meningitis of mumps might be distinguishable from meningitis caused by other organisms by response to mumps virus vaccine neutralization.

NEUTRALIZATION FOR STRAIN IDENTIFICATION

The immune mechanism is usually very specific. It can often distinguish one strain of a virus from another strain of the same species. In some of my patients who had reactions to an immunizing injection of Influenza Virus Vaccine, I tried unsuccessfully to relieve them with an Influenza Virus Vaccine containing *different* strains. When I switched back to the vaccine that contained the same strain as the one that caused the reaction, relief promptly occurred.

So another possible use of neutralization might be in distinguishing one strain from another. Early in an illness or in an epidemic, it might be important to know quickly which strain was involved in the patient and in the community.

This test would use the body's own exquisitely precise sensing mechanism in a biologic test which could be more accurate and much more rapid than viral cultures and other laboratory procedures. These laboratory procedures could still be instituted in the hope of eventually providing confirmation of the biologic neutralizing test.

USE IN ANIMALS

Veterinary medicine might also benefit by trials of neutralization in animals. I have successfully provoked and neutralized a horse to heaves, an asthma-like syndrome involving wheezing, coughing, and inability to carry a rider or pull a wagon due to shortness of breath. He is now a functionally useful animal on regular neutralizing injection therapy.

Hundreds of horses with heaves have been successfully treated by other investigators using neutralization therapy. The causative allergens in heaves have been grasses and molds predominantly but not exclusively. Other animal diseases, including virus infections, might be similarly responsive, with implications in salvaging loved, prized, or high-priced individual animals, such as pets, thoroughbred horses, and prize bulls; in meat production; and in animal models for human disease investigation.

Chapter 29

THE IMPORTANCE OF HERPES VIRUS INFECTIONS AND THE ABILITY TO NEUTRALIZE THEM

Herpes simplex virus (HSV) belongs to the group of human herpes viruses that also includes the varicella-zoster virus, Epstein-Barr virus, and cytomegalovirus. It is the varicella-zoster virus that causes both chickenpox (varicella) and shingles (herpes zoster).

More than fifty herpes viruses are known to infect more than thirty vertebrate species.[107] The ubiquitousness of the herpes virus and the intense suffering it causes underscore the need for an effective form of therapy.

HERPES SIMPLEX VIRUS I & II

In general, HSV–I causes infections above the waist, such as herpes of the lip, mouth, face, eye, ear, and brain. HSV–II usually causes infections below the waist, particularly genital herpes.[108] However, the opposite locations can occur.

Some patients are infected with both viruses. The incidence of both herpes virus infections coexisting simultaneously has been rapidly increasing with the increased incidence of orogenital sexual activities.[109]

HSV-I ("FEVER BLISTERS")

Herpes simplex infection can be mild. However, it has also been described as one of the most common, most painful, and most recurrent afflictions of mankind.[111] Some patients have attacks of severe lip and perioral lesions. For weeks they may have difficulty in eating, speaking, or swallowing. I have already described the unrelenting intense misery of patients I have seen with true chronic herpes ulcers of the mucous membranes of the mouth and throat, and their relief with Influenza Virus Vaccine neutralization.

Recurrent herpes simplex infections of the lips and perioral area are estimated to occur in 20–40 percent of the population.[110] At least 75 percent of the population is considered to have been overtly infected by this virus.[110,111] Latent HSV–I is believed to involve up to 90 percent of the population.[111,112]

HSV–I also accounts for up to 500,000 cases of ocular herpes simplex in the United States. It is the leading infectious cause of blindness in this country.[112] Further, HSV–I causes 4,000 cases of herpes encephalitis (inflammation of the brain) each year, of which more than a third die and half suffer severe permanent neurologic damage, such as cerebral palsy and mental retardation.[112]

HSV-II ("GENITAL HERPES")

The incidence of genital herpes has been increasing so rapidly that it is now considered the second most common venereal disease and a major public health problem. It was seen seven times more frequently than primary syphilis over an eighteen-month study period in the outpatient clinics of the New England Medical Center Hospitals.[109]

In a venereal disease clinic in Atlanta, virologically confirmed herpes genitalis was found in 6 percent of female patients and 0.3 percent of male patients. It was the most common cause of lesions in the genital area in females, and was second only to primary syphilis as the cause of such lesions in males.

Teenagers accounted for nearly one-half of these patients.[113] Drs. Jeansson and Molin[114] and Dr. Francis and his associates[115] reported similar figures. Dr. Olmstead[116] estimated that 200,000 new cases of genital herpes occur annually in the United States.

The isolation of HSV–II from the genitourinary tracts of 15 percent of 190 randomly selected *asymptomatic* males has been reported.[117] This asymptomatic carrier state results in the exposure of an ever-greater population to the risk of primary HSV–II infection.

Presence of HSV–II in the female genital tract results in the exposure of fetuses and newborns to this virus with a high incidence of devastating effect. Abortions, stillbirths, and premature deliveries have been reported.[118–120] Congenital malformations may also possibly be associated.[121,122]

Passage of the infant through the infected birth canal results in approximately 120 cases of neonatal herpetic infection each year.[107] At least

50 percent of newborns delivered vaginally through herpetic birth canals become infected,[118] and about 50 percent of infected infants are killed or severely damaged by the herpetic infections.[123] Caesarian section before rupture of the membranes, or possibly within four hours of rupture, may reduce these risks; but firm data on this are not yet available.[124]

Both HSV–I and HSV–II can attack the central nervous system. Encephalitis in adults is usually caused by HSV–I. However, encephalitis in newborns is usually due to HSV–II from the mother's birth canal.[125] Meningitis is caused by HSV–II.[125]

OTHER FORMS OF HERPES

Shingles accounts for 0.5–2 percent of patients seen at dermatology clinics.[126] In a study of 1,000 families the incidence of shingles was found to be 15 percent.[127] This extrapolates to 3 million cases annually in the United States.

Acute herpetic gingivostomatitis is a common, severe, prolonged, painful mouth disease of small children. Reye's syndrome is an uncommon but highly fatal disease of children, and has been associated etiologically with prior chickenpox and influenza B virus infections.[128–130]

CHICKENPOX

Chickenpox treatment has received little attention because there was no specific treatment. There was nothing much we could do except provide general supportive care. But it is a potentially much more serious disease than most people think.

It can cause severe malaise and prostration approaching stupor or coma, particularly in adults. It can cause highly fatal primary chickenpox virus pneumonia.

It can also be fatal if contracted by patients being treated for leukemia, organ transplants, and other such conditions with immunosuppressives, chemotherapeutic agents, or continuous cortisone therapy. It can be fatal in anergic conditions, which are conditions characterized by decreased numbers or inadequate functioning of microbe-destroying protective *cells,* primarily T lymphocytes. It can be fatal in patients with immunodeficiency disease, which involves low levels or poor functioning of protective *antibodies.*

It can also kill by entering through the open skin of patients with generalized skin diseases, such as eczema or burns. Children weakened by poor nutrition and other debilitating diseases may also succumb to chickenpox.

Moreover, even when a patient survives a bout of chickenpox, he is not done with the virus. It takes up permanent residence in nerve cells in certain ganglia and may surface decades later as shingles.

Chickenpox is also interesting since it is now the first virus exanthem (contagious rash-producing disease such as measles and rubella) for which an effective treatment is available, namely neutralization. When the first neutralizing dose of Influenza Virus Vaccine is administered to patients with chickenpox, the symptoms usually subside in thirty minutes; and new crops of blisters generally stop appearing almost immediately.

INFECTIOUS MONONUCLEOSIS

The Epstein-Barr virus usually causes mono in humans, and has been associated with cancer of the throat and a cancer of lymph nodes called Burkitt's Lymphoma. A unique thing about Burkitt's Lymphoma, which is global but most prevalent in central Africa, is that the virus can be carried from one patient to another by mosquitoes.

So it is possible to get this cancer from a mosquito bite! Patients with this disease who have exhausted all therapeutic methods unsuccessfully and have no hope for surviving would seem likely early candidates for neutralization therapy with Influenza Virus Vaccine.

The Epstein-Barr virus is another ubiquitous virus. Nearly all adults show positive blood tests, indicating that they have been attacked at some time by this virus. It is considered to be transmitted in children chiefly by exchange of saliva on contaminated drinking cups and other objects, and in adults by kissing.

In some patients, Epstein-Barr virus infection can become overt and chronic. Chronic Epstein-Barr virus infection can last for years or for life. It can cause severe incapacitation and require radical alteration of life styles and diminution of career and personal goals, resulting often in feelings of profound hopelessness and depression.

Infectious mononucleosis is an illness of insidious onset, characterized chiefly by vague malaise, fever, sore throat, and enlarged lymph nodes in the neck. Symptoms usually last four to six weeks but may persist for several months. Most patients recover completely; but in rare instances, serious or fatal complications may occur.

There are several new blood tests available for diagnosis, but until now there has been no specific treatment. I have provided much relief to patients with mono and patients with chronic Epstein-Barr virus infection with neutralizing doses of Influenza Virus Vaccine, using identical procedures as already discussed.

CYTOMEGALOVIRUS

The cytomegalovirus (CMV) is another ubiquitous herpes-family virus, present in virtually everyone in the world by the age of thirty. It seldom causes severe recognizable problems except in some newborns, in people who receive multiple fresh blood transfusions, and in immunosuppressed kidney transplant recipients.

However, the cytomegalovirus can cause what is known as "mono-negative mononucleosis." This is a syndrome clinically identical with infectious mononucleosis but in which it is the cytomegalovirus rather than the Epstein-Barr virus that causes the illness.

A number of research groups have reported data to indicate that in rheumatoid arthritis the basic problem is a deficiency in the suppressor T-cell system to the Epstein-Barr virus.[131,132] The suggestion has also been made that cytomegalovirus and possibly other viruses can be involved in rheumatoid arthritis in some cases. The virus antigen and the antiviral antibody combine to form antigen-antibody complexes (immune complexes) which deposit in the joints and result in joint inflammation.

Food and inhalant antigens may possibly also combine with their specific antibodies and accumulate in joints. So rheumatoid arthritis patients may reveal the clinical link between allergy, inflammation, and arthritis, and provide at least one explanation for the success of neutralization therapy in such a wide variety of allergic, nonallergic, inflammatory, and infectious diseases.

Rheumatoid arthritis may also serve as a model for the altered resistance/burden ratio I have discussed earlier as the final straw that leads to the surfacing of a clinical illness. When a patient has a lower defense level, such as inadequate suppressor T-cell function, a given total body burden is more likely to produce illness.

Since both Epstein-Barr virus and cytomegalovirus are herpes family viruses and can attack joints, neutralization with Influenza Virus Vaccine might be expected to be helpful in some patients with rheumatoid arthritis. In practice, we have noted rapid, marked relief of joint pain in some patients being treated for shingles with Influenza Virus Vaccine.

My results in rheumatoid arthritis have been generally good to excellent using neutralization against food and inhalant extracts, but have not been 100 percent effective. I am now noting similar responses as in influenza and herpes using Influenza Virus Vaccine neutralization for rheumatoid arthritis.

Recently, it has additionally been reported by several investigators that diseased arteries and atheromatous arterial placques which can lead to heart attacks and strokes often contain herpes simplex virus or cytomegalovirus, whereas normal arteries usually do not.[131–140] The relevance of this finding is not yet known.

However, it is possible that this virus may play a critical predisposing role in these major cardiovascular illnesses. If so, early neutralization with Influenza Virus Vaccine might conceivably be useful in preventing whatever adverse role these viruses might play in heart attacks and strokes.

HERPES AND CANCER

More than a dozen herpes viruses have been associated with cancer in man and various animals.[141–146] Of course, no one has caused a human cancer by deliberately injecting viruses that might cause cancer. However, this is done routinely and successfully in laboratory animals in cancer investigations.

Moreover, the Epstein-Barr virus has been consistently linked with Burkitt's Lymphoma and with nasopharyngeal carcinoma, as well as with infectious mononucleosis and chronic EB Virus Disease.[143] HSV–I has been associated with cancer of the lip.[146] HSV–II has been associated with cancer of the cervix, the second most common cancer in women.[143] Sabin and Tarro[147] have linked a herpes antigen with nine different kinds of human cancers. However, despite much suggestive evidence, herpes antigen has not yet clearly been proven to be a cause of *human* cancer.

I am not speculating that neutralization with Influenza Virus Vaccine would help in established cancer. Rather, I am wondering if early treatment and continuing control of herpes virus infections might reduce the possible tendency for herpes-infected cells to change into malignant cells.

PREDISPOSITION TO HERPES

As mentioned, HSV can cause severe localized disease or disseminated infection in immunologically impaired persons, as well as in newborns. These include patients on immunosuppressive therapy; patients with certain malignancies, such as Hodgkin's disease; and those with immune deficiency disease, such as AIDS and Wiskott-Aldrich syndrome.[148–151]

Severe herpetic disease also occurs in patients with skin impairments, such as atopic eczema and severe burns. Acutely malnourished children who are too weak nutritionally to fight off the virus are more prone to herpetic disease. It also occurs in those weakened by associated measles, whooping cough, and other debilitating diseases.[152–154]

ACCEPTABLE HERPES TREATMENT

In a comprehensive review of available therapeutic modalities for herpes virus infections, Drs. Alford and Whitley[155] listed these three requirements for an acceptable systemic treatment:

(1) Active infections should be controlled.
(2) Recurrences should be significantly reduced.
(3) There should be no acute toxicities or chronic adverse reactions from therapy.

Influenza Virus Vaccine neutralization therapy seems to satisfy all three requirements. Trial of Influenza Virus Vaccine neutralization treatment in many forms of the disease have not yet been performed. It may well not be effective in many or any of these untried conditions. However, it would be difficult to imagine a more carefully studied and more globally available vaccine than Influenza Virus Vaccine.

Therapeutic trials seem worth considering in both simple and life-threatening herpetic illnesses. This is particularly true in patients with illnesses discussed here in which all other therapeutic modalities have been utilized unsuccessfully, when the patient's health is failing, and when there is no other direction in which to turn.

IMPLICATIONS OF VIRUS NEUTRALIZATION

Influenza Virus Vaccine neutralization therapy is the first specific useful antiviral treatment for any established virus infection. It is unusually safe, highly efficient, immediately available, economical, rapidly effective, and broadly applicable.

Its discovery required absolutely no expenditure of research funds. It is particularly fortuitous that it is applicable to *two* large families of virus infection, influenza and herpes. Furthermore, it is a *killed* virus vaccine so should be safe enough to justify medical-center trials even in patients with impaired immune mechanisms.

Both influenza and herpes viruses are of major importance since they occur in *high incidence* and with *great destructive potential*. Until this breakthrough billions of dollars worth of worldwide research efforts in both fields had failed to provide the practitioner with a highly effective antiviral antibiotic, or any other specific mode of therapy, for a patient with an already-established virus infection.

In addition to potential for immediate clinical application, this is a new *concept* in medical therapy which has possible broad research implications. There are already at least twenty-five immunizing vaccines available, and the list is growing.

The successful use of a killed virus vaccine to provide *immediate relief* of active viral infections—not just preventive advance immunization—suggests clinical therapeutic trials of other killed virus vaccines. Some may be therapeutically effective for the specific virus disease (as Influenza Virus Vaccine is specifically effective for influenza virus infections),[5] and some may also be effective for some cross-responding, nonrelated virus diseases (as Influenza Virus Vaccine is for herpes virus infections).[12]

THE ERA OF IMMUNOBIOTICS

The ability to treat active infections with immunologic antibiotics or "immunobiotics" consisting of vaccines or extracts of the causative organisms opens the door to a new field of medical research concerning *immediate stimulation of the body's own natural defenses* against specific organisms. This could provide effective therapy in microbial illnesses for which no pharmacologic antibiotics are yet available.

This is not suggested as a replacement for pharmacologic antibiotics, or for any other standard treatment. It is a possible *adjunct*, an extension of our already considerable—and expanding—reach. The possibilities are exciting!

Chapter 30

ALLERGIC AND INFLAMMATORY ARTHRITIS

Although arthritis and rheumatic disorders are not top "killer" diseases in prevalence, and not major causes of mortality or hospitalization, they are *the number one cause of disability.* They are also important because they often produce much suffering over long periods and can be difficult to manage safely and effectively by commonly used methods.[156]

More than 36 million men, women, and children in this country are affected by some form of arthritis or muscle/joint inflammation. The cost of arthritis to the economy has been estimated at 13 billion dollars per year.

About 6 billion of this is from direct treatment of the arthritis, and 7 billion is from indirect factors such as lost work time.[156] The human cost in pain, functioning, impaired careers, and enjoyment of life is inestimable.

There are three main categories of arthritis. *Rheumatoid arthritis* is the type of joint inflammation that people often refer to as "crippling" arthritis. *Osteoarthritis* or degenerative arthritis is the type that comes as a normal part of aging, although in many instances immunologic or sensitivity factors play a role in the degenerative process.[157] *Nonspecific* joint and muscle pain falls into neither of these categories; but it too is often associated with swelling, inflammation, or allergic-like sensitivity.

THE IMPORTANCE OF HIDDEN FOOD SENSITIVITY IN ARTHRITIS

In recent years, there have been many publications from major research centers connecting arthritis with food sensitivity reactions in the muscles and joints.[158–176] Positive data implicating food ingestion in the flare-ups of rheumatoid arthritis have been derived from many studies. In one multicenter study, forty-four such patients were treated in environmentally controlled units where both inhalants and foods were rigidly managed.

These patients were first given a laxative and required to fast for a few days on spring water. Then they were given organically grown (less chemically contaminated) foods one at a time, as in the one-food-per-meal diet.

Reactions to each food were carefully assessed. The pain initiated by each allergenic food was measured by a pain-gauging instrument, the swelling of joints by a joint-circumference measuring instrument, and the strength of the muscles by an instrument that measures the weakness or strength of the grip. The authors concluded that there was a definite correlation between specific food and chemical sensitivities and flare-ups of rheumatoid arthritis.[175]

In my experience, *neutralization* therapy has demonstrated great efficacy in relieving some arthritis sufferers. In complex patients, providing maximum benefit may require a comprehensive approach. This may include neutralization for foods, inhalants, and chemicals. Some dietary elimination or rotation may be required, as may educated avoidance of both allergenic and nonspecific stresses.

Some patients with arthritis have told me they know from *repeated* experiences that their pain is worse after eating one or several foods. As in migraine and asthma, the symptoms may not appear until that night or the next morning. The foods they mention most frequently are wheat, pork, corn, alcoholic beverages, milk, eggs, chocolate, and sweets. However, any food can do it.

When tested and treated, some turn out to have a degree of hidden sensitivity to almost every food they eat very frequently. It is much like the long list of foods that often cause chronic migraine, chronic irritable bowel syndrome, chronic hyperactivity, and other hidden food-caused syndromes. The resistance/burden ratio seems to be thrown off balance by a summation of many factors in the external or internal environment.

As in other food-sensitivity-related stress syndromes, many arthritics with multiple hidden food sensitivities enter the office with no inkling that foods bother them at all. Further, they are not readily helped simply by diet.

This is because they are often sensitive even to the foods allowed in the restricted diet, or they are not able or willing to live on a rigid or highly restricted diet. They may also be reacting to inhalants, chemicals, infections, weather changes, chill, Candida, hormones, and other specific and nonspecific stresses.

It is significant that many patients with arthritis and other muscle/joint syndromes also suffer from migraine or other sensitivity syndromes due to environmental incitants. These incitants may also affect various other organs, such as the nose, skin, lungs, or gastrointestinal tract. Joint pain and allergic-like sensitivity, especially delayed food sensitivity, frequently coexist.

This suggests that sensitivity to environmental incitants is a common cause for multiple syndromes, only one of which is arthritis. When a patient has two or more such syndromes, neutralization therapy for one such syndrome often provides relief for the other syndromes as well.

ARTHRITIS AS A DISTURBED RESISTANCE/BURDEN RATIO

In my experience, hidden food sensitivity is often a major part of the burden in muscle/joint syndromes. On the other hand, a food-sensitive patient may also suffer a flare-up of his arthritis from an inhalant, such as the chemical odor of a new carpet installed in the bedroom or den, or a visit to a moldy basement or a dusty closet.

In such cases, sensitivity potentials from the chemical, mold, or dust add to the potential for food sensitivity. It may be the total burden that finally triggers the flare-up.

Another arthritic can flare up during atmospheric mold spore peaks, during the summer grass pollen season, during spring tree season and early fall weed season, or during winter dust/mold/chill/infection seasons. In such seasonal patients the number and degree of sensitivities usually increase as years pass. The patient may finally suffer during all seasons, more or less equally, all year around.

Yet another patient with muscle or joint pain from unrecognized food sensitivities can flare up premenstrually. Another can experience a flare-up from the added burden of a virus infection, a bacterial infection in the sinuses or bladder, or from Candida overgrowth due to the use of a necessary antibiotic for the bacterial infection.

The point is that an arthritis patient is not always suffering from a totally mysterious disease with totally unexplainable flare-ups. In some instances, he is suffering from *environmentally* induced arthritis and *environmentally* induced flare-ups. These may largely be due to causes which can be identified and controlled by neutralization, trigger and stress avoidance, and related environmental treatment.

DIFFICULTIES IN RECOGNIZING AND REMOVING CULPRIT FOODS FROM THE DIET

How can a medical history delineate the importance of food factors when the patient himself usually cannot give an accurate food allergy history? Further, there is nothing in the physical examination relevant to specific food causation, and current laboratory tests for causative hidden food factors are usually of little or no help.

Many people do not follow diets well anyway, particularly if favorite or craved foods must be totally eliminated. Paradoxically, it is often the favorite and craved foods that do much of the harm. In many patients, a very small quantity present as a hidden ingredient in another food may be sufficient to induce days of pain and swelling.

Relying solely on diets which take much of the eating pleasure out of life is almost foredoomed to failure. To make such a treatment effective, the physician must be highly motivated in this direction. He must provide hidden-food avoidance lists, frequent follow-ups, continued detailed studies of the diet diary and food ledger, and much repeated instruction. Even so, the patient must be intelligent, teachable, organized, alert, committed, and persistent.

This type of physician-patient working relationship is not easily attained. It is certainly not common practice as regards the seeking of food causation in arthritis or other muscle/joint syndromes. So even when foods are primary culprits, dietary manipulations as generally employed fail to either diagnose or relieve the condition.

In such circumstances, food neutralizing injections containing all of the hidden food culprits usually allow for a more normal life style. They also provide far superior long-term relief as compared to difficult diets alone for the multiple hidden food factors.

Despite this, some patients do obtain great relief through dietary changes if their physician can help them pinpoint some causative foods and can provide continuing support and guidance. Then it is up to the patient to exert the effort and willpower to avoid those foods meticulously and continuously.

JAMES COBURN: A DIETARY SUCCESS STORY

One of the most publicized recent examples of this is a report concerning actor James Coburn. His arthritis was reputedly so bad while making a film in Mexico that he could hardly move. It was said they were lifting him on and off horses using a crane.

After the movie was completed he apparently sought medical help, determined the causative foods, and eliminated those foods from his diet. He remarked during a Merv Griffin show in December, 1981 that the diet had "saved my life."

A BROAD VIEW OF ARTHRITIS

In my own practice, the large majority of the complex arthritics I have successfully treated have obtained greatest relief from the circumspect approach that considers both internal and external environmental incitants. Many have obtained marked relief from food extract injection therapy alone. Some have also had to eliminate a few foods, and some have had to rotate a few of their foods in addition to using food injections. Some have also had to minimize or avoid chemicalized foods, chemicalized water, and chemical inhalants.

Some have required inhalant neutralization therapy also, and others have responded to inhalants even more than to foods. Some have also had to be neutralized for progesterone for protection from premenstrual flare-ups.

AN EXAMPLE OF NEUTRALIZATION THERAPY IN ARTHRITIS

I recently had a patient, a businesswoman, with pain, swelling, stiffness, and deformity of her hands due to chronic rheumatoid inflammation. She noted beginning relief just three hours after receiving her first "single" treatment injection at the end of the first day of inhalant tests. Her "single" that day included only house dust, dust mites, molds, and epidermals. While testing, she continued improving daily after each cumulative single inhalant injection, and also later after each cumulative single food injection.

On home treatment injections her improvement continued. In four weeks she returned and demonstrated with delight the greatly decreased swelling and tenderness of her fingers and their markedly increased flexibility. This was her "best relief in years."

At eight weeks, her pain was virtually gone. She demonstrated her increased finger agility by quickly picking up a pen and writing with a free flowing hand.

She stated that she was now able to function much more efficiently in both her home and business life. She said she could type again, pick up heavy objects, and do many other things with her hands that she had not been able to do for years.

This had occurred with no need to avoid or rotate a single food or use a single drug. In fact, she was now able to do without the drugs that had formerly been a constant part of her life. This is another example of the personal, societal, occupational, and cost effectiveness of neutralization therapy.

One of the interesting points about this patient is that she had no idea that any of these inhalants or foods had ever bothered her in any way. She came to us only because her extremely hyperactive grandson had obtained such rapid and marked relief from food neutralization treatment when he had failed to improve after many previous treatments at other centers. She too had experienced repeated treatment failures, and came because she simply wanted to see if she could obtain similar help.

Unfortunately, she had not come to us until her hands were beginning to be deformed from long-continued scarring. Of course our allergy injections could not correct the deformities. However, she is free of pain and swelling, and she now has hands that she can live and work with in comfort.

COMPREHENSIVE ALLERGY MANAGEMENT OF ARTHRITIS

I do not want to give the impression that all arthritis sufferers respond, or that they always respond so well or so quickly. Arthritis patients may be slower to respond than some of the other syndromes we have discussed. Relief may come gradually but steadily over months. Some patients do not respond at all. But those who do respond have usually already exhausted all other treatment possibilities, so are very grateful patients.

Those who have had prolonged cortisone therapy seem to have a diminished capacity to respond to any treatment. Those with osteoarthritis without inflammation have also been poor responders. However, osteoarthritics who also have joint swelling and other signs of chronic inflammation often respond well.

DIETARY RELIEF

Not all patients require complete food neutralization therapy. Some have obtained marked improvement by eating simple wholesome foods; keeping careful dietary records; and meticulously eliminating such foods as milk, chocolate, egg, pork, cereal grains, alcoholic beverages, and sweets.

Others have had to eliminate all of these, plus possibly five or ten additional foods they have been eating very frequently, for a week or two. After this they usually have long enough pain-free periods that when a new pain arises, they can spot the causative food from their diet diaries.

It may be a newly eaten food, but is often a common food that they simply ate too frequently in the preceding twenty-four to forty-eight hours. They can pinpoint additional culprit foods by reintroducing or challenging one at a time the foods they initially removed from the diet. Such measures take much time and attention to detail, but are well worth it in pain relief.

I am not suggesting that exclusively dietary diagnosis and treatment are quick and easy, or can be accomplished casually. For example, the pain may not increase until long after the causative food has been eaten.

The champion of all delayed food reactions in my practice is one astute man with a joint-involving illness called Reiter's syndrome. From careful study of his own diet diary, he noted regular flare-ups of joint pain beginning *four days* after each meal containing pork. Some reactions may be even more delayed; but the longer the delay, the more difficult it is to recognize the food correlation.

NONDIETARY FACTORS

Chill prevention measures have been very helpful in some patients. Others have noted marked improvement when they put their indoor dog, cat, or bird outdoors and then cleared their homes meticulously of dusts, mites, molds, feathers, animal danders, and chemicals.

A few require all these measures plus others. And there remain some who are unhelped. We still have much to learn about the various triggers and stresses which cause arthritis.

REDUCING THE NEED FOR ARTHRITIS MEDICATIONS

Many of the medications used to treat arthritis have potentially serious side effects. Some must be given for years or a lifetime. Excluding offending foods from your diet may be inconvenient at first; but with attention paid to assure adequate nutrition, it may enable your physician to safely reduce or eliminate drug therapy.

Further, taking food extract injection therapy can diminish or eliminate the need for a diet. When it works, it is certainly safer and more pleasant than courses of potentially toxic gold injections or a lifetime of cortisones, pain relievers, and treatments for the sometimes major side effects of some therapeutic drugs.

CONFIRMATORY STUDIES

Dr. Richard Panush, Chief of the Division of Clinical Immunology, Rheumatology, and Allergy at the University of Florida, recently described two patients with rheumatoid arthritis who clearly improved on an elimination diet and experienced recurrences when deviating from the diet. He also described a patient, studied in a clinical research center, in which flare-ups of rheumatoid arthritis were induced by controlled double-blind challenges with powdered milk hidden in opaque gelatin capsules to prevent recognition of the presence of milk.[177]

Dr. Panush further cited many studies and observations by others in both humans and animals linking rheumatoid arthritis and similar joint syndromes to foods, food additives, and even to inhalants and chemicals in some instances.[161–164,170,173,178–218] These were chiefly delayed and caused by non-IgE mechanisms. Immune complexes were demonstrated in some; circulating IgE was present in some of these complexes.

IN A NUTSHELL

We do not yet know how neutralization therapy exerts its beneficial effects. We do know that neutralization therapy is effective in a wide variety of both allergic and nonallergic illnesses.

Neutralization therapy is usually effective against most antigenic substances for which we have a satisfactory extract or vaccine. We are already utilizing it successfully, as I have described, for foods, inhalants, some hormones, chemicals, contact allergens, fungi, yeasts, influenza viruses, herpes viruses, and other substances.

We have no extracts of human joint membranes, human DNA, and other self-produced substances which may be major antigens in many patients with rheumatoid arthritis and other self-allergic diseases. Possibly such extracts will become available and we can try to provide additional help by utilizing these in neutralizing doses. Clearly additional extracts, vaccines, and investigative studies are needed.

Meanwhile, reducing the total body burden through neutralization therapy in a patient with both an allergic and a nonallergic illness has often allowed the immune mechanism to function more efficiently and provide greater relief from the nonallergic illness, as well as the allergic one.

Chapter 31

COMING REVOLUTIONS IN MEDICINE

Today we hear with astonishment how "hackers," bright youngsters with small home computers, have been able to break into the programs of huge multimillion dollar mainframe computers of giant corporations, the federal government, and even the defense department.

The body contains what is analogous to a gargantuan mainframe computer. This includes billions of nerve cells in the central nervous system, and billions of lymphocytes which can circulate through the brain and all other organs. It also includes the billions of other circulating and fixed cells of the body.

CHEMICAL MESSENGERS AND THEIR SPECIFIC CELL RECEPTORS

These cells are in constant communication with each other through the hormones, chemical mediators, or other *messenger* molecules they produce and send out to other specific cells. The messenger molecules combine with specific antenna-like *receptor* molecules, located chiefly on the surfaces of the "receiving" cells.

This allows the receiving cells to "hear" only the specific messages which are meant for them. It is like tuning in to the broadcast signal of a single radio or television station although the air is full of invisible waves from many such stations, ham transmitters, CB radios, airplanes, control towers, ships at sea, etc.

It is also like the natural olfactory sensitivity of bloodhounds, deer, and many other animals and insects. This enables them to detect a faint though specific odor from a great distance and distinguish it from the myriad stronger odors simultaneously impinging on their sensory nervous systems.

In other words, gene-produced specific circulating chemical messengers from some cells can combine only with certain gene-produced specific receptors on other cells which are programmed to receive these specific messages. The receiving cells may be nearby or in a distant part of the body from the sending cells. The match between messenger and receptor is precise, like a specific key for a specific lock or an antibody for its antigen.

Homeostatic balance and health are dependent on the close interaction in perfect harmony of the cells of the nervous system, the immune system, and the hormonal system. In addition, there are many other chemical systems in the body whose harmonious interactions are necessary to maintain body functions.

Obviously, the whole human body is extremely complex. It is marvelously and delicately balanced.

However, the very complexity of the system is predictive of a great many ways in which it might be thrown off balance. Tilting one isolated mechanism may produce an illness. Restoring balance to this mechanism can eliminate or control the illness.

Increased sensitivity to a substance in the internal or external environment may reflect such a tilt. Rebalancing the specifically tilted mechanism may be the rationale of neutralization with specific extracts.

NEUTRALIZATION MAY REPROGRAM THE SYSTEM

The neutralizing system of testing can then be visualized as analogous to the small home computers of hackers. Neutralization provides a fairly simple procedure for breaking into the homeostasis-maintaining programs of our complex mainframe protective mechanism.

Neutralizing testing and treatment for specific substances such as allergens, hormones, or viruses may reprogram isolated bits of the main frame. This may restore proper regulation of the body's response to each of these specific substances.

Let us carry this limited analogy a bit further. Let us consider that flaws in the programs of the defense department's mainframe system could result in the inappropriate firing off of destructive missiles.

One human defense system analogy is the inappropriate firing off of chemical mediators from basophils and mast cells. Another is the firing off of excessive antibodies by B cells which have escaped suppressor control, resulting in excessive mediators or immune complexes. Others consist of the firing off of chemical missiles from complement and other potentially harmful molecules in blood serum; and also from other cells involved in allergy and inflammation, such as neutrophils. Reprogramming faulty mechanisms in any case could cause cessation of potentially destructive processes.

NEUTRALIZATION IS IMMUNORESTORATIVE, NOT IMMUNOSUPPRESSANT

Currently available immunosuppressive drugs employed in many illnesses attack and weaken the entire immune apparatus. The hope is that the harmful part of the immune system will be affected most, and that the beneficial parts will survive or regenerate best.

This can be a risky business. It may impair the *beneficial* parts of the immune system beyond recovery. The result of such therapy can be immune deficiency, not strength. It may leave the patient dangerously susceptible to a great many serious illnesses which are kept in check by an effective immune mechanism.

By contrast, neutralization therapy is specific and immunorestorative. Each extract used merely pushes a specific immune imbalance back toward normality.

The general immune system remains intact. In fact, it is strengthened by being released from the need to be diverted into expending metabolic energy fighting these specific imbalances.

NEUTRALIZATION PROVIDES NEW METHODOLOGY, DIRECTIONS, LOGIC, AND HOPE

I sincerely believe that the discovery of neutralization therapy will soon be recognized as a major milestone in medical history. It constitutes a method of providing relief in myriad allergic and nonallergic illnesses. For many of these illnesses, no comparable treatment was previously available.

Neutralization testing and treatment attacks environmentally-induced illnesses at their precise source, namely the specific causes of the impaired resistance/burden balance. More importantly, it determines immediately the precise dose of each antigen needed for correcting each impaired balance.

Neutralization thus supplies the methodology, the direction, and the logic for diminishing harmful responses in many known illnesses. It also strongly suggests the hope of doing so in a great many related illnesses for which, to my knowledge, it has not yet even been tried.

WITH HELP, THE BODY CAN HEAL ITSELF

When an environmentally-induced illness occurs, some incitant has *temporarily* thrown some previously balanced specific offensive/defensive equation slightly out of equilibrium. Although unbalanced, *both sides of the equation for the specific antigen are still present and active.* Immune balance simply has been tilted into immune imbalance.

In neutralization therapy, the situation apparently is brought from an equation of abnormality toward one of normality. When this is accomplished, both the incitant and the defense against the incitant are still present, *but in better proportions.* This greatly decreases or eliminates symptoms of illnesses.

In these diseases, the body contains the basic mechanisms with which to heal itself! All it needs is a little nudge in the proper direction to make things better.

REGAINING AND MAINTAINING IMMUNE BALANCE

Most antigens enter the body through the mucous membranes of the respiratory, digestive, and genitourinary tracts. It is the antigen entering the body that drives the system, for good or for ill. The body simply responds to the antigen.

This relationship is quantitative. A harmful response may be corrected by altering the quantity of antigen added to the system. Neutralization testing determines how much of a specific antigen should be added to improve the equilibrium for that antigen throughout the entire body.

Regular neutralization treatment injections keep the favorable equilibrium response going. Better immune balance is regained and maintained.

CONTROLLING THE AMPLIFICATION SYSTEM

The mediator-releasing system is among the most important and sophisticated of the body's defense mechanisms. Mediators can amplify their damaging effects tremendously by stimulating or "turning on" other powerful immune processes and potentially harmful cells such as neutrophils. So a small amount of mediator release can result in severe consequences.

Therefore, the body invests a great deal of its physiologic and metabolic resources to keep mediator release suppressed and under control.

Even so, the balance is delicate; and suppression and regulation of mediator release is not always successful.

This seems particularly true when those of us who are genetically prone are exposed to large or frequent contacts with certain substances. These include both natural materials and new man-made materials not anticipated by evolution.

Even fluctuations in our own hormones, day/night changes in our defensive capacities, chilling, exercise, and many other factors can upset the delicate balance. It is this balance that seems to be restored by neutralization therapy.

Chapter 32

BROADENING HEALTH HORIZONS

You yourself can control some nonspecific mediator releasing factors, such as exercise, diet, and exposure to chill, and by educated avoidance of specific suspected allergens. Now that physicians have the neutralizing system, which turns off harmful responses caused by non-Ige factors as well as by IgE, we should all broaden our view and work together to achieve relief for the many who are not now receiving it.

Not only sick people, but the knowledge base of the medical profession itself, will benefit from a deeper study of this procedure and its mechanism of action. Broader understanding holds the potential for benefiting more suffering patients than we can now imagine. This includes patients who fit into such specialties as allergy, immunology, environmental medicine, otolaryngology, rheumatology, oncology, infectious diseases, endocrinology, gynecology, neurology, psychiatry, dermatology, and gastroenterology.

NEUTRALIZATION GREATLY INCREASES THE NUMBER OF PEOPLE WHO CAN BE HELPED

We are told by the Institute of Allergic and Infectious Diseases that there are approximately 35 million allergic people in the United States. Nine million of these have asthma. Most of the rest have nose or skin allergies and their sequelae.[219]

This is the population considered to be made ill by direct IgE mechanisms alone. Until now, these were the only individuals thought capable of responding to allergy immunotherapy. The neutralizing system makes it obvious that this group is a drop in the bucket of the population we can really help.

ALLERGIC HEADACHE

The simple recognition of the existence and importance of *food and chemical sensitivity* and of the benefits of *neutralization therapy* will enable us to help many additional patients.

For example, there are said to be 44 million people in the United States with migraine.[31] Thus, migraine alone represents a larger field than the entire "allergic" population. But migraine is only one of a great number of illnesses that can be helped by neutralization therapy and other procedures described in this book.

GASTROINTESTINAL ALLERGY

The same procedures can be applied effectively to the additional millions of people with food allergy syndromes referable to the gastrointestinal tract (canker sores, nervous stomach, spastic colon, irritable bowel, chronic ulcerative colitis, and Crohn's Disease). The National Commission on Digestive Diseases states that nearly 18 million Americans are affected by digestive diseases.

Digestive diseases rank second only to cardiovascular diseases in leading causes of visits to physicians. They are the leading cause of hospitalization in the United States, the second leading cause of disability and lost work days, and the third leading cause of death.[220,221] They rank with the common cold as one of the leading causes of recurrent minor disability.[222]

Irritable bowel syndrome affects 9 million Americans, equal to the number with asthma. It is usually caused by food sensitivity and relieved by food extract injection therapy.

Furthermore, approximately 2 million young Americans are affected by such severe digestive diseases as chronic ulcerative colitis or Crohn's ileocolitis, with 100,000 new victims annually.[223] About half of all patients with chronic ulcerative colitis of thirty-five years' duration develop cancer of the bowel from the prolonged irritative and inflammatory process.[224]

If treated in time, both of these serious illnesses usually respond extremely well to food neutralization therapy. So here is a situation in which early and continued neutralization therapy might prevent a highly prevalent form of cancer.

SKIN ALLERGY

Skin diseases in which foods are rapidly becoming recognized as major causes are atopic dermatitis (eczema), neurodermatitis, urticaria, angioedema, and adult acne. Figures are not available for all these syndromes, since some never come to medical attention and some are not tabulated.

However, the National Institute of Allergic and Infectious Diseases estimates that there are approximately 6 million patients with eczema in the United States, and that approximately 45 million people have had urticaria at some time.[219]

Although no figures are available for adult acne, it is very common. My experience has been that it has almost always been neutralizable by either food or progesterone neutralization.

Poison ivy/oak/sumac dermatitis is also usually neutralizable, using appropriate extracts and doses of these plants. It is the most common cause of contact dermatitis, and is among the greatest public health problems associated with environmental agents.

It is usually an acute temporary problem, but repeated attacks are common. It may also become disabling, and it may require job changes. A study in California revealed that poison oak dermatitis was the number one cause of lost work days in that state.[219]

Contact dermatitis can be caused by many substances other than poison ivy, oak, and sumac. Contact allergy is a tremendous field. If one form of contact dermatitis is neutralizable, perhaps many others are also. This opens a whole new area for investigation and potential relief.

ARTHRITIS

The National Institute for Allergic and Infectious Diseases states that there are approximately 12 million people in the United States with arthritis.[225] More than 36 million are affected by some form of muscle/joint syndrome. About 5 million have rheumatoid arthritis.[226]

Osteoarthritis can be demonstrated by x-ray in 90 percent of the population by age forty.[194] Although only a small proportion of these have symptoms by then, advancing age, inflammation, and degenerative changes are common causes of chronic disability.

Degenerative osteoarthritis has not usually responded to neutralization therapy. Inflammatory osteoarthritis often has. There are no figures available on the number of patients with inflammatory osteoarthritis, but joint swelling and other signs of the presence of inflammation in osteoarthritis have become more emphasized recently.[194]

Patients with inflammatory osteoarthritis as well as inflammatory rheumatoid arthritis who have allergic or sensitivity illnesses of other types for which neutralization therapy has been employed (for example, migraine or spastic colon) have often noted marked improvement in their arthritis as well. Patients treated with neutralizing injections of Influenza Virus Vaccine for shingles have frequently exclaimed that their arthritis was markedly benefited at the same time as their shingles.

BRAIN ALLERGY

The number of patients with brain dysfunction due to foods and other antigens is very difficult to estimate. Figures range up to 9 million children, and there are probably at least an equal number of adults.[33,227] Some of the diagnostic labels used are hyperactivity, learning disability, behavior disorder, dyslexia, minimal brain dysfunction, and attention deficit disorder.

In adults as well as in children, hyperactivity, learning disability, episodic bizarre behavior, brain fogginess, unusual fatigue, and compulsive drowsiness must be far more common than would likely come to medical attention or be recognized for what they are. The same can be said for periodic spells of impaired capacity to think, remember, analyze, and create.

RESPIRATORY ALLERGY

Even some patients with respiratory syndromes, such as resistant asthma and resistant nasal symptoms with their many serious throat, sinus, ear, head pain, and other complications, can be helped by the addition of *food* neutralization therapy. Furthermore, the *inhalant* factors in these syndromes can usually be helped extraordinarily well by inhalant neutralization therapy.

YEASTS, HORMONES, VIRUSES

Add also the millions with chemical sensitivities, Candida yeast sensitivity, Candida yeast infection, premenstrual and menstrual problems, endometriosis, and the nausea and vomiting of pregnancy. Further add all those who can be relieved of reactions to immunizing doses of Influenza Virus Vaccine or from live-virus influenza infections.

Add the millions more who can be relieved of herpes family virus infections of the many varieties described in this book (Herpes Simplex I and II, shingles, postherpetic neuralgia, chickenpox, infectious mononucleosis, and chronic Epstein-Barr Virus infection), and possibly cytomegalovirus infection.

THE LARGER VIEW

The disciplines of allergy, immunology, and environmental medicine are in a potentially explosive growth position. Even so, this is a small glimpse of a still larger potential vista.

CANCER

Creative thinking about potential new uses of extracts and vaccines *already available* might lead to additional applications. We have mentioned that early and prolonged food neutralization therapy might prove useful in preventing cancer from chronic ulcerative colitis. In addition, by early treatment of the herpes factor with Influenza Virus Vaccine neutralization *before* malignant changes occur in various herpes-associated cancers, the tendency to malignant change might be dampened. Herpes-associated cancers include Burkitt's Lymphoma; and carcinoma of the cervix, lip, and nasopharynx.

THE PROMISE OF NEW EXTRACTS AND NEW APPLICATIONS

The future production of many *new* extracts and vaccines would be greatly stimulated by the recognition of the value of neutralization therapy. This could result in an effective system of therapy for an additional host of currently difficult or incurable diseases.

Drug sensitivities; autoimmune diseases; occupational diseases; and globally prevalent diseases due to viruses, bacteria, rickettsiae, protozoa, insects, worms, and other parasites constitute a few of many vast unexplored areas. People who have *already* contracted serious illnesses and are therefore no longer capable of being protected by newly developed preventive vaccines might be candidates for neutralizing *therapy* when the newly developed vaccines become available.

AGING

The aging process itself seems to be at least partially related to the wearing down of organ functions through the adverse effects of repeated and chronic immunologic stresses and immune imbalances. Maintaining homeostasis to the maximum degree possible might conceivably result in improved and more vigorous longevity.

CLINICAL OBSERVATIONS AND LABORATORY CORRELATIONS

Practicing physicians making clinical observations that seem to run counter to traditional teachings have great problems. "Radical" new concepts tend to send shock waves through the ranks of the orthodox. Throughout medical history, the establishment has characteristically reacted defensively, protecting the status quo and making difficult the lives of observers, thinkers, and constructive innovators.

Everyone recognizes that reality is often first noted in the trenches of patient care, rather than in laboratories. Medical history is replete with instances of breakthroughs made by individuals which were not accepted for decades or centuries, after which these concepts became the new orthodoxy.

THE PROMISING FUTURE

The science of immunology is still in an early though dynamic stage of development. Many gaping holes yet exist in our knowledge of immunologic mechanisms and in applications of existing bits of discrete immunologic data to practical clinical needs.

When clinical discoveries precede scientific explanations, as they commonly do in all branches of medical practice, we must as *scientists* be patient while awaiting the filling in of intellectual gaps in our knowledge.

However, as *practicing physicians* we are acutely aware that our patients need and can be provided help now with beneficial procedures at hand. Our patients do not want to continue to suffer and deteriorate while we spend decades working our way through the tedious process of ferreting out all the immunochemical minutiae and convincing every last one of our naturally skeptical colleagues.

All physicians know that we can control many diseases for which we do not know all or any of the causes or mechanisms. Every day we use many approved drugs whose mechanisms of action have not yet been delineated. We use them because we know they work.

In diseases of immune imbalance, practitioners can continuously correlate and interpret the laboratory studies already available, draw analogies, and even speculate about mechanisms. However, we cannot in good conscience withold relief until all the scientific i's are dotted and t's crossed.

EXPANDING THE HEALTH REVOLUTION

This book is a sincere effort to transmit a valuable message to millions of suffering people with a wide variety of "difficult" diseases. It describes precise methods for dietary self-help, as well as powerful new diagnostic and treatment procedures by which physicians can provide relief not previously available.

The number of illnesses which have been found to respond to these new methods has been growing rapidly over the past two decades, and new discoveries continue to be made.

Practicing physicians and investigators who are openminded, positive, and diligent in their pursuit of scientific truth and improvement of the human condition may well study and build on these beginnings. The result could be a greatly expanded revolutionary health boon for much of mankind.

God speed!

REFERENCES

1. Bookman R: "Observations and reflections of a practicing allergist." Annals of Allergy 45:4, pp 264–266, 1980.
2. Patterson R: *Allergic Disease,* JB Lippincott Company, Philadelphia, p 295, 1972.
3. Lee C: "A new test for diagnosis and treatment of food allergies." Buchanan County Medical Bulletin Vol. 25, p 9, 1961.
4. Miller JB: "Relief of premenstrual symptoms, dysmenorrhea, and contraceptive tablet intolerance." The Journal of the Medical Association of the State of Alabama 44:2, pp 57–60, 1974.
5. Miller JB: "Influenza: Rapid relief without drugs." Clinical Medicine 81:9, pp 16–19, 1974.
6. Miller JB: "Influenza neutralization." Transactions of the American Society of Ophthalmologic and Otolaryngologic Allergy 14:1, pp 159–168, 1974.
7. Miller JB: "Food allergy: Technique of intradermal testing and subcutaneous injection therapy." Transactions of the American Society of Ophthalmologic and Otolaryngologic Allergy 16:1, pp 154–168, 1976.
8. Miller JB: "A double-blind study of food extract injection therapy: A preliminary report." Annals of Allergy 38:3, pp 185–191, 1977.
9. Miller JB: "Optimal dose method of food allergy management." The Journal of Continuing Education in O.R.L. and Allergy 40:5, pp 37–50, 1978.
10. Miller JB: "Hidden food ingredients, chemical food additives, and incomplete food labels." Annals of Allergy 41:2, pp 93–98, 1978.
11. Miller JB: "Immunotherapy of virus infections." Transactions of the American Society of Ophthalmologic and Otolaryngologic Allergy 18:1, pp 144–148, 1978.
12. Miller JB: "Treatment of active herpes virus infections with influenza virus vaccine." Annals of Allergy 42:5, pp 295–305, 1979.
13. Miller JB: "Herpes: Rapid relief with influenza virus vaccine." The Journal of the Alabama Dental Association 68:3, pp 17–23, 1984.
14. Miller JB: *Food Allergy: Provocative Testing and Injection Therapy,* Charles C Thomas, Springfield, Illinois, 1972.
15. Miller JB: Special techniques of aerosol therapy for infants and children, in *Somatic and Psychiatric Treatment of Asthma,* Abramson HA (Editor), Williams and Wilkins Company, New York, pp 520–539, 1951.
16. Miller JB: Management of migraine headaches, in *Current Therapy of Allergy,* Frazier CA (Editor), Medical Examination Publishing Company, Inc., New York, pp 224–225, 1974.
17. Miller JB: Virus and hormone neutralization, in *Clinical Ecology,* Dickey LD (Editor), Charles C Thomas, Springfield, Illinois, pp. 597–605, 1976.

18. Miller JB: Management of migraine headaches, in *Current Therapy of Allergy,* Frazier CA (Editor), Medical Examination Publishing Company, Inc., New York, pp 307–320, 1978.
19. Miller JB: Management of food allergy, in *Food Allergy: New Perspectives,* Gerrard JW (Editor), Charles C Thomas, Springfield, Illinois, 1980.
20. Miller JB: The optimal dose method of food allergy management, in *Otolaryngologic Allergy,* King HC (Editor), Symposia Specialists, Inc., pp 253–283, 1981.
21. Miller JB: Neutralization therapy update, in *Allergy-Immunologic and Management Considerations,* Spencer JT (Editor), MEDED Publishers, Inc., Miami, Florida, 1982.
22. Miller JB: Audio cassette course entitled *Food Allergy: Provocative Testing and Injection Therapy.* Insta-Tape, Inc., 810 South Myrtle Avenue, Monrovia, California 91016-5729.
23. Miller JB: Allergy seminar audio track of video cassette course entitled *Food and Chemical Sensitivity in Human Disease.* Insta-Tape, Inc., 810 South Myrtle Avenue, Monrovia, California 91016-5729.
24. May CD: "Objective clinical and laboratory studies of immediate hypersensitivity reactions to foods in asthmatic children." J Allergy Clin Immunol 58:4, 500–515, 1976.
25. Randolph TG: "Masked food allergy as a factor in the development and persistence of obesity." J. Lab Clin Med Vol. 32, p 1547, 1947.
26. Alvarez WC: Foreword from Speer F: *Allergy of the Nervous System,* Charles C Thomas, Springfield, Illinois, 1970.
27. Randolph TG: The role of specific sugars, in *Clinical Ecology,* Dickey LD (Editor), Charles C Thomas, Springfield, Illinois, pp 313–314, 1976.
28. Randolph TG: The role of specific alcoholic beverages, in *Clinical Ecology,* Dickey LD (Editor), Charles C Thomas, Springfield, Illinois, pp 321–333, 1976.
29. Friedman AP: "Current concepts in the diagnosis and treatment of chronic recurring headache." Med Clin North Am Vol.56, pp 1257–1271, 1972.
30. Saper JR: "Migraine. I. Classification and pathogenesis." J Am Med Assoc Vol.239, p 22, 1978.
31. Dalessio DJ: *Wolff's Headache and Other Head Pain,* 4th Edition, Oxford University Press, New York, pp 56–130, 1980.
32. Wender EH: "Hyperactivity and the food additive free diet." Journal of Florida Medical Association 66:4, p 466, 1979.
33. Tryphonas H and Trites R: "Food allergy in children with hyperactivity, learning disabilities and/or minimal brain disfunction." Annals of Allergy 42:1, pp 22–27, 1979.
34. Rapp DJ: *Allergies and the Hyperactive Child,* Sovereign Books, New York, 1979.
35. DRAFT National Institute of Health Consensus Development Conference Statement. "Defined Diets and Childhood Hyperactivity." January 13–15, 1982.
36. Adams F: *The Genuine Works of Hippocrates,* The Williams and Wilkins Company, Baltimore, Maryland, 1939.
37. Lucretius: De Rerum Natura IV:637, 95–55 B.C. Cited in Talmage DW: Ann Rev Med Vol.8, p 239, 1957.
38. *The Living Bible.* Tyndale House Publishers, Wheaton, Illinois, 1971.
39. Speer F: *Allergy of the Nervous System,* Charles C Thomas, Springfield, Illinois, 1970.

40. Williams JI and Cram DM: "Diet in the management of hyperkinesis." Can Psych Assoc J 23:4, pp 241–248, 1978.
41. Baker S: "Fatigue in school children." Education Review Vol.15, p 34, 1898.
42. Schofield AT: "A case of egg poisoning." Lancet Vol.1, p 716, 1908.
43. Rinkel HJ, Randolph TG, and Zeller M: *Food Allergy.* Charles C Thomas, Springfield, Illinois, 1951.
44. Vaughan WT and Black JH: *Practice of Allergy,* 3rd Edition. CV Mosby, St. Louis, Missouri, pp 321–323, 1954.
45. Speer F: "Allergic tension-fatigue in children." Annals of Allergy Vol.12, p 168, 1959.
46. Crook WG, Harrison WE, Crawford SE, and Emerson BS: "Systemic manifestations due to allergy." Pediatrics Vol.27, p 790, 1961.
47. Kittler FJ: The effect of allergy on children with minimal brain damage, in *Allergy of the Nervous System,* Speer F (Editor), Charles C Thomas, Springfield, Illinois, 1979.
48. Kittler FJ and Baldwin DG: "The role of allergic factors in the child with MBD." Annals of Allergy Vol.28, p 203, 1970.
49. Rowe A and Rowe A Jr: *Food Allergy,* Charles C Thomas, Springfield, Illinois, 1972.
50. Brutten M, Richardson SO, and Mangel C: *Something Is Wrong With My Child,* Harcourt Brace, New York, 1973.
51. Levy HB: *Square Pegs—Round Holes,* Little-Brown, Boston, 1973.
52. O'Brian JF: Foreword from Stevens LJ and Stoner RB: *How To Improve Your Child's Behavior Through Diet,* Harcourt Brace, New York, 1973.
53. Tuft L: *Allergy Management in Clinical Practice,* CV Mosby, St. Louis, Missouri, p 311, 1973.
54. Wunderlich RC: *Allergy, Brains, and Children Coping,* Johnny Reads, Inc., St. Petersburg, Florida, 1973.
55. Crook WG: *Can Your Child Read? Is He Hyperactive?* Professional Books, Jackson, Tennessee, 1973.
56. Feingold BF: *Why Your Child Is Hyperactive,* Random House, New York, 1975.
57. Palmer S, Rapoport JL, and Quinn PO: "Food additives and hyperactivity." Clin Pediatrics Vol.14, p 956, 1975.
58. Conners CK, Goyette CH, Southwick DA, Lees JM, and Andrulonis PA: "Food additives and hyperkinesis: A controlled double-blind experiment." Pediatrics Vol.58, p 154, 1976.
59. Cook PS and Woodhill JM: "The Feingold dietary treatment of the hyperkinetic syndrome." Med J Aust Vol.2, p 85, 1976.
60. Ross DM and Ross SA: *Hyperactivity: Research, Theory and Action,* John Wiley, New York, pp 1–228, 1976.
61. Barkely RA and Cunningham CE: "Do stimulant drugs improve the academic performance of hyperkinetic children?" Clin Pediatrics 17:1, pp 85–92, 1978.
62. Harley JP, Matthews CG, and Eichman P: "Synthetic food colors and hyperactivity in children: A double-blind challenge experiment." Pediatrics Vol.62, pp 975–983, 1978.
63. Levy F, Dumbrell S, Hobbes G, Ryan M, Wilton N, and Woodhill JM: "Hyperkinesis and diet: A double-blind crossover trial with tartrazine challenge." Med J Aust Vol.1, p 61, 1978.
64. O'Leary KD, Rosenbaum A, and Hughes PC: "Fluorescent lighting: A pur-

ported source of hyperactive behavior." J Abnor Child Psychol Vol.6, pp 285–289, 1978.

65. Rapp DJ: "Double-blind confirmation and treatment of milk sensitivity." Med J Austr Vol.1, p 571, 1978.
66. Swanson J and Kinsbourne M: "Artificial food colors impair the learning performance of hyperactive children: Laboratory evaluation of in-patients." Presented at the American College of Allergists, Second International Food Allergy Symposium, Mexico City, 1978.
67. Bosco JJ and Robin SS: Hyperkinesis: How common is it and how is it treated? in *Hyperactive Children: The Social Ecology of Identification and Treatment,* Whalen CH and Henker B (Editors), Academic Press, Inc., New York, 1979.
68. Cantwell DP: "The hyperactive child." Hospital Practice 14:1, p 65, 1979.
69. Rapp DJ: "Food allergy treatment for hyperkinesis." J Learn Disab Vol.12, p 608, 1979.
70. Swidler HJ and Walson PD: "Hyperactivity: A current assessment." J Fam Pract Vol.9, pp 601–608, 1979.
71. Conners CK: *Food Additives and Hyperactive Children,* Plenum Press, New York, 1980.
72. Crook WG: "Can what a child eats make him dull, stupid or hyperactive?" J Learn Disab 13:5, pp 53–58, 1980.
73. Levine MD and Oberklaid F: "Hyperactivity: Symptom complex or complex symptom?" American Journal of Diseases Of Children Vol.134, pp 409–414, 1980.
74. Randolph TG and Moss RW: *An Alternative Approach to Allergies,* Lippincott and Crowell, New York, 1980.
75. Rapp DJ: Hyperactivity and the tension fatigue syndrome, in *Food Allergy: New Perspectives,* Gerrard JW (Editor), Charles C Thomas, Springfield, Illinois, pp 186–208, 1980.
76. Schauss A: *Diet, Crime and Delinquency,* Parker House, Berkeley, California, 1980.
77. Stevens LJ and Stoner RB: *How to Improve Your Child's Behavior Through Diet,* Doubleday and Company, Inc., New York, 1979.
78. May CD and Bock SA: Adverse reactions to food due to hypersensitivity, in *Allergy Principles and Practice,* 1st Edition, Middleton E Jr, Reed CE, Ellis EF (Editors), CV Mosby, St. Louis, Missouri, Vol.2, pp 1159–1169, 1983.
79. Schloss OM: "A case of allergy to common foods." Am J Dis Child Vol.111, p 341, 1912.
80. Fries JF: "Peanuts: Allergic and other untoward reactions." Annals of Allergy 48:4, pp 220–226, 1982.
81. Randolph TG: *Human Ecology and Susceptibility to the Chemical Environment,* Charles C Thomas, Springfield, Illinois, pp 115–116, 1962.
82. Billman A: *Guidelines: A Compilation of Products and Resources for the Chemically Sensitive,* Human Ecology Research Foundation of the Southwest, 12110 Webbs Chapel Road, Suite 305E, Dallas, Texas 75231, 1981.
83. *Wholesalers of Organic Produce and Products Directory,* California Agrarian Action Project, P.O. Box 464, Davis, California 95617, 1984.
84. Considine GM and Considine GD: *Foods and Food Production,* Van Nostrand Reinhold Company, New York, 1982.

85. "Food Technology." A Publication of the Institute of Food Technologists, 221 N. LaSalle Street, Suite 2120, Chicago 60601.
86. *Handbook of Food Additives,* Furia TE (Editor), The Chemical Rubber Company, Cleveland, Ohio, 1968.
87. Schweigert BS: "The food ingredients dilemma in the modern marketplace." Food Technology 38:1, pp 54–56, 1984.
88. Odds FC: *Candida and Candidosis,* University Park Press, Baltimore, Maryland, 1979.
89. Romney SL: *Gynecology and Obstetrics: The Health Care of Women,* McGraw Hill Book Company, New York, 1975.
90. Truss CO: *The Missing Diagnosis,* P.O. Box 26508, Birmingham, Alabama, 35226, 1983.
91. Crook W: *The Yeast Connection,* Professional Books, P.O. Box 3494, Jackson, Tennessee, 38301, 1983.
92. Mabray CR, Burditt ML, Martin TL, Jaynes CR, and Hayes JR: "Treatment of common gynecologic-endocrinologic symptoms by allergy management procedures." Obstetrics and Gynecology 59:5, pp 560–564, 1982.
93. Dalton K: *Once a Month,* Hunter House Incorporated, 748 East Bonita Avenue, Suite 105, Pomona, California 91767, 1979.
94. Miller JB, Lee C, Binkley EL, and Hardt SH: "Relief of influenza symptoms by the provocative-neutralizing method—a preliminary report." Journal of the Medical Association of the State of Alabama 41:7, pp 493–502, 1972.
95. Hirsch A: *Handbook of Geographical and Historical Pathology,* Vol. 1, translated from the Second German Edition by Charles Creighton, New Sydenham Society, London, pp 7–17, 1883.
96. Thomson D and Thomson R: "Influenza." Ann Pickett-Thomson Res Lab Vol.9, p 4, 1933.
97. Crosby AW: *Epidemic and Peace,* 1918. Part IV, Greenwood Press, Westport, Connecticut, pp 203–226, 1976.
98. Hers JFP, Masurel N, and Mulder J: "Bacteriology and histopathology of the respiratory tract and lungs in fatal Asian influenza." Lancet Vol.2, p 1141, 1958.
99. Mulder J and Hers JFP: *Influenza,* Woltoers-Noordhoff, Gronigen, Netherlands, 1972.
100. Rogers DE, Louria DB, and Kilbourne ED: "The syndrome of fatal influenza virus pneumonia." Trans Assoc Am Phys Vol.71, p 260, 1958.
101. Walsh JJ, Dieptlein LF, Low FN, Burch GE, and Mogabgab WJ: "Bronchotracheal response in human influenza." Arch Intern Med Vol.108, p 376, 1961.
102. Scadding JG: "Lung changes in influenza." QJ Med Vol.6, p 425, 1937.
103. Stuart-Harris CH and Schild GC: *Influenza, the Viruses and the Disease,* Publishing Sciences Group, Inc., Boston, 1976.
104. Davenport FM: *Influenza Viruses: Viral Infections of Humans, Epidemiology and Control,* Evans AS (Editor), Plenum Publishing Co., New York, 1976.
105. Fox JP and Kilbourne ED: "Epidemiology of influenza—summary of influenza workshop. IV." J Infect Dis Vol.128, p 361, 1973.
106. *The Influenza Virus,* Kilbourne ED (Editor), Academic Press Inc., New York, 1975.
107. Nahmias AJ and Roizman B: "Infection with herpes-simplex viruses I and II, Part I." New Eng J Med Vol.289, p 719, 1973.

108. Nahmias AJ and Roizman B: "Infection with herpes-simplex viruses I and II, Part II." New Eng J Med Vol.289, p 719, 1973.
109. Chang T, Fiumara NJ, and Weinstein L: "Genital herpes: Some clinical and laboratory observations." J Am Med Assoc Vol.229, p 544, 1974.
110. Spruance SL, Overall JC Jr, Kern ER, Krueger GG, Pliam VP, and Miller W: "The natural history of recurrent herpes simplex labialis." New Eng J Med Vol.297, p 72, 1977.
111. Rytel MW: "Herpes simplex infections." Drug Thera Vol.6, p 27, 1976.
112. Sugar A: "Managing herpes eye infections." Drug Thera Vol.7, p 85, 1977.
113. Nahmias AJ, Dowdle WR, Naib ZM, Josey WE, McLone D, and Domescik G: "Genital infection with type II herpes virus hominis, a commonly occurring venereal disease." Br J Ven Dis Vol.45, p 294, 1969.
114. Jeansson S and Molin L: "Genital herpes virus hominis infection: A venereal disease?" Lancet Vol.1, p 1064, 1970.
115. Francis DP, Herrmann KL, MacMahon JR, Chavigny KH, and Sanderlin KC: "Nosocomial and maternally acquired herpes-virus hominis infections." Am J Dis Child Vol.129, p 889, 1975.
116. Olmstead CB: "Genital herpes: The newest venereal disease: Report of a case associated with aseptic meningitis." Cutis Vol.20, p 113, 1977.
117. Centifanto YM, Drylie DM, Deardourff SL, and Kaufman HE: "Herpesvirus type II in the male genito-urinary tract." Science Vol.178, p 318, 1972.
118. Nahmias AJ, Josey WE, Naib ZM, Freeman WG, Fernandez RJ, and Wheeler JH: "Perinatal risk associated with maternal genital herpes simplex virus infection." Am J Obst Gyn Vol.110, p 825, 1971.
119. Nahmias AJ, Josey WE, and Naib ZM: "Significance of herpes simplex virus infection during pregnancy." Clin Obst Gyn Vol.15, p 929, 1972.
120. Naib ZM, Nahmias AJ, Josey WE, and Wheeler JH: "Association of maternal genital herpetic infection with spontaneous abortion." Obst and Gyn Vol.35, p 260, 1970.
121. Nahmias AJ, Alford CA, and Korones SB: "Infection of the newborn with herpesvirus hominis." Advances in Pedia Vol.17, p 185, 1970.
122. Florman A, Gershon AA, Blackett PR, and Nahmias AJ: "Intrauterine infection with herpes-simplex virus—resultant congenital malformations." J Am Med Assoc Vol.225, p 129, 1973.
123. St. Geme JW Jr, Bailey SR, Koopman JS, Oh W, Hobel CJ, and Imagawa DT: "Neonatal risk following late gestational genital herpesvirus hominis infection." Am J Dis Child Vol.129, p 342, 1975.
124. Hanshaw JB: "Herpesvirus hominis infections in the fetus and the newborn." Am J Dis Child Vol.126, p 546, 1973.
125. Nahmias AJ and Roizman B: "Infection with herpes-simplex viruses I and II, Part III." New Eng J Med Vol.289, p 781, 1973.
126. Miller LH: "Herpes zoster in the elderly." Cutis Vol.18, p 427, 1976.
127. Brown GR: "Herpes Zoster: Correlation of age, sex distribution, neuralgia, and associated disorders." So Med J Vol.69, p 576, 1976.
128. Landay SE: "Varicella hepatitis and Reye's syndrome: An interrelationship?" Pediatrics Vol.60 746, 1977.
129. Corey L, Rubin RJ, Thompson T, Noble GR, Cassidy E, Hattwick MAW, Gregg MB, and Eddins D: "Influenza-B associated with Reye's syndrome:

Incidence in Michigan and potential for prevention." J Infect Dis Vol.135, p 398, 1977.
130. Linnemann CC, Shea L, Kauffman CA, Schiff GM, Partin JG, and Schubert WK: "Association of Reye's syndrome with viral infection." Lancet Vol.2, p 179, 1974.
131. Purchase HG: "Role of herpesvirus of Marek's disease, a malignant lymphoma of chickens." Federal Proc Vol.31, p 1634, 1972.
132. Benditt E, Barrett T, and Mc Dougall J: Proceedings of the National Academy of Sciences Vol.80, pp 6386–6389, 1983.
133. Melnick JL: "Herpes, heart disease linked," as quoted by Paul Raeburn in Mobile Register, Tuesday Jan.17, 1984, p 7-A.
134. Melnick JL: Virus and host factors in cytomegalovirus infections, in *Transplantation and Clinical Immunology* XII. Touraine JL et al (Editors), Excerpta Medica 3–9, Amsterdam, 1980.
135. Smith KO, Gehle WD, and Sanford BA: "Evidence for chronic viral infections in human arteries." Proc Soc Exp Biol Med, Vol.147, pp 357–360, 1974.
136. Burch GE: "Viruses and arteriosclerosis." Am Heart Journal Vol.87, pp 407–412, 1974.
137. Fabricant CG, Fabricant J, Littenta MM, and Minick CR: "Virus induced atherosclerosis." J Exp Med Vol.148, pp 335–340, 1978.
138. Minick CR, Fabricant CG, Fabricant J, and Littenta MM: "Atherosclerosis induced by infection with a herpes-virus." Am J Pathol Vol.96, pp 673–706, 1979.
139. Fabricant CG, Fabricant J, Minick CR, and Littenta MM: Herpesvirus induced atherosclerosis, in *Cold Spring Harbor Conference on Cell Proliferation: Viruses in Naturally Occurring Cancers,* Vol.VII, Cold Spring Harbor Laboratory Press, pp 1251–1257, 1980.
140. Fabricant CG, Hajjar DP, Minick CR, and Fabricant J: "Herpesvirus infection enhances cholesterol and cholesteryl ester accumulation in cultured arterial smooth muscle cells." Am J Pathol Vol.105, pp 176–184, 1981.
141. Biggs PM, de The G, and Payne LN (Editors): *Oncogenesis And Herpesvirus.* International Agency for Research on Cancer, France, 1972.
142. Symposium. "Herpesvirus and cervical cancer." Key Biscayne, Florida. Dec. 8–10, 1972. Reported in Cancer Research Vol.33, 1973.
143. Klein G: "Herpesvirus and oncogenesis." Proc of National Acad of Sci Vol.69, p 1056, 1972.
144. Sabin A: "Commentary: Varicella-zoster virus vaccine." J Am Med Assoc Vol.238, p 1731, 1977.
145. Wyburn MR: "Malignant changes following herpes-simplex." Br Med J Vol.2, p 615, 1957.
146. Kvasnicka A: "Relationship between herpes simplex and lip carcinoma. IV. Selected cases." Neoplasma Vol.12, p 61, 1965.
147. Sabin AB and Tarro G: "Herpes-simplex and herpes genitalis viruses in etiology of some human cancers." Proc Natl Acad Sci USA Vol.70, p 3225, 1973.
148. Logan WS, Tindall JP, and Elson ML: "Chronic cutaneous herpes simplex." Arch Dermatol Vol.103, p 606, 1971.
149. Nahmias AJ: "Disseminated herpes-simplex virus infections." New Eng J Med Vol.282, p 684, 1970.

150. Muller SA, Herrmann EC Jr, and Winkleman RK: "Herpes simplex infections in hematologic malignancies." Am J Med Vol.52, p 102, 1972.
151. St. Geme JW Jr, Prince JT, Burke BA, Good RA, and Krivit W: "Impaired cellular resistance to herpes-simplex virus in Wiskott-Aldrich syndrome." New Eng J Med Vol.273, p 229, 1965.
152. Becker WB, Kipps A, and McKenzie D: "Disseminated herpes-simplex virus infection: Its pathogenesis based on virological and pathological studies in 33 cases." Am J Dis Child Vol.115, p 1, 1968.
153. Nash G and Foley FD: "Herpetic infection of the middle and lower respiratory tract." Am J Clin Pathol Vol.54, p 857, 1970.
154. Wheeler CE Jr and Abele DC: "Eczema herpeticum, primary and recurrent." Arch Dermatol Vol.93, p 162, 1966.
155. Alford CA and Whitley RJ: "Treatment of infections due to herpesvirus in humans: A critical review of the state of the art." J Infect Dis (Supplement) Vol.33, p A192, 1976.
156. Fry J: *Common Diseases,* 2nd Edition, JB Lippincott Co., Philadelphia, pp 257, 269, 1979.
157. *Cecil Textbook of Medicine,* 16th Edition, Wyngaarden JB and Smith LH (Editors), WB Saunders Co., Philadelphia, 1982.
158. Denman AM, Mitchell B, and Ansell BM: "Joint complaints and food allergic disorders." Annals of Allergy 51:2, pp 260–263, 1983.
159. Peskett SA, Platts-Mills TAE, Ansell BM, and Stearns GN: "The incidence of atopy in rheumatic disease." J Rheumatol Vol.8, pp 321–324, 1981.
160. Russel AS: "Arthritis, inflammatory bowel disease and histocompatibility antigens." Ann Int Med Vol.86, pp 820–821, 1977.
161. AAAI and NIAID report: "Adverse reactions to foods." U.S. Dept of Health and Human Services National Institute of Health. NIH Pub. No. 82-2442, pp 84–85, July, 1984.
162. Coombs RRA and Oldham G: "Early rheumatoid-like joint lesions in rabbits drinking cow's milk." Int Arch Allergy Appl Immunol Vol.64, pp 287–292, 1981.
163. Zeller M: "Rheumatoid arthritis—food allergy as a factor." Annals of Allergy Vol.7, pp 200–239, 1949.
164. Rowe AH and Rowe A Jr: Food allergy and the arthropathies, in *Food Allergy: Its Manifestations and Control and the Elimination Diets,* Charles C Thomas, Springfield, Illinois, pp 435–443, 1972.
165. Criep LH: "Allergy of joints." J of Bone Joint Surg Vol.28, pp 276–279, 1946.
166. Tisscher: Discussion, in *The Mast Cell: Its Role in Health and Disease,* Pepys J and Edwards AM (Editors), Pittman Medical, Kent, England, p 475, 1979.
167. Randolph TG: *Human Ecology and Susceptibility to the Chemical Environment,* Charles C Thomas, Springfield, Illinois, p 148, 1962.
168. Delire M: Detection of circulating immune-complexes in infants fed on cow's milk, in *The Mast Cell: Its Role in Health and Disease,* Pepys J and Edwards AM (Editors), Pittman Medical, Kent, England, pp 375–379, 1979.
169. Moment GB: "Editorial: Aging, arthritis and food allergies: A research opportunity revisited." Growth Vol.44, pp 155–159, 1980.
170. Parke AL and Hughes GRV: "Rheumatoid arthritis and food: A case study." British Medical Journal Vol.282, pp 2027–2029, 1981.
171. Williams R: "Rheumatoid arthritis and food: A case study." British Medical Journal Vol.283, p 363, 1981.

172. Jones V, Jacoby R, Wellington T, and Holt P: "Immune complexes in early arthritis I: Detection of immune complexes before rheumatoid arthritis is definite." Clin Exp Immunology Vol.44, pp 512–521, 1981.
173. Skoldstam L, Larson L, and Lindstrom F: "Effects of fasting and lactovegetarian diet on rheumatoid arthritis." Ann of Rheum Dis Vol.42, pp 45–51, 1983.
174. Feinberg SM: Miscellaneous manifestations, in *Allergy in Practice,* The Year Book Publishers, Inc., Chicago, pp 771–772, 1944.
175. Stroud RM, Kroker G, Marshall RT, Carroll FM, Bullock JD, Greenberg M, Rea W, Smiley R, and Randolph TG: "Comprehensive environmental control and its effect on rheumatoid arthritis II: Food and chemical challenges." Presented at the Third International Food Allergy Symposium of the American College of Allergists, Boston, 1980.
176. Little CH, Stewart AG, and Fennessy MR: "Platelet serotonin release in rheumatoid arthritis: A study in food intolerant patients." Lancet Vol.2 pp 297–299, 1983.
177. Panush RS: "Food-induced (allergic) arthritis. I. Rheumatoid arthritis exacerbated by milk." (in preparation)
178. Paganelli R, Levinsky RJ, Brostoff J, and Wraith DG: "Immune complexes containing food proteins in normal and atopic subjects after oral challenge and effect of sodium cromoglycate on antigen absorption." Lancet Vol.1, pp 1270–1272, 1979.
179. Paganelli R, Levinsky R, and Atherton D: "Detection of specific antigen within circulating immune complexes: Validation of the assay and its application to food antigen-antibody complexes formed in healthy and food-allergic subjects." Clin Exp Immunol Vol.46, pp 44–53, 1981.
180. Brostoff J (Editor): "Food allergy." Clinics Immunol Allergy Vol.2, pp 1–260, 1982.
181. Panush RS: "Controversial arthritis remedies." Bulletin Rheumatic Diseases (in press)
182. Panush RS and Webster EM: Adverse reactions to foods, in Immunologic Disorders. Corman LC (Editor), Med Clin N Amer (in press)
183. Webster EM and Panush RS: Nutrition and arthritis, in *Rehabilitation Management of Rheumatic Conditions,* Erlich GE (Editor). (in press)
184. Walker WA and Isselbacher KJ: "Uptake and transport of macromolecules by the intestine. Possible role in clinical disorders." Gastroenterology Vol.67, pp 531–550, 1974.
185. Cunningham-Rundles C, Brandeis WE, Good RE, and Day NK: "Bovine antigens and the formation of circulating immune complexes in selective immunoglobulin A deficiency." J Clin Invest Vol.64, pp 272–279, 1979.
186. Cunningham-Rundles C, Brandeis WE, Pudifin DJ, Day NK, and Good RA: "Autoimmunity in selective IgA deficiency: Relationship to anti-bovine protein antibodies, circulating immune complexes, and clinical disease." Clin Exp Immunol Vol.45, pp 299–304, 1981.
187. Rooney PJ, Jenkins RT, Goodacre RL, and Sivakumaran T: "Gut permeability of small molecules in rheumatoid disease." Clin Res Vol.31, p 160A, 1983 (abstract)
188. Sundqvist T, Linstrom F, Magnusson KE, Skoldstom L, Stjernstom I, and Tagesson C: "Influence of fasting on intestinal permeability and disease activity in patients with rheumatoid arthritis." Scand J Rheum Vol.11, pp 33–38, 1982.

189. Lockshin MD: "The unproven remedies committee." Arthritis Rheum Vol.24, pp 1188–1190, 1981.
190. Robinson WD: Nutrition and rheumatoid diseases, in *Textbook of Rheumatology*, Kelley WN, Harris ED, Ruddy S and Sledge CS (Editors), WB Saunders, Philadelphia, pp 337–349, 1980.
191. Fernandes G, Yunis EJ, Jose DG, and Good RA: "Dietary influence on antinuclear antibodies and cell-mediated immunity in NZB mice." Int Arch Allergy Vol.44, pp 770–782, 1973.
192. Weatherbee M: "Chronic arthritis. The clinical analysis of three hundred and fifty cases." AMA Arch Intern Med Vol.50, pp 926–944, 1932.
193. Minot GR: "General aspects of the treatment of chronic arthritis." New Eng J Med Vol.208, pp 1285–1290, 1933.
194. Bauer W: "What should a patient with arthritis eat?" J Am Med Assoc Vol.104, pp 1–6, 1935.
195. Hench BS, Bauer W, Dawson MH, Hall F, Holbrook WP, Key JA, and McEwen C: "The problem of rheumatism and arthritis. Review of American and English Literature, 1983 (6th Rheumatism Review)." Ann Intern Med Vol.13, pp 1838–1990, 1940.
196. Hench BS, Bauer W, Boland E, Dawson MH, Freyberg RH, Holbrook WP, Key JA, Locke LN, and McEwen C: "Rheumatism and arthritis. Review of the American and English Literature, for 1940 (8th Rheumatism Review)." Ann Intern Med Vol.15, pp 1002–1108, 1941.
197. Rosenberg EF: Diet and vitamins in rheumatoid arthritis, in *Comroe's Arthritis and Allied Conditions.* Fifth Edition. Hollander JL (Editor), Lea and Febiger, Philadelphia, pp 542–546, 1954.
198. Turnbull JA: "Changes in sensitivity to allergenic foods in arthritis." Amer J of Digestive Diseases Vol.15, pp 182–190, 1944.
199. Pottenger RT: "Constitutional factors in arthritis with special reference to incidence and role of allergic disease." Ann Int Med Vol.12, pp 323–333, 1928.
200. Kaufman W: "Food induced allergic musculoskeletal syndromes." Ann Allergy Vol.11, pp 179–184, 1953.
201. Zussman BM: "Food hypersensitivity simulating rheumatoid arthritis." Southern Med J Vol.59, pp 935–939, 1966.
202. Millman M: "An allergic concept of the etiology of rheumatoid arthritis." Ann Allergy Vol.30, pp 135–141, 1972.
203. Lewin P and Taub SJ: "Allergic synovitis due to ingestion of English walnuts." J Am Med Assoc Vol.106, p 2144, 1936.
204. Berger H: "Intermittent hydroarthrosis with an allergic basis." J Am Med Assoc Vol.112, pp 2402–2405, 1939.
205. Hench PS and Rosenberg EF: "Palindromic rheumatism." Proc Staff Meetings Mayo Clinic Vol.16, pp 808–815, 1941.
206. Vaughn WT: "Palindromic rheumatism among allergic persons." J Allergy Vol.14, pp 256–263, 1943.
207. Randolph TG: Ecologically oriented rheumatoid arthritis, in *Clinical Ecology*, Dickey LD (Editor), Charles C Thomas, Springfield, Illinois, pp 201–212, 1976.
208. Uden AM, Trang L, Venizelos N, and Palmbad J: "Neutrophil functions and clinical performance after total fasting in patients with rheumatoid arthritis." Annals Rheum Dis Vol.42, pp 45–51, 1983.

209. Prickett JD, Robinson DR, and Steinberg AD: "Effects of dietary enrichment with eicosapentaenoic acid upon autoimmune nephritis in female NZB X NZW/F_1 mice." Arthritis Rheum Vol.26, pp 133–139, 1983.
210. Levy JA, Ibrahim AB, Shirai T, Ohta K, Nagasawa R, Yoshida H, Estes J, and Gardner M: "Dietary fat affects immune response, production of antiviral factors, and immune complex disease in NZB/NZW mice." Proc Natl Acad Sci USA Vol.79, pp 1974–1978, 1982.
211. Epstein S: Hypersensitivity to sodium nitrate: "A major causative factor in cases of palindromic rheumatism." Annals of Allergy Vol.27, pp 343–349, 1969.
212. Marguardt JL, Snyderman R, and Oppenheim JJ: "Depression of lymphocyte transformation and exacerbation of Behcet's syndrome by ingestion of English walnuts." Cellular Immunology Vol.9, pp 263–272, 1973.
213. Mandell M and Conte A: "The role of allergy in arthritis, rheumatism, and associated polysymptomatic cerebro-viscero-somatic disorders: A double-blind provocation test study." Annals of Allergy Vol.44, p 51, 1980.
214. Darlington LE and Mansfield JR: "Food allergy and rheumatoid disease." Ann of Rheum Dis Vol.42, p 219, 1983 (abstract)
215. Stroud RM: The effect of fasting followed by specific food challenge on rheumatoid arthritis, in *Current Topics in Rheumatology,* Hahn BH, Arnett FC, Zizic TM, and Hochberg MC (Editors), Upjohn Institute, Kalamazoo, Michigan, pp 145–157, 1983.
216. Wraith DG: "Allergic joint symptoms." Presented at the Fourth International Food Allergy Symposium of the American College of Allergists, Vancouver, Canada, July 25–29, 1982.
217. Brostoff J: "IgE complexes and auto-antibodies to IgE in patients with food allergies and rheumatoid arthritis." Presented at the Fourth International Food Allergy Symposium of the American College of Allergists, Vancouver, Canada, July 25–29, 1982.
218. Panush RS, Carter RL, Katz P, Kowsari B, Longley S, and Finnie S: "Diet therapy for rheumatoid arthritis." Arthritis Rheum Vol.26, pp 462–471, 1983.
219. NIAID Task Force Report. "Asthma and the Other Allergic Diseases." U.S. Dept. of Health, Education, and Welfare. NIH Pub. No. 79-387, May, 1979.
220. Fact Sheet: National Commission on Digestive Diseases. September 15, 1977.
221. Greenberger NJ: *Gastrointestinal Disorders: A Pathophysiological Approach,* 2nd Edition, Yearbook Medical Publishers, Inc., Chicago, pp 211, 214, 1981.
222. *Cecil-Loeb Textbook of Medicine* VII. 12th Edition, Beeson and McDermott (Editors), WB Saunders Co., Philadelphia, p 850, 1967.
223. National Commission on Digestive Diseases, as quoted in Mobile Press Register, p 51-A, December 4, 1977.
224. Hales, D: "Chronic GI disorders in children said to carry serious risks, sequelae." Medical Tribune, p 18, December 12, 1979.
225. NIAID Task Force Report. U.S. Dept. of Health, Education, and Welfare and National Institute of Health, 1975.
226. Rowland HS (Editor): *The Nurses' Almanac,* Aspen Publication Systems Inc., Maryland (The Arthritis Foundation and National Institute of Health), p 612, 1978.
227. Shaywitz SE, Cohen DJ, and Shaywitz BA: "The biochemical basis of minimal brain dysfunction." J of Pedia 92:2, 1978.

APPENDICES

APPENDIX I
ROTARY DIET CHARTS

The number preceding each food or family in Appendix I corresponds to the numbers in the Food Family Classification (Appendix II) and the Individual Simple Foods (Appendix III). Foods included within a given box are members of a family.

ROTARY DIET DAY 1

BREAKFAST	*LUNCH*	*DINNER*
111. Atlantic halibut Pacific halibut plaice right eye flounder turbot winter flounder	77. duck goose	115. chicken *egg* peafowl pheasant quail
32-C. *oat*	107. oyster	109. walleye pike yellow perch
73. American grapes European grapes muscadines raisins	105. scallop	88. dolphin fish
8. cabbage palm coconut (meal, oil, nut) date date sugar Sago starch	125. clam	90. common dolphin; 76. honey
60. *black guava* *coffee* *woodruff*	115. croaker freshwater drum King whiting redfish squeteague weakfish	22. broccoli, Brussels sprouts, cabbage, cauliflower, Chinese cabbage, collard, horseradish, kale, kohlrabi, mustard, radish, rape, rutabaga, turnip, watercress, wintercress
	121. porgy	2. mushroom truffle yeast
	100. North American squid	30. cassava meal (yuca) tapioca
	65. bell pepper, cape gooseberry, cayenne pepper, chili (paprika), eggplant, ground cherry, melon pear, potato (white, Irish), strawberry tomato, tomato, tree tomato	32-A. *barley rye wheat*
	15. caper	49. olive (ripe, black), (oil)
	43. American gooseberry	62. litchi nut
	44. breadfruit, fig, *hops*, mulberry	10. filberts, hazelnuts *oil of birch (wintergreen flavor)*
	52. sesame seed, oil	58. apple (*vinegar*), crabapple, loquat, pear, quince, redhaw, rosehips
	51. poppyseed	

DAY 1

BREAKFAST	*LUNCH*	*DINNER*
Broiled flounder Fresh grapes Coffee with date sugar	Potato soup, chili pepper seasoning with oysters Redfish or croaker dipped in potato flour, fried in sesame oil Baked potato with pepper and salt Eggplant strips dipped in potato flour fried in sesame oil Sliced tomato Tomato juice or water	Chinese cabbage, radish, apple wedges, cauliflower salad with apple vinegar and olive oil Baked or broiled chicken Mushroom gravy thickened with tapioca Homemade bread with wheat, honey, yeast, and water Broccoli Rutabaga Tapioca and apple dessert with honey or deep dish apple pie with honey Apple juice or water
Fried flounder (dipped in coconut meal, fried in coconut oil) Oatmeal with raisins and date sugar Coffee with date sugar	Roast duck Bell pepper stuffed with eggplant seasoned with cayenne pepper Layers of sliced potato and tomato, sesame seed and oil as casserole Tomato juice or water Figs	Cabbage slaw, radish, watercress, olives, hardboiled eggs with olive oil and cider vinegar Chicken dipped in cassava meal or wheat flour and fried in olive oil Turnips or rutabaga Baked apple with honey and filberts
Oatmeal with chopped dates Fresh coconut wedges Coconut milk or coffee	Oysters dipped in potato flour, fried in sesame oil French fried potatoes in sesame oil Sliced tomato and bell peppers Tomato juice or water Figs	Fried yellow perch using cassava meal or wheat flour and olive oil Cauliflower Collards or mustard Radishes and olives Pear

ROTARY DIET DAY 2

BREAKFAST	*LUNCH*	*DINNER*
114. salmon trout	99. hare rabbit / 95. abalone	80. beef
79. California halibut left eyed flounder southern flounder summer flounder	117. mackerel tuna bonita	104. guinea fowl
32-D. *corn (grits, starch, vegetable, oil, meal syrup)* *popcorn*	120. sole	87. whitefish
61. citron grapefruit kumquat lemon lime orange tangelo tangerine	91. anchovy	106. common smelt
64. currant English gooseberry	75. beluga sturgeon	82. amberjack pompano jack mackerel yellow jack
6. American pawpaw	96. edible snail	21. sweet potato (vine tuber)
55. macadamia nut	41. cottonseed (meal, oil) okra	40. asparagus *sarsaparilla* chives shallot garlic Welsh onion leek yucca onion
	71. *angelica* *cumin* *anise* *dill* *caraway* *fennel* carrot *lovage* celeriac parsley celery parsnips *chervil* *sweet cicily* *coriander* *sweet fennel*	24. Florida arrowroot
	45. banana plantain	32-B. *rice* *wild rice*
	26. persimmon	50. *vanilla bean*
	9. malanga poi taro	12. pineapple
	11. comfrey (vegetable, *tea*)	38. Brazil nut paradise nut
	69. *basswood* *linden (tea)*	20. juniper pine nut
	31. beechnut chinquapin chestnut	
	70. water chestnut	

DAY 2

BREAKFAST	*LUNCH*	*DINNER*
Trout (mealed)/fried in corn oil Grapefruit and orange sections/ corn syrup Hot lemonade/corn syrup	Tuna/water chestnuts Okra (fry in cottonseed meal & oil) Carrot sticks/celery Banana	Roast beef/garlic Wild rice (plain gravy) Boiled small onions Asparagus Baked sweet potato
Tangerine/orange sections/corn syrup Corn meal pancakes/corn syrup Grapefruit or orange juice	Baked mackerel Parsnips Boiled okra Carrot/celery Baked banana	Steak/sliced onions Rice/steak gravy Asparagus Brazil nuts/sweet potato/pineapple Pineapple juice
Grits Salmon/lemon juice Half grapefruit/corn syrup Juice	Rabbit (cottonseed meal and fried in cottonseed oil) Okra (boiled or fried) Baked plantain Carrots Persimmon	Casserole ground beef, onion slices, chives, rice Asparagus Sliced pineapple Sweet potato custard with pure vanilla

ROTARY DIET DAY 3

BREAKFAST	*LUNCH*	*DINNER*
118. ocean perch rosefish	80. goat	80. lamb
103. mullet silversides	102. turkey	116. squirrel
113. North American paddlefish	83. buffalofish, chub, hag, lumpfish, sucker, white sucker	101. red snapper
54. buckwheat garden sorrel rhubarb sea grapes	85. herring, menhaden, pilchard (sardine), shad	94. grunt (common, gray and yellow)
57. blackraspberry boysenberry burnet dewberry loganberry red raspberry strawberry	32-G. *bamboo shoots, sprouts*	92. muskellunge, northern pike, pickerel
32-F. *sorghum* *sugar cane*	23. cantaloupe, casaba melon, chayote, cucumber, gherkin, honeydew melon, muskmelon, Persian melon, pumpkin (seed, meal, vegetable), squash (all kinds), watermelon	27. American yam (plant tuber, not vine) Chinese potato Indian yam
68. *tea*	67. Fiji arrowroot	14. Queensland arrowroot
	74. *cardamom*, *East Indian arrowroot*, *ginger*, *tumeric*	19. burdock root, *camomile*, celtuce, chicory, dandelion, endive, escarole, French endive, globe artichoke, Jerusalem artichoke, *kaffir (tea)*, lettuce, safflower (oil), sunflower (seed, meal, oil), *tansy*, *tarragon*, *yarrow*, salsify
	46. *mace*, *nutmeg*	36. artichoke-Chinese and Japanese, *balm*, *basil*, *bergamot*, *catnip*, *clary*, *horehound*, *hyssop*, *lavender*, *marjoram*, *mint: common, horse, round leaf, curled*, *oregano*, *pennyroyal*, *peppermint*, *rosemary*, *sage*, *savory*, *spearmint*, *thyme*
	16. elderberry	
	1. black walnut, butternut, English walnut, hickory nut, pecan	

DAY 3

BREAKFAST	*LUNCH*	*DINNER*
Broiled mullet Rhubarb sauce/cane sugar Black raspberries/cane sugar Raspberry juice or water Hot tea	Sardines or other allowed fish Bamboo sprouts Baked chayote Cucumbers Cantaloupe Arrowroot custard/maple syrup, nutmeg and pecans	Baked red snapper or other allowed fish Globe artichokes/herbed safflower oil Baked American yams Salad of lettuce, endives, escarole/safflower oil and oregano, thyme and savory Kaffir tea or water Dandelion tea
Buckwheat pancakes/sorghum syrup Strawberries/cane sugar Pan-broiled ocean perch Hot tea/cane sugar	Baked turkey Stewed zucchini squash with turmeric Baked pumpkin with nutmeg, maple syrup and pecans Cucumber slices Watermelon or honeydrew melon	Lamb/mint Heart of lettuce/herbed sunflower oil Fried American yam slices Globe artichokes/safflower oil and herbs Camomile tea or water
Buckwheat groats/sorghum syrup Raspberries/cane sugar Mullet or ocean perch Hot tea	Baked turkey with gravy or natural juices Acorn squash with nutmeg, walnuts and maple sugar Bamboo shoots Cantaloupe	Squirrel (boiled) with oregano American yams/peppermint Chopped lettuce, sunflower seed, Jerusalem artichoke slices, escarole, dandelion leaves with safflower oil and herbs Globe artichokes Yarrow tea or water Dandelion tea

ROTARY DIET DAY 4

BREAKFAST	*LUNCH*	*DINNER*
122. butterfish	81. crab	123. pork
93. cod haddock pollock silver hake	97. crayfish lobster prawn	84. black bass (largemouth, smallmouth, spotted) blue gill longeared sunfish sunfish pumpkinseed
32-E. *millet*	108. shrimp	119. grouper white bass rockfish white perch
59. almond apricot cherry (fresh) nectarine peach plum prunes sloes wild cherry	98. catfish Mississippi catfish	37. avocado *cinnamon* bay leaf *sassafras*
72. *lemon verbene (tea)*	113. bluefish	42. West Indian arrowroot (maranta starch)
33. *maté (yerba maté)*	78. common eel	47. *allspice* jambolan *cloves* roseapple guava Surinam cherry
	39. acacia gum lima bean adsuki bean navy bean *alfalfa* peanut (nut, oil) asparagus bean peas (all kinds) carob pinto bean English pea snapbean fava bean soybean (flour, nut, oil, milk) *fenugreek* stringbean garbanzo bean tamarind (fruit) *guar* tepary jack bean tonka bean kidney bean *(imitation vanilla)* lablab bean *tragacanth gum* lentil yambean *licorice*	53. *black and white pepper*
	17. papaya	34. *saffron* *orris root*
	56. pomegranate	28. black huckleberry lingonberry blueberry wintergree cranberry berries
	13. prickly pear	18. beet spinach *beet sugar* Swiss chard
	3. *carrageenan* *kelp (seaweed)*	4. agave
		7. *ginseng*
		25. Chinese water chestnut chufa (groundnut)
		5. cashew mango pistachio

DAY 4

BREAKFAST	*LUNCH*	*DINNER*
Millet cereal Prunes Broiled peaches Lemon verbena tea or maté Allowed fruit juice	Crab claws or lobster English peas Peanut butter (pure) Papaya Carob	Pork chops with black pepper Sliced beets with bay leaf Avocado Spinach
Codfish Allowed fresh fruit (apricots, peach, cherries) Juice of fruit Millet bread (cook millet, allow to get cold and slice)	Catfish fried with soy flour and oil Lentil soup with shrimp Salad of navy, pinto, kidney, stringbeans with soy oil Pomegranate Fenugreek tea	Fresh pork ham with cloves and beet sugar Swiss chard Avocado and cashews Cranberry sauce and beet sugar Cranberry juice
Allowed fish, baked or broiled Prunes Millet cakes (pancakes) Fresh fruit (nectarines, plums, peach, etc.) Hot fruit juice	Boiled shrimp Stringbeans Soy crackers with peanut butter (pure) Prickly pear Carob	Allowed fish, broiled or baked with saffron Chinese water chestnuts Beets Spinach Blueberries with beet sugar Sassasfras tea, beet sugar

APPENDIX II
FOOD FAMILIES

The number preceding each food family in Appendix II corresponds to the numbers in the Rotary Diet Charts (Appendix I) and the Individual Simple Foods (Appendix III).

The food family classification is adapted from the following references:

1. Corwin AH: The Rotating Diet and Taxonomy, in *Clinical Ecology,* Dickey LD (Editor), Charles C Thomas, Springfield, Illinois, pp 122–147, 1976.
2. Speer F and Dockhorn RJ: *Allergy and Immunology in Childhood,* Charles C Thomas, Springfield, Illinois, pp 277–282, 288, 1973.
3. Golos N: *Management of Complex Allergies,* New England Foundation of Allergic and Environmental Diseases, Norwalk, Connecticut, pp 50–53, 1975.

Plant Family Classification

1. Aceraceae (maple): maple sugar and syrup
2. Agaricaceae (fungi): mushroom, truffle, yeast
3. Algae (algae): carrageen, kelp or seaweed
4. Amaryllis (amaryllis): agave
5. Anacardiaceae (cashew): cashew, mango, pistachio
6. Annonaceae (buttercup): American pawpaw
7. Araliaceae (ginseng): ginseng
8. Arecaceae (palm): cabbage palm (oil), coconut (meal, milk, oil), date (date sugar), Sago starch
9. Araceae (Arum): malanga, poi, taro
10. Betulaceae (birch): filbert, hazel nut, oil of birch (wintergreen flavoring)
11. Boraginaceae (borage): comfrey
12. Bromeliaceae (pineapple): pineapple
13. Cactaceae (cactus): prickly pear
14. Cannaceae (canna): Queensland arrowroot
15. Capparidaceae (caper): caper

16. Caprifoliacea (honeysuckle): elderberry

17. Caricaceae (papaya): papaya

18. Chenopodiacea (goosefoot): beet (beet sugar), spinach, Swiss chard

19. Compositae (sunflower): burdock leaves, burdock root, celtuce, chamomile, chicory, dandelion, endive, escarole (French endive), globe artichoke, Jerusalem artichoke, kaffir, lettuce, safflower (oil), salsify, sunflower (meal, oil, seed), tansy, tarragon, yarrow

20. Coniferae (conifer): juniper, pine nut or pinon

21. Convoluculaceae (sweet potato): sweet potato (vine tuber, Ipomoea batatas species)

22. Cruciferae (mustard): broccoli, Brussels sprouts, cabbage (Chinese, common, savoy), cauliflower, collards, horseradish, kale, kohlrabi, mustard, radish, rape, rutabaga, turnip, watercress, wintercress

23. Cucurbitateae (gourd): cantaloupe, casaba melon, chayote, cucumber, gherkin (Indian), honeydew melon, muskmelon, Persian melon, pumpkin (meal, seed), squash (all kinds), watermelon

24. Cycadaceae (cycad): Florida arrowroot (Zamia)

25. Cyperaceae (sedge): Chinese water chestnuts, chufa or groundnut

26. Ebenaceae (ebony): American persimmon, Oriental persimmon

27. Dioscoreaceae (yam): American yam, Chinese potato, Indian yam

28. Ericaceae (heath): black huckleberry, blueberry, cranberry, lingonberry, wintergreen berry

29. Erythrosylaceae (coca): coca leaf (flavor, Coca Cola)

30. Euphorbiaceae (spurge): cassava, tapioca, yuca

31. Fagaceae (beech): beechnut (American, European), chestnut (American, Chinese, Spanish), chinquapin

32-A. Graminneae, Hordeae (grass): barley, rye, wheat

32-B. Graminneae, Oryzeac (grass): rice, wild rice

32-C. Graminneae, Aveneae (grass): oats

32-D. Graminneae, Maydeae (grass): corn (grain, oil, starch, sugar, syrup, vegetable), popcorn

32-E. Graminneae, Paniceae (grass): millet (browntop, common, ditch, finger, foxtail, Japanese, pearl)

32-F. Graminneae, Andropogoneae (grass): cane syrup, sorghum, sugar cane

32-G. Graminneae, Bambuseae (grass): bamboo (shoots and sprouts)

33. Iliacaceae (holly): mate' (Yerba mate')

34. Iridaceae (iris): orris root, saffron (flavors)

35. Juglandaceae (walnut): black walnut, butternut, English walnut, hickory nut, pecan, white walnut

36. Labiatae (mint): balm, basil, bergamot, catnip, Chinese artichoke, clary, common mint, curled mint, hoarhound, horse mint, hyssop, Japanese artichoke, lavender, marjoram, oregano, pennyroyal, peppermint, rosemary, round-leafed mint, sage, savory, spearmint, spike lavender, thyme, water mint

37. Lauraceae (laurel): avocado, bay leaf, cinnamon, sassafras

38. Lecythiadaceae (sapucaya): Brazil nut, paradise nut

39. Leguminosae (legume): acacia gum, adsuki bean, alfalfa (tea), asparagus bean, beans (all varieties), carob bean, fava bean, fenugreek, garbanzo pea, guar, gum arabic, jack bean, lablab bean, lentil, licorice, peanut, peas (all varieties), soybean tamarind, tepary bean, tonka bean, tragacanth, yambean

40. Liliaceae (lily): asparagus, chives, garlic, leek, onion, sarsaparilla, shallot, Welsh onion, yucca

41. Malvaceae (mallow): cottonseed (meal, oil), okra

42. Marantaceae (arrowroot): West Indian arrowroot (Maranta starch)

43. Melostomadaceae (melostomad): American gooseberry

44. Moraceae (mulberry): breadfruit, fig, hops, mulberry

45. Musaceae (banana): banana, dwarf banana, plantain

46. Myristiceae (nutmeg): mace, nutmeg

47. Myrtaceae (myrtle): allspice, clove, guava, jambolan, roseapple, Surinam cherry

48. Nymphaeaceae (water lily): Chinese lotus

49. Oleaceae (olive): olive (oil)

50. Orchidaceae (orchid): vanilla bean

51. Papaveraceae (poppy): poppyseed

52. Pedaliaceae (pedalium): sesame seed and oil

53. Piperaceae (pepper): black and white pepper

54. Polygonaceae (buckwheat): buckwheat, garden sorrel, rhubarb, sea grape

55. Proteaceae (protea): macadamia nut

56. Punicaceae (pomegranate): pomegranate

57. Rosaceae, Rosoideae (berries): blackberry, black raspberry, boysenberry, burnet, dewberry, loganberry, red raspberry, strawberry

58. Rosaceae, Pomoideae (pomes): apple, crabapple, loquat, pear, quince, redhaw, rose hips

59. Rosaceae, Prunoideae (stone fruits): almond, apricot, nectarine, peach, plum, prune, sloe, sweet cherry, wild cherry

60. Rubiaceae (madder): black guava, coffee, woodruff

61. Rutaceae (citrus): citron, grapefruit, kumquat, lemon, lime, orange, tangelo, tangerine

62. Sapindaceae (soapberry): litchi nut

63. Sapotaceae (sapodilla): chicle

64. Saxifragaceae (saxifrage): currant, English gooseberry

65. Solanaceae (nightshade): bell pepper, cape gooseberry, cayenne pepper, chili (paprika), eggplant, garden peppers, ground cherry, melon pear, potato (white), strawberry tomato, tomato, tree tomato

66. Sterculiaceae (cola nut): chocolate, cocoa, cola, karaya gum

67. Taccaceae (tacca): Fiji arrowroot (Tacca)

68. Theaceae (tea): tea

69. Tiliaceae (linden): basswood, lime or linden (for tea)

70. Trapaceae (water chestnut): water chestnut

71. Umbelliferae (parsley): angelica, anise, black cumin, caraway seed, carrot, celeriac, celery, chervil, coriander, cumin, dill, fennel, lovage, parsley, parsnip, sweet cicily, sweet fennel

72. Verbenaceae (verbena): lemon verbena (tea)

73. Vitaceae (grape): American grape, European grape, muscadines, raisins, scuppernongs

74. Zingiberaceae (ginger): cardamom, East Indian arrowroot, ginger, turmeric

Animal Family Classification

75. Acipenseridae: beluga, sturgeon

76. Apidea (bee): honey

77. Anatidae: duck, goose

78. Anguillidae: common eel

79. Bothidae: California halibut, left-eyed flounder, southern flounder, summer flounder

80. Bovidae: African buffalo, American bison, Brahman, cattle (cow's milk), goat, sheep

81. Cancridae: crab

82. Carangidae (jack): amberjack, jack mackerel, pompano, yellow jack

83. Catostomidae (sucker): buffalofish, chub, hag, lumpfish, sucker, white sucker

84. Centrarchidae (sunfish): bluegill, largemouth black bass, longeared sunfish, pumpkinseed, smallmouth black bass, spotted black bass, sunfish

85. Clupeidae: herring, menhaden, pilchard (sardine), shad
86. Columbidae: pigeon
87. Coregonidae: lake whitefish
88. Coryphaenidae: dolphin fish
89. Cyprinidae: carp
90. Delphinidae: common dolphin
91. Engraulidae: anchovy
92. Esocidae (pike): muskellunge, northern pike, pickerel
93. Gadidae: cod, haddock, pollock, silver hake, tomcod
94. Haemulidae: common grunt, gray grunt, yellow grunt
95. Haliotidae: red, pink and green abalone
96. Helicidae: edible snail
97. Homaridae: crayfish, lobster, prawn
98. Ictaluridae: catfish, Mississippi catfish, yellow bullhead
99. Leporidae: Belgian hare, cottontail, domestic rabbit, jackrabbit, snowshoe rabbit
100. Loliginidae: North American squid
101. Lutjanidae: red snapper
102. Meliagridae: turkey
103. Mugilidae: mullet, silversides, white bait
104. Numididae: guinea fowl
105. Pectenidae: scallops
106. Osmeridae: common smelt
107. Ostreidae: oyster
108. Peneidae: shrimp

109. Percidae: walleye pike, yellow perch

110. Phasianidae: chicken (egg), domestic pheasant, Indian pheasant, peafowl, quail

111. Pleuronectidae: Atlantic halibut, Pacific halibut, plaice, right-eyed flounder, turbot, winter flounder

112. Polydonitdae: North American paddlefish

113. Pomatomidae (bluefish): bluefish

114. Salmonidae: salmon, trout

115. Sciendidae: croaker, freshwater drum, king whiting, redfish, squeteague, weakfish

116. Sciuridae: prairie dog, squirrel, woodchuck

117. Scombridae: albacore, Atlantic mackerel, bluefin tuna, bonita, king mackerel, skipjack tuna, Spanish mackerel

118. Scorpaenidae: ocean perch, rosefish

119. Serranidae: black sea bass, brown grouper, Oriental spotted bass, red grouper, rockfish, speckled hind, white bass, white perch

120. Soleidae: common sole, European sole

121. Sparidae: porgy

122. Stromateidae: butterfish

123. Suidae: pig

124. Tetraonidae: prairie chicken, ruffled grouse (partridge)

125. Veneridae: clams

Uncommon Animal Foods

126. Antilocapridae: pronghorn antelope

127. Castoroidae: beaver

128. Cervinae: American elk, European red deer

129. Chelidridae: snapping turtle

130. Didelphidae: opossum

131. Equidae: horse

132. Musticeiti: blue whale, fin whale, Greenland whale, humpback whale, North Atlantic whale, Pacific gray whale, sperm whale, white whale

133. Odocoileinae: caribou, moose, reindeer, white tailed deer

134. Phocidae: common seal

135. Procyoninae: raccoon

136. Ranidae: American bullfrog, European edible bullfrog

137. Ursidae: black bear, brown bear, grizzly bear

APPENDIX III
INDIVIDUAL SIMPLE FOODS

The number preceding each food in Appendix III corresponds to the numbers in the Food Family Classification (Appendix II) and the Rotary Diet Charts (Appendix I).

INDIVIDUAL SIMPLE FOODS

MEATS

80 Beef
80 Goat
99 Hare
80 Lamb
123 Pork
99 Rabbit
116 Squirrel
128 Venison, European red
133 Venison, white tailed

FOWL

110 Chicken
77 Duck
77 Goose
104 Guinea fowl
110 Peafowl
110 Pheasant
110 Quail
102 Turkey
110 Egg (chicken, duck, etc.)

SCALEFISH

82 Amberjack
91 Anchovy
119 Bass, Oriental spotted
119 Bass, white
75 Beluga
84 Black bass, largemouth
84 Black bass, smallmouth
84 Black bass, spotted
113 Bluefish
84 Bluegill
117 Bonita
83 Buffalofish
122 Butterfish
89 Carp
98 Catfish
98 Catfish, Mississippi
83 Chub
93 Cod
115 Croaker
90 Dolphin, common
88 Dolphin fish
115 Drum, freshwater
78 Eel, common
79 Flounder, left-eyed
111 Flounder, right-eyed
79 Flounder, southern
79 Flounder, summer
111 Flounder, winter
119 Grouper
94 Grunt, common
94 Grunt, gray
94 Grunt, yellow
93 Haddock
83 Hagfish
111 Halibut, Atlantic
79 Halibut, California
111 Halibut, Pacific
85 Herring
83 Lumpfish
117 Mackerel, Atlantic
117 Mackerel, frigate
82 Mackerel, jack
117 Mackerel, king
117 Mackerel, Spanish
85 Menhaden
103 Mullet, gray
103 Mullet, striped
103 Mullet, white
92 Muskellunge
112 Paddlefish, North American
118 Perch, ocean

119 Perch, white
109 Perch, yellow
92 Pickerel
92 Pike, northern
109 Pike, walleye
85 Pilchard (sardine)
111 Plaice
93 Pollock
82 Pompano
121 Porgy
84 Pumpkinseed
115 Redfish
101 Red snapper
119 Rockfish
118 Rosefish
114 Salmon, Atlantic
114 Salmon, coho
114 Salmon, pink
119 Sea bass, black
85 Shad
93 Silver hake
103 Silversides
106 Smelt, common
120 Sole
115 Squeteague
75 Sturgeon
83 Sucker
83 Sucker, white
84 Sunfish
84 Sunfish, longeared
114 Trout, brook
114 Trout, brownlake
114 Trout, rainbow
117 Tuna, bluefin
117 Tuna, skipjack
111 Turbot
115 Weakfish
87 Whitefish
115 Whiting, king
82 Yellow jack

CRUSTACEANS

81 Crab
97 Crayfish
97 Lobster
97 Prawn
108 Shrimp

MOLLUSKS

95 Abalone
125 Clam
107 Oyster
105 Scallop
96 Snail, edible
100 Squid, North American

VEGETABLES

36 Artichoke, Chinese
19 Artichoke, globe
36 Artichoke, Japanese
19 Artichoke, Jerusalem
40 Asparagus
32-G Bamboo shoots
32-G Bamboo sprouts
39 Beans
- acacia
- adsuki
- alfalfa
- asparagus
- black
- broad
- bush
- butterbean, calico
- butterbean, white
- carob
- fava
- fenugreek
- frijole
- guar gum
- gum arabic
- jack
- kidney, red
- kidney, white
- lablab
- licorice
- lima
- navy
- pinto
- pole
- snapbean
- soybean
- stringbean
- tamarind
- tepary
- tonka
- tragacanth

wax
yambean
18 Beets
22 Broccoli
22 Brussels sprouts
19 Burdock leaves
19 Burdock root
22 Cabbage, Chinese
22 Cabbage, common
22 Cabbage, savoy
8 Cabbage palm
39 Carob
71 Carrot
22 Cauliflower
71 Celeriac
71 Celery
19 Celtuce
18 Chard, Swiss
71 Chervil
19 Chicory
40 Chives
22 Collards
11 Comfrey
32-D Corn
19 Dandelion
65 Eggplant
19 Endive, common
19 Endive, French (escarole)
71 Fennel, sweet
22 Horseradish
22 Kale
22 Kohlrabi
19 Lettuce
2 Mushroom
41 Okra
71 Parsnip
39 Peanut
39 Peas
blackeye
butterpeas
chick (garbanzo)
cowpea
creme
crowder
English
field
green split
lady finger
lentil
pigeon pea, common
purplehull
snow
Spanish
yellow eye
yellow split
32-D Popcorn
21 Potato, sweet
65 Potato, white
22 Radish
22 Rape
54 Rhubarb
22 Rutabaga
19 Salsify
3 Seaweed
18 Spinach
23 Squash
65 Tomato
65 Tomato, strawberry
65 Tomato, tree
2 Truffle
22 Turnip
22 Watercress
22 Wintercress
27 Yam, American
27 Yam, Chinese
27 Yam, Indian
19 Yarrow
40 Yucca

FRUITS & BERRIES

58 Apple
59 Apricot
45 Banana
57 Blackberry
28 Blueberry
57 Boysenberry
44 Breadfruit
23 Cantaloupe
15 Caper
23 Chayote
65 Cherry, ground
47 Cherry, Surinam
59 Cherry, sweet
59 Cherry, wild
61 Citron

58 Crabapple
28 Cranberry
64 Currant
8 Dates
57 Dewberry
16 Elderberry
44 Fig
43 Gooseberry, American
65 Gooseberry, cape
64 Gooseberry, English
73 Grape, American
73 Grape, European
61 Grapefruit
47 Guava
60 Guava, black
44 Hops
28 Huckleberry, black
47 Jambolan
20 Juniper
61 Kumquat
61 Lemon
61 Lime
28 Lingonberry
57 Loganberry
58 Loquat
48 Lotus, Chinese
5 Mango
23 Melon, casaba
23 Melon, honeydew
23 Melon, Persian
44 Mulberry
73 Muscadine
23 Muskmelon
59 Nectarine
61 Orange, common
61 Orange, mandarin
61 Orange, sour
17 Papaya
6 Pawpaw, American
59 Peach
58 Pear
65 Pear, melon
26 Persimmon, American
26 Persimmon, Oriental
12 Pineapple
45 Plantain
59 Plum, American
59 Plum, beach
59 Plum, common
59 Plum, Damson
59 Plum, Oriental
59 Plum, Pacific
56 Pomegranate
13 Prickly pear
59 Prune
23 Pumpkin
58 Quince
73 Raisin
57 Raspberry, black
57 Raspberry, red
58 Redhaw
47 Roseapple
58 Rose hips
73 Scuppernong
54 Sea grape
59 Sloe
57 Strawberry, beach
57 Strawberry, cultivated
57 Strawberry, meadow
39 Tamarind
61 Tangelo
61 Tangerine
23 Watermelon
28 Wintergreen (berry)

MEALS, STARCHES & CEREALS

74 Arrowroot, East Indian
67 Arrowroot, Fiji
24 Arrowroot, Florida
14 Arrowroot, Queensland
42 Arrowroot, West Indian
32-A Barley
54 Buckwheat
39 Flour, carob
39 Flour, lima bean
39 Flour, soybean
9 Malanga
42 Maranta
30 Meal, cassava
32-D Meal, corn
41 Meal, cottonseed
23 Meal, pumpkin
19 Meal, sunflower
32-E Millet
32-C Oats

9 Poi
32-B Rice
32-B Rice, wild
32-A Rye
32-D Starch, corn
8 Starch, Sago
30 Tapioca
9 Taro
32-A Wheat
2 Yeast (in bread)
30 Yuca
40 Yucca

SALADS

19 Artichoke, Jerusalem
37 Avocado
65 Bell pepper
19 Burdock leaves
22 Cabbage, Chinese
22 Cabbage, common
22 Cabbage, savoy
71 Carrot
22 Cauliflower
71 Celeriac
71 Celery
19 Celtuce
71 Chervil
19 Chicory
40 Chives
23 Cucumber
19 Dandelion leaves
19 Endive, French (escarole)
54 Garden sorrel
23 Gherkin, Indian
40 Leek
19 Lettuce
2 Mushroom
49 Olive
40 Onion
71 Parsley
65 Pepper, garden varieties
22 Radish
40 Shallot
18 Spinach
65 Tomato (all varieties)
70 Water chestnut
22 Watercress
22 Wintercress

OILS

8 Coconut
32-D Corn
41 Cottonseed
49 Olive
8 Palm
39 Peanut
19 Safflower
52 Sesame seed
39 Soybean
19 Sunflower seed

VINEGAR

58,2 Apple
32,2 Grain
32A,2 Malt
73,2 Wine

SPICES, FLAVORINGS & SEASONINGS

47 Allspice
71 Angelica
71 Anise
36 Balm
36 Basil
37 Bay leaf
36 Bergamot
57 Burnet
71 Caraway
74 Cardamom
36 Catnip
19 Chamomile
65 Chili (paprika)
71 Cicily, sweet
37 Cinnamon
36 Clary
47 Clove
29 Coca leaf
66 Cola
71 Coriander
71 Cumin, black
71 Cumin, common
71 Dill

71 Fennel
71 Fennel, sweet
39 Fenugreek
40 Garlic
74 Ginger
36 Hoarhound
36 Hyssop
36 Lavender oil
40 Leek
39 Licorice
71 Lovage
46 Mace
36 Marjoram
36 Mint
22 Mustard, black
22 Mustard, Indian
22 Mustard, white
46 Nutmeg
10 Oil of birch (wintergreen)
40 Onion
40 Onion, Welsh
36 Oregano
34 Orris root
71 Parsley
36 Pennyroyal
53 Pepper, black
65 Pepper, cayenne
65 Pepper, chili (paprika)
65 Pepper, garden
53 Pepper, white
36 Peppermint
51 Poppyseed
36 Rosemary
34 Saffron
36 Sage
40 Sarsaparilla
37 Sassafras
36 Savory
52 Sesame seed
40 Shallot
36 Spearmint
19 Tansy
19 Tarragon
36 Thyme
39 Tonka bean
74 Turmeric
50 Vanilla bean
60 Woodruff

NUTS & SEEDS

59 Almond
31 Beechnut
38 Brazil nut
35 Butternut
5 Cashew
31 Chestnut, American
31 Chestnut, Chinese
31 Chestnut, Spanish
31 Chinquapin
25 Chufa (ground nut)
8 Coconut
10 Filbert
10 Hazelnut
35 Hickory nut
62 Litchi nut
55 Macadamia nut
38 Paradise nut
39 Peanut
35 Pecan
20 Pine nut (pinon)
5 Pistachio
52 Sesame seed
19 Sunflower seed
39 Tepary
35 Walnut, black
35 Walnut, English
35 Walnut, white
70 Water chestnut
25 Water chestnut, Chinese

SWEETS

76 Honey
32-F Sorghum
18 Sugar, beet
32-F Sugar cane
32-D Sugar, corn
8 Sugar, date
1 Sugar, maple
32-F Syrup, cane
32-D Syrup, corn
1 Syrup, maple

BEVERAGES

4 Agave
69 Basswood fruit
66 Chocolate
66 Cocoa
8 Coconut milk
60 Coffee
7 Ginseng, American
7 Ginseng, Asian
33 Mate' (Yerba)
80 Milk: cow, goat, etc.
58 Rose hips
39 Soybean milk
68 Tea
39 Tea, alfalfa
11 Tea, comfrey
19 Tea, kaffir
72 Tea, lemon verbena
69 Tea, linden lime (flower)

GUMS

39 Acacia
3 Carrageen
63 Chicle
39 Guar
39 Gum arabic
66 Karaya
3 Kelp
39 Tragacanth

APPENDIX IV
DIET DIARY

Name ______________

14 DAY DIET DIARY

Date ______________

1st DAY	2nd DAY	3rd DAY	4th DAY	5th DAY	6th DAY	7th DAY
SYMPTOMS						
MEDICATION						
BREAKFAST						
SYMPTOMS						
MEDICATION						
LUNCHEON						
SYMPTOMS						
MEDICATION						
DINNER						
SYMPTOMS						
MEDICATIONS						

RECORD FOODS AND MEDICATIONS IN BLUE AND SYMPTOMS IN RED, (over)

8th DAY	9th DAY	10th DAY	11th DAY	12th DAY	13th DAY	14th DAY
SYMPTOMS						
MEDICATION						
BREAKFAST						
SYMPTOMS						
MEDICATION						
LUNCHEON						
SYMPTOMS						
MEDICATION						
DINNER						
SYMPTOMS						
MEDICATIONS						

RECORD FOODS AND MEDICATIONS IN BLUE AND SYMPTOMS IN RED.

APPENDIX V
FOOD TOLERANCE LEDGER

FOOD TOLERANCE LEDGER

TOLERATED *(Live on These)*	*POSSIBLE MILD SYMPTOMS* *(Try Again)*	*DEFINITE MILD SYMPTOMS* *(Avoid if Possible)*	*POSSIBLE OR DEFINITE SEVERE SYMPTOMS* *(Avoid!)*

AUTHOR INDEX

SUBJECT INDEX

I

J

K